Philosophical Foundations of Quality of Life

Alex C. Michalos

Philosophical Foundations of Quality of Life

The Selected Works of Alex C. Michalos

Springer

Alex C. Michalos
University of Northern British Columbia
Prince George, BC
Canada

ISBN 978-3-319-50726-2 ISBN 978-3-319-50727-9 (eBook)
DOI 10.1007/978-3-319-50727-9

Library of Congress Control Number: 2017934319

Printed on acid-free paper

This Springer imprint is published by Springer Nature
The registered company is Springer International Publishing AG
The registered company address is: Gewerbestrasse 11, 6330 Cham, Switzerland

Other Books by Alex C. Michalos

North American Social Report, 5 volumes
Global Report on Student Well-Being, 4 volumes
Essays on the Quality of Life
Ancient Views on the Quality of Life
Militarism and the Quality of Life
Foundations of Decision Making
Trade Barriers to the Public Good
Good Taxes
A Pragmatic Approach to Business Ethics
Principles of Logic
Improving Your Reasoning
The Popper-Carnap Controversy

For Deborah, with love

Acknowledgements

Most of the previously published papers in this set of four volumes (and most of my books) appeared in a publication of Springer, Kluwer, Reidel or Nijhoff, a chain of publishers that I have had the opportunity to work with since the 1960s. Since the original source of each paper in the collection is given on its first page in this collection, there is no need to repeat all these sources and express my thanks for permission to reprint them in each occurrence. I am happy to express here my gratitude for the lot and for the many years of our pleasant and productive work together.

In each of the volumes in this set, I will acknowledge permission to reprint each of the previously published papers appearing in scholarly journals, books or newspapers apart from the chain of publishers listed above. In this first volume, I would like to thank Victoria University of Wellington, Australia for Chap. 2. Weijers, D. (2014). An interview with Alex C. Michalos. *International Journal of Wellbeing*, 4: 1–6.; UNESCO Publishers for Chap. 5. Michalos, A.C. (2006). Logic, philosophy of science and the quality of life. In Philosophy and World Problems, John McMurtry (Ed.). *Encyclopedia of Life Support Systems (EOLSS)*, Developed under the Auspices of the UNESCO, Eolss Publishers, Paris, France (http://www.eolss.net); University of Chicago Press for Chap. 6. Michalos, A.C. (1979). Philosophy of Social Science. In P.D. Asquith & H. Kyburg (Eds.). *Current Research in Philosophy of Science*, (pp. 463–502). Baltimore: Philosophy of Science Association; Philosophy of Science Association for Chap. 7. Michalos, A.C. (1967). Postulates of rational preference. *Philosophy of Science*, 34: 18–22; University of Illinois Press for Chap. 8. Michalos, A.C. (1970). Decision making in committees. *American Philosophical Quarterly*, 7: 91–106; Oxford University Press for Chap. 9. Michalos, A.C. (1970). Analytic and other 'dumb' guides of life. *Analysis*, 30: 121–123; Canadian Philosophical Association for Chap. 11. Michalos, A.C. (1988). Meeting current needs. *Dialogue*, 27: 507–515.

In the Appendix of each volume, I included some photographs and pictures to provide a somewhat different kind of historical context to my narrative. What I have been able to contribute over the past 50 years or so have been influenced by many more people than I have been able to picture here, but when I reflect on what I have done, most of the people pictured here are very much a part of the story. Most of the photographs and pictures are from my family albums, but some have come from friends and a couple newspapers. I would like to express my thanks to the following for allowing me to reprint their items: Wolfgang Glatzer for photographs in How Good Policies and Business Ethics Enhance Good Quality of Life, numbered v2.1 (short for photo #1, volume 2), in Development of the Quality of Life Theory and its Instruments (v3.3, v3.5, and v3.6), and in Connecting the Quality of Life Theory to Health, Well-Being and Education (v4.1); to Ferran Casas for photographs v2.6, v3.1, v3.2 and v3.4; to Filomena Maggino for v4.4, v4.5 and v4.6; to Anna L.D. lau and Roberty A. Cummins for v4.3, v4.8 and v4.9; to Valerie Moller for v3.7 and v3.8; to Joanna Kit-Chun Lam for v3.11; to Daniel T.L. Shek for v4.2; to the *Cleveland Plain Dealer* for Philosphical Foundations of Quality of Life (v1.4), and to the *Detroit Free Press* for v1.7.

Contents

1 Alex C. Michalos: Pioneer of Quality of Life and Social Indicators Research 1
Bruno D. Zumbo

2 Interview by Dan Weijers 5
Dan Weijers
What Got You Interested in Wellbeing Research? 5
What Do You Take "Wellbeing" to Mean? 6
Why Is Wellbeing Research Important? 6
What Is the Most Important Wellbeing-Related Finding from Your Research? 6
What Are You Working on Right Now? 7
What Do You Think the Next Big Thing in Wellbeing Research Will Be? 8
What Are the Main Benefits of Interdisciplinary Research on Wellbeing? 8
What Would the Ideal Census Question on Wellbeing Be and Why? 8
What Parts of Your Research Have Brought You the Most Enjoyment and/or Satisfaction? 9
What Parts of Your Research Have Brought You the Most Dissatisfaction and/or Displeasure? 9
Is There Anything Else You Would like to Comment on? 10
References 11

3 The Best Teacher I Ever Had Was … J. Coert Rylaarsdam 13
Alex C. Michalos

4 The Case for Atheism 17
Alex C. Michalos
Introductory Comments 17

The General Argument . . . 18
Examples of a Creation at War with Itself . . . 23
Summary of the Last 7 Arguments . . . 24

5 **Logic, Philosophy of Science and the Quality of Life** . . . 25
Alex C. Michalos
Introduction . . . 25
Logical Foundations . . . 26
Philosophy of Science . . . 30
Scientific Significance . . . 31
Theory and Observation . . . 33
Discovery and Growth . . . 37
Explanation . . . 42
Induction . . . 47
Probability . . . 49
Utility . . . 51
Social Responsibility . . . 52
Quality of Life . . . 55
Glossary . . . 59
Bibliography . . . 64

6 **Philosophy of Social Science** . . . 67
Alex C. Michalos
Introduction . . . 67
Aspects of the Problem . . . 67
Part One of the Solution: Dissertations . . . 70
Part Two of the Solution: Articles . . . 72
Part Three of the Solution: Books . . . 75
Suggestions for the Future . . . 78
The Future Following Past Performance . . . 78
The Future Beyond the Present Main Stream . . . 80
Appendix 1: Issues Discussed or Theses Defended in Recent Dissertations in Philosophy of Social Science . . . 82
Appendix 2: Dissertation Bibliography. Philosophy of Social Science 1961–1977 . . . 86
Appendix 3: Proceedings and Colloquia Volumes . . . 91
References . . . 93

7 **Postulates of Rational Preference** . . . 97
Alex C. Michalos
References . . . 101

8 **Decision-Making in Committees** . . . 103
Alex C. Michalos
Introduction . . . 103

The Problem 104
Criteria of Adequacy 105
Weighting Voters 108
Weighted Voting 113
Objections and Replies: Weighting Voters 118
Objections and Replies: Weighted Voting 126
Conclusion 129

9 Analytic and Other "DUMB" Guides of Life 131
Alex C. Michalos

10 The Morality of Cognitive Decision-Making [Ethics of Belief] 135
Alex C. Michalos
Introduction 135
The Question 135
The Case for a Negative Ethics of Belief 138
The Case Against a Negative Ethics of Belief 141
The Case for a Positive Ethics of Belief 144
The Case Against a Positive Ethics of Belief 146
The Case Against Any Ethics of Belief 146
Conclusion 149

11 Meeting Current Needs 151
Alex C. Michalos

12 A Reconsideration of the Idea of a Science Court 159
Alex C. Michalos
Outline of the Science Court Experiment 160
Initiation 160
Organization 160
Suggested Procedures 160
Conclusion 176

13 Technology Assessment, Facts and Values 177
Alex C. Michalos
Introduction 177
Fact and Value: Ontology 178
Fact and Falsehood: Epistemology 180
From Ontology to Epistemology 181
From Ontology to Methodology 185
Theories of Value 187
Naturalistic Objectivism 191
Naturalistic Subjectivism 191
Nonnaturalistic Objectivism 192
Nonnaturalistic Subjectivism 192
Emotivism 193

Prescriptivism. 194
Rational Decision-Making 195
Conclusion 196

14 A Pragmatic Theory of Value 197
Alex C. Michalos
Introduction 197
Satisfaction 199
Criteria of Adequacy 201
Generic Value. 203
Objective Value 205
Moral Value 210
Objections to Consequentialism 212
Epistemic Value 223
Rationality 226
References 226

15 Creating a Culture of Support for the Social Sciences: Lessons from the First Forty Years of the Social Science Federation of Canada 229
Alex C. Michalos
Introduction 229
Ad Hoc Meeting 1 230
Ad Hoc Meeting 2 232
Ad Hoc Meeting 3 233
Ad Hoc Meeting 4 235
Ad Hoc Meeting 5 237
Ad Hoc Meeting 6 237
Reflections on Directions 240
Canadian Research Council in the Social Sciences, First Meeting 242
CRCSS, Second Meeting 243
The Official First Annual Meeting of the CRCSS. 244
CRCSS Executive Meeting, November 4, 1944 245
CRCSS Annual Meeting, December 15, 1945 245
CRCSS Annual Meeting, November 1, 1946 246
CRCSS Annual Meeting, October 25, 1947 246
CRCSS Annual Meeting, June 12, 1948. 247
CRCSS Executive Meeting, January 22, 1949 247
CRCSS Annual Meeting, October 29, 1949 248
Executive Meeting, February 25, 1950. 249
Annual Meeting, June 3, 1950 250
Annual Meeting, June 3, 1951 250
Meetings from November 1952 to March 1956 252
Meetings, June 9, 1956 to November 30, 1957 254

Meetings, 1958 256
Meetings, 1960–1962 257
Meetings, 1963–1965 261
Meetings, 1966–1968 263
The Social Sciences in Canada (Timlin-Faucher Report) 265
Meetings in 1968 269
Meetings in 1969–1970 272
1970–1973 277
Critical Choices 285
Conclusions 287
References 288

16 Notes for a System of Scientific Research Reports Accounts 291
Alex C. Michalos

Appendix 299

Overview of the "The Selected Works of Alex C. Michalos"

How Good Policies and Business Ethics Enhance Good Quality of Life

1 **Social Sciences and Business Ethics** ... 1
Alex C. Michalos

2 **Business Ethics and the Quality of Life** ... 5
Alex C. Michalos

3 **The Costs of Decision-Making** ... 13
Alex C. Michalos

4 **Efficiency and Morality** ... 27
Alex C. Michalos

5 **Rationality Between the Maximizers and the Satisficers** ... 35
Alex C. Michalos

6 **The Loyal Agent's Argument** ... 53
Alex C. Michalos

7 **Moral Responsibility in Business, or Fourteen Unsuccessful Ways to Pass the Buck** ... 63
Alex C. Michalos

8 **A Case for a Progressive Annual Net Wealth Tax** ... 81
Alex C. Michalos

9 **Militarism and the Quality of Life** ... 111
Alex C. Michalos

10 **The Impact of Trust on Business, International Security and the Quality of Life** ... 127
Alex C. Michalos

11 **Ethical Considerations Regarding Public Opinion Polling During Election Campaigns** . . . 155
Alex C. Michalos

12 **Brief to the Ontario Cabinet Committee on North American Free Trade** . . . 185
Alex C. Michalos

13 **Issues for Business Ethics in the Nineties and Beyond** . . . 197
Alex C. Michalos

14 **Observations on Performance Indicators and Performance-Based Management in Public Administration** . . . 213
Alex C. Michalos

15 **The Integration of Public Policy-Making with Outcomes Measurement** . . . 235
Alex C. Michalos

16 **A Handful of Sand in the Wheels of Financial Speculation** . . . 251
Alex C. Michalos

17 **Ethics Counselors as a New Priesthood** . . . 273
Alex C. Michalos

18 **Observations on the Proposed BC—STV Voting System** . . . 293
Alex C. Michalos

19 **Ancient Observations on Business Ethics: Middle East Meets West** . . . 297
Alex C. Michalos

20 **The Monster of Supercapitalism** . . . 313
Alex C. Michalos

21 **The Business Case for Asserting the Business Case for Business Ethics** . . . 329
Alex C. Michalos

22 **Public Policy Letters to Editors 1989–2001** . . . 343
Alex C. Michalos

Appendix . . . 377

Development of Quality of Life Theory and Its Instruments

1 **Quality of Life, Two-Variable Theory** . . . 1
Alex C. Michalos

2 **Satisfaction and Happiness** 5
Alex C. Michalos

3 **Multiple Discrepancies Theory (MDT)** 39
Alex C. Michalos

4 **A Feminist View of Women and Development** 97
Alex C. Michalos

5 **Highlights of Four Volume Global Report on Student Well-Being** 103
Alex C. Michalos

6 **Comments on Papers for the Special Issue on Global Report on Student Well-Being** 111
Alex C. Michalos

7 **Aspects of the Quality of Life in Prince George: A Case Study in Canada** 117
Alex C. Michalos

8 **Quality of Life in Jasper, Alberta** 137
Bruno D. Zumbo and Alex C. Michalos

9 **British Columbians' Expectations and Attitudes Going into the Third Millennium** 157
Alex C. Michalos and Bruno D Zumbo

10 **Identifying The Horse, The Cart and Their Proper Order in Sustainable Development** 175
Alex C. Michalos

11 **Connecting Communities with Community Indicators** 185
Alex C. Michalos

12 **Stability and Sensitivity in Perceived Quality of Life Measures: Some Panel Results** 199
Alex C. Michalos and P. Maurine Kahlke

13 **Arts and the Perceived Quality of Life in British Columbia** 241
Alex C. Michalos and P. Maurine Kahlke

14 **What Did Stiglitz, Sen and Fitoussi Get Right and What Did They Get Wrong?** 287
Alex C. Michalos

15 **Progress in Measuring Knowledge, Attitudes and Behaviours Concerning Sustainable Development Among Tenth Grade Students in Manitoba** 301
Alex C. Michalos, P. Maurine Kahlke, Karen Rempel, Anu Lounatvuori, Anne MacDiarmid, Heather Creech and Carolee Buckler

16 **Social Indicators Research: The Little Red Hen 40 Years Later** 337
Alex C. Michalos

17 **Michalos-Zumbo Well-Being Index** 341
Bruno D. Zumbo and Alex C. Michalos

Appendix 347

Connecting the Quality of Life Theory to Health, Well-Being and Education

1 **Cost-Benefit Versus Expected Utility Acceptance Rules** 1
Alex C. Michalos

2 **Social Indicators Research and Health-Related Quality of Life Research** 25
Alex C. Michalos

3 **Culture as a Moderator of Overall Life Satisfaction—Life Facet Satisfaction Relationships** 59
Alison G.C. Mallard, Charles E. Lance and Alex C. Michalos

4 **Determinants of Health and the Quality of Life in the Bella Coola Valley** 81
Alex C. Michalos, Harvey V. Thommasen, Rua Read, Nancy Anderson and Bruno D. Zumbo

5 **Health and Quality of Life of Aboriginal Residential School Survivors, Bella Coola Valley, 2001** 123
Sylvia S. Barton, Harvey V. Thommasen, Bill Tallio, William Zhang and Alex C. Michalos

6 **Comparing Self-rated Health, Satisfaction and Quality of Life Scores Between Diabetics and Others Living in the Bella Coola Valley** 137
Angela Grigg, Harvey V. Thommasen, Hugh Tildesley and Alex C. Michalos

7 The Relationship Between Health Survey and Medical Chart Review Results in a Rural Population 151
Donald C. Voaklander, Harvey V. Thommasen and Alex C. Michalos

8 Health and Quality of Life of Older People, a Replication After Six Years 165
Alex C. Michalos, P. Maurine Hatch, Dawn Hemingway, Loraine Lavallee, Anne Hogan and Bev Christensen

9 Good Health is Not the Same as a Good Life: Survey Results from Brandon, Manitoba 201
Alex C. Michalos, Douglas Ramsey, Derrek Eberts and P. Maurine Kahlke

10 A Note on Student Quality of Life 247
Alex C. Michalos and Julie Anne Orlando

11 Quality of Life of Some Under-Represented Survey Respondents: Youth, Aboriginals and Unemployed 255
Alex C. Michalos and Julie Anne Orlando

12 Education, Happiness and Wellbeing 277
Alex C. Michalos

13 A Developmental View of Liberal Education 301
Alex C. Michalos

14 Einstein, Ethics and Science 313
Alex C. Michalos

15 Observations on Unacknowledged Authorship from Homer to Now 327
Alex C. Michalos

16 Building the Encyclopedia of Quality of Life and Well-Being Research 335
Alex C. Michalos

17 Milestones of Quality of Life Research in Canada, 1960s to 2014 347
Alex C. Michalos

Appendix 397

Introduction to "Selected Works of Alex C. Michalos"

Biographical Notes

The central aim of this set of volumes is to describe and explain the context and connections among a subset of papers and books produced over the past 50 years. Rather than a mere reproduction of work already published, this will be an attempt to disclose the productive processes in their various historic contexts that led to the various research projects and publications. In Michalos (2003a), I published a collection called *Essays on the Quality of Life* containing 20 articles focused on the quality of life, 3 of which appear in other volumes of this set because they seemed to be so central to the array of issues in the 70 articles in these volumes. For completeness, I mention articles from the earlier collection and books that are directly relevant to the themes in these volumes.

Some years ago (these days it seems that most things begin with "some years ago", unfortunately), in a debate about the existence of God, a member of the audience put a question to us "Why would God want to watch re-runs?" The question made sense from the point of view of one of the debaters, since God was supposed to know everything that is going to happen before it happens. As the atheist in the debate, I could only say that I have no idea why, although a lot of people seem to enjoy them.

While I also enjoy some re-runs, I would not find much joy in re-binding some old papers for a new audience. I do, however, find the idea of describing the historical context in which similar research questions more or less simultaneously appeared to people in diverse parts of the globe and were addressed first individually and then collectively. Here, the historical context includes some of my own biographical material. This is offered as a kind of second-best effort substituting for an autobiography that I have never had the courage to write, notwithstanding having thought about it many times.

My father ended his formal education in the sixth grade and my mother ended hers in the eighth grade. As far as I have been able to discern, in 1917, when he was about 17, my father, Charles K. Michalos, emigrated from the island of Chios,

Greece, to work in the steel mills of Gary, Indiana. He arrived with a pocket-sized Greek–English dictionary, learned to speak English with a heavy Greek accent, moved from the mills to driving a Nabisco bread and pastry truck for another 17 years, bought a small hamburger joint, then a somewhat bigger one and finally something more like a diner on Euclid Avenue in Cleveland, Ohio. Its claim to fame was the fact that many of the Cleveland Browns ate there, which was quite a big deal in 1947 when the Browns were the All American Football Conference champions, and I was one of their biggest junior high school fans. My father died in January 1951, at about 51. We were never sure, because he was never sure, how old he was. I was daddy's boy, and his loss was a great loss to me.

My mother, Josephine Pucci, was born in Akron, Ohio, one of eight children of immigrants from Palermo, Sicily. She worked at the May Company department store, sang in the chorus of the Cleveland Opera Company, married my father in 1931, produced my brother in 1932 and me in 1935, and provided the mom part of our mom-and-pop diner. Unlike my dad, she was not a particularly happy person, but she lived to be 93 years old, dying in June 1998. Like my dad, and the rest of us I guess, she did the best she could with what she had.

I was generally an above average but not outstanding primary and secondary school student. In secondary school and the first half of university, I was more interested in sports and girls than scholarship, though I enjoyed mathematics and history. I went to what was then Western Reserve University (now Case-Western Reserve University) in 1953, majoring in history with minors in philosophy and religion. When I read Plato's *Republic*, I felt as if he was talking directly to me. It had never occurred to me to ask what a good life might be, but the more I thought about it, the more I *had* to think about it.

I grew up in a very mixed religious family. The story my mother told was that her family were Catholics until the local priest did something that led my grandfather to tell him to go to hell and he took the whole gene pool into a more friendly Baptist church. My father seemed to practice the religion of washing his car on Sundays, but he thought his sons had to be baptized Greek Orthodox in order to preserve something or other that was important to him. So, we were. However, because our house was one block away from a small Quaker church, my brother, Chuck Michalos, and I were sent off together as soon as we were old enough to find our way there and back. I have a gold medal showing that I accumulated three years of Sundays without missing Quaker Sunday school.

Given this background, when I began to think seriously about a good life, I thought I should make my peace with God if there were one. So, besides studying philosophy, I studied the history of religions. Then I went to graduate school at the University of Chicago. Because I was what one would have called a doubter, I wanted to study religion in a school of believers, assuming that if anyone could convince me that I was wrong, they could. At least they would be inclined to try. So, in 1957 I enrolled in the Divinity School, which seemed to have the most diverse faculty, including visiting experts in Buddhism, which especially interested me.

I also married in the summer of 1957, a marriage that lasted about 23 years and produced Cyndi (1960), Ted (1961) and Stephanie (1963). In 1985, I married the love of my life, Deborah Poff, a lucky break for both of us at the time and ever since.

While studying the history of religions, I took courses in philosophy and it seemed to me that philosophers had more precise and decisive methods of pursuing the truth than theologians. The University of Chicago had a wonderfully flexible approach to higher education, allowing students to pursue more than one degree at a time. To get a Bachelor of Divinity degree, a student was required to pass 7 comprehensive exams and have a year internship in some relevant field of practice. I took some courses designed to prepare one to take the exams and some courses in philosophy that I found interesting. At the 1961 convocation, I received a B.D. and an M.A. in philosophy, and then proceeded to pursue a Ph.D. in philosophy of science. I completed the latter in 1965 with a dissertation on a dispute between Rudolf Carnap and Karl Popper on the nature and use of probability theory in the assessment of scientific theories (Michalos 1971).

Many of the most salient and important features of the following 50 years of research and other activities may be regarded as relatively natural developments of these earlier initiatives. In a memorable essay on the best teacher he ever had, Keyfitz (2003) said that scholars should replace the metaphor of providing building blocks for a relatively durable corporate body of knowledge with that of providing biodegradable nutrition out of which new knowledge would grow. In a sense, today's nutrient is tomorrow's fertilizer. What I did until 1965 provided the ingredients for what followed, just as the latter will feed what comes afterward. Most importantly, I think my general approach has been informed by a pragmatic and philosophic interest in a holistic, comprehensive understanding of any particular object of investigation. I will try to explain this approach in the next few paragraphs.

Broadly speaking, there are two ways to define "*philosophy*". From a *functional* point of view, philosophy may be identified as critical thinking about anything at all, from asphalt to zebras. From a *content* point of view, philosophy may be identified as a body of knowledge answering three questions. What is it? What good is it? How do you know?

Answering the question "What is it?" gives one a discussion of the nature or being of something. In short, it gives one an *ontology*, a word derived from the Greek "on" meaning nature or being, and logos, meaning discourse (among other things). Descriptions of the nature of things, ontologies, have at least two aspects. Everything has, after all, a form, structure, morphology or anatomy on the one hand, and a function, activity or physiology on the other. A duck, smile or football game, for example, can be described at a minimum by describing their structural parts and how the parts function. What Isaac Newton might have referred to as natural philosophy and we now would call natural science is close to what philosophers would call ontology.

Answering the question "What good is it?" gives one a discussion of the value, worth or goodness in some sense of something. In short, it gives one an *axiology*, a word derived from the Greek "axios" meaning worthy or valuable, and logos. Of the variety of kinds of value that may be described, it is most useful to distinguish intrinsic from instrumental value. *Intrinsic value* refers to the worth or goodness of a thing in itself, its value as an end in itself rather than as a means to something else. *Instrumental value* refers to the worth or goodness of a thing as a means to something else, not as a thing in itself. Standard examples include things such as eating an apple or throwing a ball at a target having instrumental value insofar as the former produces nutrition and the latter scores points, which in this context have intrinsic value.

Since practically anything might be a useful means to something else for someone in some circumstances for some purposes, practically anything can have instrumental value. However, some people believe that all alleged sorts of intrinsic value may be reduced to a single one. For example, they would argue that the nutrition obtained from eating an apple is really only instrumentally valuable as a means to good health, which is itself instrumentally valuable for a life of pleasure, happiness or satisfaction. Those who believe that there is finally only one intrinsically valuable thing such as pleasure, happiness or satisfaction may be called monists with respect to the ultimate nature (ontological status) of value, while those who believe that there are many intrinsically valuable things may be called *pluralists*.

For a monist, then, it may be said that ontologically distinct things such as music, cheese and justice have different degrees of some sort of value such as pleasure, happiness or satisfaction, while for a pluralist, such ontologically distinct things have ontologically distinct values (music value, cheese value and justice value) regardless of how much pleasure, happiness or satisfaction these things produce. From an ontological point of view, then, a monist would have a numerically smaller number of ontologically distinct things in his or her world (e.g. music, cheese, justice and some degree of pleasure, happiness or satisfaction generated by the other three), while a pluralist's world would have music, cheese, justice plus music value, cheese value and justice value.

For a monist, the task of measuring the total value of something, a person, event, object, attitude, belief, proposition, action or life itself, is in principle straightforward. One simply needs to measure the degree of intrinsic value generated by that thing in terms of or operationalized as pleasure, happiness or satisfaction. For pluralists, the task of measuring the total value of something is not at all straightforward because there may be no way to compare ontologically distinct values like the value of music versus the value of cheese or justice. There does not appear to be any common measure, scale or instrument available to answer questions such as "How much is music worth compared to the value of justice or cheese?" or "What is the value of this piece of music in terms of the value of justice or cheese?"

Given the severe comparability problems faced by all value pluralists, it is not surprising that the most frequently studied theories of economists and decision theorists, namely preference theory, choice theory, utility theory and game theory, and one of the most popular ethical theories studied by philosophers, utilitarianism, assume value monism of some sort. As we will see in many of the papers in this collection and many more cited in those papers, scholars have invented a great variety of methods for living in and managing a world apparently containing a plurality of values. In particular, I will describe my own efforts over about 50 years, which have been interesting but largely unsuccessful.

Answering the question "How do you know?" gives a discussion of one's knowledge of something. In short, it gives one an *epistemology*, a word derived from the Greek "episteme" meaning knowledge and logos, hence, a theory of knowledge. Strictly speaking one ought, prudentially and morally, to have a fairly clear answer to the epistemological question before one attempts to answer the ontological and axiological questions. Since a philosopher aims to obtain a body of knowledge about the nature and value of things to be used in the practice of living a good life, a patently necessary condition of achieving that aim is clarity with respect to knowledge itself and its production. That is why the earliest essays in these 4 volumes concern epistemological issues.

Comments on the Articles

All of the papers in this set of volumes are arranged partly in chronological order and partly by their logical connections. Each volume has its own major themes and within those themes articles have been selected and arranged to provide some idea of the time at which they appeared and its relation to my own and others' research agendas around that time.

In this volume, we begin with three biographical articles. Chapter 1 is a biographical sketch written by Bruno Zumbo for a series of similar articles on pioneers of quality of life research in the journal *Applied Research in Quality of Life*, the official journal of the International Society for Quality of Life Studies. This is followed by a transcript of an interview I gave to Dan Weijers for a similar kind of series in the *International Journal of Wellbeing*. While Zumbo's chapter is a relatively objective overview of my professional life described in his voice, Weijers's chapter gives someone a more subjective overview in my own voice. The website of ISQOLS has a number of videos of interviews of pioneers in its series, one by Michael B. Frisch covering Michalos.

Since I was a university professor for 40 years, I spent a lot of time reading and thinking about teaching, observing and talking to other teachers, preparing to teach, trying to teach, teaching, evaluating my teaching, trying to improve my teaching, succeeding and failing probably in equal measure. As part of this lifelong interest, in Michalos (2003b) I put together 124 essays written by Fellows of the Royal Society of Canada, an honorary association of Canada's most productive scholars, describing the best teacher they ever had. Chapter 3 below, on J. Coert Rylaarsdam, was originally published in *Teaching Business Ethics*, a scholarly journal that I co-founded and edited with Deborah Poff. (I founded or co-founded 7 scholarly journals, including *Social Indicators Research*, *Journal of Business Ethics*, *Teaching Business Ethics*, *Journal of Happiness Studies*, *Journal of Academic Ethics*, *Applied Research on the Quality of Life* and the *Asian Journal of Business Ethics*.) It was reproduced in the Royal Society collection. If I was ever any good as a teacher, I owe much of it to Rylaarsdam.

After leaving Divinity School, I seldom gave any thought to theological issues except when I was teaching introductory philosophy courses or asked to participate in public panel discussions. Chapter 4 is a set of notes I used in a panel discussion on the question of the existence of God.

Chapter 5 provides a summary of some of my basic epistemological beliefs, including elementary principles of logic and fundamental issues in the philosophy of science, e.g. the nature of scientific explanation, theories, laws and probabilistic assessment of the acceptability of scientific theories. These are the subjects I taught every year of the 40 years I worked in universities. Following this review, I address the axiological question of the contribution these subjects can make to the definition, measure and living a life of a morally good quality. Within the limits of a relatively brief essay, this chapter connects much of what I routinely taught my whole career with what became my primary research field across most of the period. My first three books and two anthologies were on logic and the philosophy of science: *Principles of Logic* (1969), *Improving Your Reasoning* (1970), *The Popper-Carnap Controversy* (1971), *Philosophic Problems of Science and Technology* (1974) and *Boston Studies in the Philosophy of Science, Vol. 32, Proceedings of the 1974 Biennial Meeting of Philosophy of Science Association* (1976, co-edited with R.S. Cohen, C.A. Hooker and J.W. Van Evra).

A shorter version of Chap. 6 was presented at a conference in Reston, Virginia, in October 1977 on Critical Research Problems organized by a committee of the Philosophy of Science Association and sponsored by the US National Science Foundation. The committee consisted of Henry E. Kyburg, Peter Asquith, Arthur Burks, David Hull, Alex Michalos and Ernan McMullin. After the conference, authors were asked to produce longer versions that included information obtained from conference discussions. Twenty-eight essays were then published in a volume edited by Asquith and Kyburg in 1979. Each essay was supposed to provide readers with a guide to the current problems being researched in the field and to suggest problems for research in the future. My contribution covered roughly 20 years of research in the philosophy of social sciences. A review of 571 abstracts from social science journals showed that "more work was put on decision-making than on anything else. Forty-nine articles were devoted to this subject. Moreover, since most of the articles on values (46), rationality (25) and utility (21) are related to decision making, this subject easily dominates the literature in the philosophy of social science". Readers of this chapter will find a good illustration of one piece of the sort of research field review often called for by the founders of the Social Sciences Federation of Canada in Chap. 15.

Chapters 7–11 all deal with some features of decision-making. My fourth book, *Foundations of Decision Making* (1978), contains my most comprehensive and considered views about this topic, some of which are also represented in How Good

Policies and Business Ethics Enhance Good Quality of Life of this collection. In Chap. 7, I showed that the postulates of rational preference used by decision theorists most famously since the classic treatise of John Von Neumann and Oskar Morgenstern, *Theory of Games and Economic Behavior* (1944) are "inaccurate empirical generalizations and unacceptable normative principles". In Chap. 8, I proposed and evaluated a type of group decision-making procedure "distinguished by the fact that inequalities in the 'weight' of individual voters *and* their votes are permitted". The upshot of the discussion is that it seems to be the case that the standard democratic procedure with each person having one equally weighted vote is at least as good as any of the systems considered.

In his classic *Logical Foundations of Probability* (1950), Rudolf Carnap reiterated a traditional positivist view that, because it is impossible to completely verify any empirical claim, statements about the probability of such claims should be a "guide of life". In Chap. 9, I showed that some fine contemporary philosophers of science (A.J. Ayer, P.K. Feyerabend, W.C. Salmon and W.C. Kneale) who challenged this view were mistaken. Some logically true or analytic probability statements can, should and do function as guides to human action, and some are better than others.

In Chap. 10, I describe and analyze a dispute that arose in 1886 between the British philosopher W.K. Clifford and the American philosopher William James over the question whether or not someone could be morally praiseworthy or blameworthy for deciding that something is true or false. Nobody doubts that people's actions are always subject to moral appraisal, but many people believe that decisions made merely about beliefs or what to believe, so-called cognitive decisions, are not subject to such appraisal. Briefly, this disagreement is traditionally known as the problem of an ethics of belief. James and Clifford both believed that there is an ethics of belief, but they disagreed on its content and prescriptions. I evaluate the arguments of each philosopher and show that James had a more plausible case.

Chapter 11 is a critical review of David Braybrooke's *Meeting Needs* (1987), including some comments from an exchange we had in a panel discussion of the book at the 1987 annual meeting of the Canadian Philosophical Association. It is included here because concepts of needing and wanting are basic elements in my *Foundations of Decision Making* and because many people have suggested that a system of social indicators or social accounts should be based on a hierarchy of human needs as explained in, for example, A.H. Maslow's *Motivation and Personality* (1954). The suggestion is typically made by people who assume that needs provide a relatively objective basis for such systems, and Braybrooke's explication of the concept or concepts of needs makes a similar assumption. I show that any plausible explication of a concept of needs is essentially evaluative and contingent upon someone's subjective assessments, implying that it would be a mistake to search for a completely objective basis for systems based on needs.

In the 1970s, the Philosophy of Science Association began to make room in its annual conferences for sessions on philosophy of technology. Lines between technology and science are a bit fuzzy, but philosophers interested primarily in the former seemed to be concerned with axiological/ethical issues while those interested primarily in the latter were concerned with epistemological issues. By 1976, philosophers of technology became convinced that their interests would always only be marginally represented at philosophy of science conferences. So the Society for Philosophy and Technology was born. Since I had interests and friends in both areas of research, I became active in the new organization, serving a term as President in 1983–85. Chapters 12 and 13 were written in the context of developing this organization.

Chapter 12 begins with the sentence "In August 1976 the U.S. Task Force of the Presidential Advisory Group on Anticipated Advances in Science and Technology published an interim report on something they called 'The Science Court Experiment'". The aim of the Court was to provide an unbiased, transparent and decisive adjudication procedure for public policy making concerning scientific and technological innovations. I thought the idea promised some relief from the frequently occurring problem of experts routinely appearing for and against innovations with no mutually agreed-upon set of rules for deciding which experts were right. My paper reviewed all the arguments of proponents and opponents of the Court, with the aim of clearing its path for future development. As it turned out, it had no future.

The thesis defended in Chap. 13 is a product of considerations that arose in my analysis of the Science Court. In this chapter, I show that "there are good theoretical and practical reasons to avoid any appeals to a fact-value distinction in the assessment of technology". After drawing an ontological distinction between facts and values versus an epistemological distinction between facts (truths) and falsehoods, I analyze five types of unsound arguments used in technology assessment and other public policy making based on confusing the ontological and epistemological distinctions. Then, I sketch 6 theories of value, i.e. theories designed to reveal its nature or ontological structure. One of these theories, that I call *naturalistic subjectivism*, has driven a great deal of my research.

Chapter 14 contains my most ambitious effort to construct a naturalistic subjectivist theory of value building on the work of American pragmatists, mostly Ralph Barton Perry *General Theory of Value* (1926), John Dewey *Theory of Valuation* (1939) and Clarence Irving Lewis *An Analysis of Knowledge and Valuation* (1946). The general plan was to define value in a naturalistic way as the human psychological attribute, satisfaction. So, briefly, following the traditional monistic position, something would have value just so far as it produced satisfaction for someone, and the more satisfaction produced in more people, the more valuable anything would become. A detailed set of proposed definitions for the foundation of such a theory is presented in the chapter, awaiting only an empirical theory of satisfaction to complete the story. Armed with such an empirically based theory of value, in principle it would be possible to scientifically and relatively objectively evaluate every aspect of our world and measure its total worth. Multiple discrepancies theory (MDT) was supposed to be the empirical theory of satisfaction (Michalos 1985) required for the empirically based theory of value, and *North American Social Report* (1980a, b, 1981a, b, 1982) was supposed to be an empirical assessment of the quality of life in Canada and the USA in the 1964–74 period based on that naturalistic subjectivist theory. An overview of the *North American Social Report* is presented in the fourth volume (Connecting the Quality of Life Theory to Health, Well-Being and Education) of this collection with other Canadian milestones. As it turned out, MDT involves some circularity preventing it from providing a thoroughly empirical basis of value, there is no generally accepted set of purely descriptive features of any country and no known way to evaluate such features using MDT. So, the grand plan could not be implemented although, hopefully, the articles and discussions in these 4 volumes will reveal something useful for the next person with some such plan.

Chapter 15 is a historical account of the development of what was the Social Sciences Federation of Canada from 1938 to 1980. Since 1996, the organization has been the Federation for the Humanities and Social Sciences, representing "over 80 scholarly associations, 79 institutions and six affiliate organizations, representing 85,000 researchers, educators and students across Canada" (http://www.ideas-idees.ca/about/about-the-federation). The history is written as a story of how an ad hoc group of relatively far-sighted social scientists collaborated to build an institution designed to nurture a culture of support for social scientific research in Canada. The focus is on the variety of players over the period, their views about what should and could be done, what actually was done and what were the important lessons for the future.

The final article, appearing as Chap. 16, is a brief sketch of the flow of research reports representing the most visible output of scientific investigation mapped onto the scheme of the National Income and Product Accounts. The aim was to try to craft a kind of input–output system that would allow something like an accounting system for a country's scientific research.

References

Braybrooke, D. (1987). *Meeting needs.* Princeton, NJ: Princeton University Press.

Carnap, R. (1950). *Logical foundations of probability*. Chicago: University of Chicago Press.

Dewey, J. (1939). *Theory of valuation*. Chicago: University of Chicago Press.

Keyfitz, N. (2003). Nathan Keyfitz on Mr. Somerville and others. In A. C. Michalos (Ed.). *The best teacher I ever had: Personal reports from highly productive scholars* (pp. 126–131). London, Ontario: Althouse Press.

Lewis, C. I. (1946). *An analysis of knowledge and valuation*. LaSalle: The Open Court Pub. Co.

Maslow, A. H. A. (1954). *Motivation and personality*. New York: Harper and Row.

Michalos, A. C. (1969). *Principles of logic*. Englewood Cliffs: Prentice-Hall, Inc.

Michalos, A. C. (1970). *Improving your reasoning*. Englewood Cliffs: Prentice-Hall, Inc.

Michalos, A. C. (1971). *The Popper-Carnap controversy*. Hague: Martinus Nijhoff.

Michalos, A. C. (Ed.). (1974). *Philosophic problems of science and technology*. Boston: Allyn and Bacon.

Michalos, A. C. (1978). *Foundations of decision making*. Ottawa: Canadian Library of Philosophy.

Michalos, A. C. (1980a). *North American social report, vol. 1: Foundations, population and health*. Dordrecht: D. Reidel.
Michalos, A. C. (1980b). *North American social report, vol. 2: Crime, justice and politics*. Dordrecht: D. Reidel.
Michalos, A. C. (1981a). *North American social report, vol. 3: Science, education and recreation*. Dordrecht: D. Reidel.
Michalos, A. C. (1981b). *North American social report, vol. 4: Environment, transportation and housing*. Dordrecht: D. Reidel.
Michalos, A. C. (1982). *North American social report, vol. 5: Economics, religion and morality*. Dordrecht: D. Reidel.
Michalos, A. C. (1985). Multiple discrepancies theory (MDT). *Social Indicators Research, 16*, 347–413.
Michalos, A. C. (2003a). *Essays on the quality of life*. Dordrecht: Kluwer Academic Publishers.
Michalos, A. C. (Ed.). (2003b). *The best teacher I ever had: Personal reports from highly productive scholars*. London, Ontario: The Althouse Press.
Michalos, A. C., Cohen, R. S., Hooker, C. A., & Van Evra, J. W. (Eds.). (1976). *Boston studies in the philosophy of science, vol. 32: Proceedings of the 1974 Biennial Meeting of the Philosophy of Science Association*. Dordrecht: D. Reidel.
Perry, R. B. (1926). *General theory of value*. Cambridge: Harvard University Press.
Von Neumann, J., & Morgenstern, O. (1944). *Theory of games and economic behavior*. Princeton: Princeton University Press.

Chapter 1
Alex C. Michalos: Pioneer of Quality of Life and Social Indicators Research

Bruno D. Zumbo

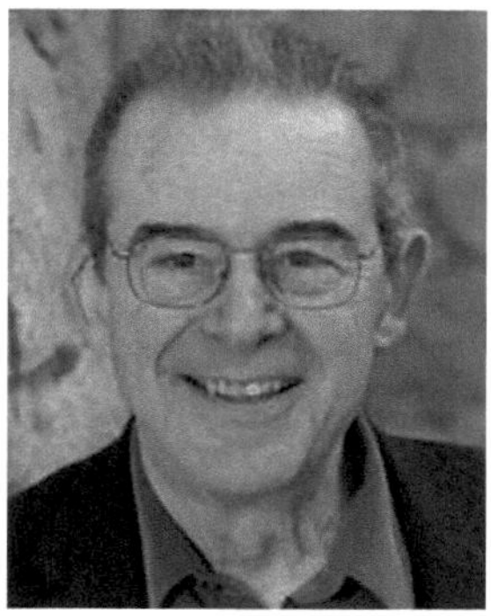

When I think of *pioneers* I imagine a hardy people traveling from a former life to a new unsettled place full of unknowns. My image of pioneers is influenced by John Wayne movies and the TV show *Bonanza.* These pioneers are, of course, not starting from nothing because they bring with them their tools, ideas, and beliefs from their earlier lives. I imagine life as a pioneer to be risky, exhausting, and chalk full of prospecting.

These images capture some of the main features of what I imagine to be my friend and longtime research collaborator Alex C. Michalos' pioneering life in quality life and social indicators research. He traveled from the comforts of a

Zumbo, B.D.: 2014. Alex C. Michalos: Pioneer of Quality of Life and Social Indicators Research. Applied Research in Quality of Life, 9, pp. 457–459. © Springer Science+Business Media Dordrecht and The International Society for Quality-of-Life Studies (ISQOLS) 2013.

B.D. Zumbo (✉)
Department of ECPS, The University of British Columbia,
Scarfe Building, 2125 Main Mall, Vancouver, BC V6T 1Z4, Canada
e-mail: bruno.zumbo@ubc.ca

A.C. Michalos, *Philosophical Foundations of Quality of Life*,
DOI 10.1007/978-3-319-50727-9_1

well-established and highly successful life well known for his work in philosophy of science, logic, and ethics to break new ground in social indicators and quality of life research. He brought with him his tools of theorizing and formalism as well as a love for data, surveys, evaluation and decision making, data analysis and a deep foundation in philosophical Pragmatism that can be evidenced in all of his work.

Although I will focus on Alex's work in quality of life and social indicators, his influence continues to be felt in academic philosophy where he is well known as the founder and Editor in Chief of the oft-cited *Journal of Business Ethics.* When I first met Alex, I knew him as a philosopher having read his *Principles of Logic* (1969), and *The Popper-Carnap Controversy* (1970). His reviews in philosophical journals were always incisive and very interesting to read, and a gold mine for graduate students interested in broad perspective on philosophical problems.

Alex is currently Emeritus Professor in Political Science at the University of Northern British Columbia, where he taught from 1994 to 2001 and served as Chancellor from 2007 to 2010. He was Professor of Philosophy at University of Guelph from 1966 to 1994, and Assistant Professor at State University of New York (1964–1966) and at State College, St. Cloud (1962–1964). Alex earned his Ph.D. in Philosophy of Science (1965), B.D. in history of religions and M.A. in logic (1961) all from the University of Chicago, and his B.A. from Western Reserve University (1957).

One can imagine how precarious it feels to try and capture such a productive and influential scholarly life as Alex's in a limited number of words so I will relieve myself of any such aspirations and give you what I believe are his most impactful contributions to quality of life and social indicators research and make him an unprecedented pioneer in the field.

1. His creation and ongoing editorship of the journal *Social Indicators Research.* Alex, and a small band of fellow pioneers, founded the journal in 1974. Alex has remained at the helm of the journal through its 114 volumes and 3149 articles published to date. The journal is important in the history of the discipline because it gave scholars an identity as well a place to publish (and read) work in the field. The journal, like Alex himself, takes a broad view of the field and includes empirical, philosophical and methodological studies.
2. His 1985 paper introducing, describing, and empirically testing Multiple Discrepancies Theory (MDT) is developed with an eye to conceptual detail and is an exemplar of solid theory building and testing. In the paper, Alex clearly states six basic hypotheses, extensive supporting evidence, and how the basic hypotheses yield five derived hypotheses that lend themselves to empirical test. The clarity and rigorous account, including the historical antecedents, is what makes the paper a required reading, and a lovely exemplar of how a seasoned philosopher of science builds and empirically tests theories in the social sciences.
3. His comprehensive 1991 four-volume *Global Report on Student Well-being.* The data are rich and the analyses are detailed.

4. His embracing of a life well lived that includes scholarship that impacts the community. There are many examples of this but my personal favorite is our joint creation of the University of Northern British Columbia *Institute for Social Research and Evaluation.* The institute is a partnership with the community to gain greater understanding of the social issues of central British Columbia.
5. His work with emerging scholars locally, nationally and internationally. Alex is well-known for his support of emerging scholars by way of working with them to publish their papers and encouraging them to contribute to conferences and associations.
6. His tireless work as the Editor of the soon to be published 12 Volume *Encyclopedia of Quality of Life and Well-Being Research.* At last count, there will be 2053 entries ranging in length from a few hundred words to several thousand words per entry. This monumental task is the first comprehensive multi disciplinary reference work on scientific and other scholarly research in the social, behavioral and health sciences on quality of life and well-being. The encyclopedia alone is sufficient for pioneer status.
7. It is breath-taking to imagine how one person could have done so much, and so well. He has published 26 books and over 115 refereed articles and founded or cofounded seven scholarly journals. In addition, he is general editor and founder of the *Social Indicators Research Book Series* (having published 52 volumes). He has served as president of the Canadian Commission for UNESCO's Sectoral Commission on Natural, Social and Human Sciences (2004–2008), Academy II (Humanities and Social Sciences) of the Royal Society of Canada (2000–2002), Society for Philosophy and Technology (1983–1985) and the International Society for Quality of Life Studies (1998–2000), and has served as director of research for the Canadian Index of Wellbeing (2006–2011).
8. Not surprisingly, given his tremendous career, he has won several awards of distinction, including most notably the Gold Medal for Achievement in Research (2004) from the Social Sciences and Humanities Research Council of Canada (the Council's highest honor), Member of the Order of Canada, C.M. (2010), Queen Elizabeth II Diamond Jubilee Medal (2012), Award for the Betterment of the Human Condition (2003) from the International Society for Quality of Life Studies (ISQOLS), the ISQOLS Award for Extraordinary Contributions to Quality of Life Research (1996), the Secretary of State's Prize for Excellence in Interdisciplinary Research in Canadian Studies (1984) for his five-volume treatise *North American Social Report: A Comparative Study of the Quality of Life in Canada and the USA from 1964 to 1974.*

My eight favorites of Alex's many accomplishments are but a few select ones from a very long list. As a pioneer, at least in my TV image of one, Alex continues to ride high in the saddle.

Chapter 2
Interview by Dan Weijers

Dan Weijers

What Got You Interested in Wellbeing Research?

I began my academic career in philosophy of science, with a dissertation on the Popper/Carnap controversy on measuring the acceptability of scientific theories. So I did a lot of work on probability theory. Then I moved on to decision and voting theory. Somewhere along the way I read the pragmatists William James, Ralph Barton Perry, John Dewey and Clarence Irving Lewis, and I got intrigued with the idea of a rigorous pragmatic naturalistic theory of value along the lines of Perry (1926) and Lewis (1946) in particular.

I was a visiting professor at the University of Pittsburgh in 1969 and my friend there, Nicholas Rescher, was preparing a manuscript for his book on welfare. I was struck by the way he integrated statistical data and philosophical analysis. At the same time I was reading about practical decision making from Simon (1945, 1957) and the new social indicators movement. I became a charter member of the Public Choice Society, met Mancur Olson and was convinced that if I worked with people in that movement, I could mix my philosophical and statistical interests perfectly.

What I have been doing since the late 60s, as a pragmatist and consequentialist from a philosophical point of view, is trying to define and measure the dependent variable in searches for a good life or a good quality of life, what some people call general wellbeing now.

Weijers, D.: 2014. An interview with Alex C. Michalos. International Journal of Wellbeing, 4, pp.1–6. © The Author(s).

D. Weijers (✉)
University of Northern British Columbia, Prince George, BC, Canada
e-mail: michalos@brandonu.ca

A.C. Michalos, *Philosophical Foundations of Quality of Life*,
DOI 10.1007/978-3-319-50727-9_2

What Do You Take "Wellbeing" to Mean?

I identify wellbeing with a life of good quality, all things considered. There is no rule book about what should be included in the "all things considered". So it takes a lot of conceptualizing and measuring to get a generic package that will be acceptable to most individuals and societies. When I started back in the 60s, I thought it might take 25 years or so before the world would reach some agreement on what elements to include in the dependent variable. Then in the 80s the sustainable development movement came along and it became clear to me that 25 years would not be enough. Maybe it's a totally open-ended human quest, altering a bit with time and across cultures. Certainly the root issues driving what we have been doing for the past 50 years can be traced back to ancient scholars in the fifth and fourth centuries BCE, i.e., the search for a clear view of a good life and a good way to live.

I am convinced that a good quality of life or wellbeing is precisely the dependent variable needed to measure sustainable development. It is precisely what we want or should want to sustain. We are a long way from agreement on the dependent variable and most people do not even seem to see the connection between quality of life research and sustainable development. Although in the crucial parts of the Brundtland Commission report, where it talks about satisfying current needs without reducing options for the next generation, a few sentences down on the same page it also talks about improving quality of life as the important thing; not just satisfying needs, but meeting aspirations for a good life. Something like that.

Why Is Wellbeing Research Important?

For a pragmatist and consequentialist, it is impossible to assess the value of our lives, decisions we make about good and evil, about a good life and a good society unless we have a good understanding of the dependent variable. We need a clear vision of where we want to go, how we think things should be and the best way to get there in a sustainable way.

What Is the Most Important Wellbeing-Related Finding from Your Research?

I think there are two. First, I assume that robust theories are important for driving scientific research and I still think multiple discrepancies theory points the way toward a more comprehensive, coherent, integrated, conceptually sound and empirically well-supported theory of subjective wellbeing. When I invented it, I thought I was giving a new foundation to classical utility theory, an empirical foundation in the tradition of Perry and Lewis for defining naturalistic value and through it satisfaction and happiness. I later realized that there was circularity built into the theory. So it could not deliver a purely naturalistic theory. Besides, I no longer believe in a naturalistic theory. I think we always smuggle in some a priori stuff when we define value, wellbeing, or quality of life.

People working in the logical positivist tradition have been quite happy to conduct research with a relatively slim understanding of 'theory' and little emphasis on it, and I do believe that a lot of good research can be done with such understanding. Generally speaking, positivists adopt a rigid distinction between facts and values, and between observation terms and theoretical terms, the need for value-free science and scientific research, scientific explanation based on the model of sound arguments, clearly distinguishable scientific laws and theories, and the possibility of theory-free measurement. I confess to being a teenage positivist and some of the boy remains in the man, but I am convinced that robust theories are still important and should be high on our research agendas. Such theories provide context and allow us to see not only essential elements but the need to find relationships, making some elements more influential than others and some lines of investigation particularly helpful for breaking new ground.

Second, there is a so-called gold standard self-report measure of overall health status in the health-related quality of life research tradition called Short Form 36 (SF-36), which is also used by many people as a measure of quality of life. I demonstrated in a few publications with survey data that there is a huge difference between good health and a good life. The explanatory predictors of both things are clearly distinct. So people should stop using SF-36 to measure quality of life. I don't think it will change anyone's behaviour, but I do think what I demonstrated is very important. Life is like that sometimes.

What Are You Working on Right Now?

Well, the 12 volume *Encyclopedia of Quality of Life and Well-Being Research* (Springer) came out in March and I am working a bit to get the word out through various outlets, newspapers, newsletters, listservs. Along with a couple dozen others, I am working on parts of a history of wellbeing. I think I will use some of what I am writing about ancient views of wellbeing for a short monograph and I will use some of what I am writing on North American research for an article on Canadian milestones. I have a province-wide survey of 15-year-olds' knowledge, attitudes and behaviours around sustainable development. I am still editor in chief of the *Journal of Business Ethics,* the most frequently cited journal in the world devoted to business ethics. I started it over 30 years ago to pick up research being done on quality of work life and on corporate social accounting. I have never given business ethics more than about 10 or 15% of my research time, but that journal is much larger than *Social Indicators Research.*

What Do You Think the Next Big Thing in Wellbeing Research Will Be?

I don't know what it will be but I think what it should be is continuing to get agreement on the nature of the dependent variable and on its connection to sustainable development. Once we get clear about what it is we want to sustain, we can measure what it takes to keep the thing going given the rates of change of required inputs to desired outputs.

Judging from the report by Stiglitz, Sen and Fitoussi, I think we are still held back by economists and policy makers who can't see much beyond what economists say. With some exaggeration I think that in part one of their report they told us what we already knew (limits of GDP), in part two they told us quite a bit less than we know (about quality of life) and in part three they told us to ask someone else (about sustainable development). A pretty disappointing result from some first-rate economists.

What Are the Main Benefits of Interdisciplinary Research on Wellbeing?

There is no other or more promising way. Regarding the quantity of life we are notoriously limited to one per person, but the quality of life is as varied as there are perspectives from which it can be assessed. No one discipline can capture all the elements and their relationships.

What Would the Ideal Census Question on Wellbeing Be and Why?

If we are limited to only one, I think we will be in dangerous territory. In several publications I have shown that measures of health, standard of living, quality of life, life satisfaction and happiness do not capture exactly the same things. If we use only one measure for our dependent variable, we are bound to get distorted views about what is most important and how all the important things are related. I suppose most money is behind a single life satisfaction or happiness question, but these are very limited in what they capture. We really do need subjective and objective indicators in order to distinguish real paradise and hell from a fool's paradise and hell. Either one sort of indicator alone cannot do the work of adequately measuring quality of life or wellbeing.

The *World Happiness Report,* edited by John Helliwell, Richard Layard and Jeffrey Sachs, had five measures of their dependent variable presumed to capture overall wellbeing of some sort, namely, Cantril's ladder, life satisfaction, happiness, positive affect and negative affect. Examining their list of explanatory variables, one finds very few if any measures of human agency, e.g., measures of people's perceived wants and needs, of their expectations, hopes and fears, efforts, equity, past experiences, constraints and resources. A lot of resources were invested in measuring relatively objective features of people's lives to explain their perceived wellbeing, but what people tried to make or made of those features was largely neglected.

What Parts of Your Research Have Brought You the Most Enjoyment and/or Satisfaction?

What I like most about research is learning new things. I especially like discovering things that, so far as I know, nobody else has found. I suspect this view would be similar to most scholars as far back as Anaxagoras. I also enjoy expressing my views in sentences that I think are particularly graceful, if that's the right word. T.S. Eliot talked about the music of prose and I think there is something to that. Sometimes the ideas turn into sentences that are quite pleasant to read. If you look at Bertrand Russell's manuscripts, you find that he usually hit the expressions he wanted on the first shot. If you looked at mine, before computers, you would find writes and re-writes. I usually have a hard time getting the right expression first time around, although I must say that the older I get, the easier it gets to hit the right mark first off. Hopefully, this is not a sign that I am losing my taste or standards, though that would not surprise me given all the other things I have lost to age. The other thing I like most about my research is the opportunity it has given me to know and work with people all over the world with similar interests. There is something special, I think, about working with a team or another person. Maybe it is related to the essential sociality of our species, although I know of several good scholars who work on their own and prefer that. In fact, for some, it is best for all of us if they keep to themselves.

What Parts of Your Research Have Brought You the Most Dissatisfaction and/or Displeasure?

Writing proposals for research funding against very bad odds of success. Then not getting funded. Having my work evaluated by people who clearly know less than I do about the subject. Having papers submitted to journals and having them neglected by editors who were not managing the store well. The worst case I experienced was with a paper I wrote called 'Efficiency and morality'. Thirteen months after submitting the paper, I wrote to find its status. The editor said he mislaid it and asked me to re-submit. I wrote back that I did not think he understood either efficiency or morality, and published the paper somewhere else.

I have always found longer works more satisfying than shorter ones. However, with long works I always have had a troublesome feeling that I would drop dead before finishing the piece. Then, when it is finished, I am troubled by the thought that no one will read it or that those who do read it will find it stinks. I am pretty sure some of my work has met both fates. When I was working on my 5-volume *North American Social Report* (1980–82), I started looking for a publisher after I finished the first 2 volumes. After 57 rejections, I really worried a lot about the time I was investing and the likelihood that nothing would come of it. Then Riedel accepted it and I worried about finishing it, etc. It took me 12 years to write that treatise. It did win the Secretary of State's Award for Interdisciplinary Research, but I doubt that anyone has read the whole thing. Still, it was a great learning experience.

After I published my *Citation Classics from Social Indicators Research* (2005), I had a look at the 168 or so citations to my paper on multiple discrepancies theory (1985). I found that about 70% of the citations were perfunctory. Some authors clearly had never read my paper. Some reported that I said exactly the opposite of what I did say. I still think citation analysis has some validity and proper uses. My wife had the impression that I did a lot of self-citing and I had been convinced that I did too. Then I found I self-cited about 5% of the time compared to something like 22% for average authors. That kind of thing is nice to know.

Is There Anything Else You Would like to Comment on?

For years I preferred the spelling 'wellbeing' to the longer 'well-being'. After we gathered up most of the 2200 or so articles for the encyclopedia, my friend at Springer did some citation research and discovered that there was something like 6 times more citations to well-being than to quality of life, and more citations to well-being than to wellbeing. So we added 'and WellBeing' to the name of the encyclopedia. Although I think of well-being and quality of life as pretty much synonyms, a lot of people apparently don't. So we went for the bigger pool. The Oxford English Dictionary uses well-being, but other dictionaries use wellbeing. We also noticed that some people use 'quality of life' and others 'quality-of-life' more or less inconsistently. So we just stayed with quality of life.

About Alex C. Michalos (provided by Alex C. Michalos, April 2014)

Alex is Emeritus Professor in Political Science from the University of Northern British Columbia, where he taught from 1994 to 2001. He was Professor of Philosophy at the University of Guelph (Ontario) from 1966 to 1994, and has held positions at several other universities. His awards include a Gold Medal for Achievement in Research (2004) from the Social Sciences and Humanities Research Council of Canada (the Council's highest honour), and he is a Member of the Order of Canada, C.M. (2010).

References

Lewis, C. L. (1946). *Analysis of knowledge and valuation*. LaSalle: Open Court Publishing Co.
Perry, R. B. (1926). *General theory of value*. Cambridge: Harvard University Press.
Simon, H. A. (1945). *Administrative behavior*. New York: MacMillan Co.
Simon, H. A. (1957). *Models of man*. New York: Wiley.

Chapter 3
The Best Teacher I Ever Had Was … J. Coert Rylaarsdam

Alex C. Michalos

Because *Teaching Business Ethics* is designed for those with a special interest in teaching, it seems appropriate to devote some space in every issue to some reflections on teachers who have made a difference to people who, probably in most cases for readers of this journal, later became teachers themselves. The hope of the Co-Editors of the journal is that the short essays describing people's best teachers will provide instruction and inspiration to other teachers. The aim here is not to present research studies on good teachers, but to try to bring readers close to those teachers who for one reason or another had a significant positive impact on the writers' lives and work. In general, we anticipate on average perhaps two or three pages per article, and perhaps more than one article per issue, depending on how much material we attract. We hope that many readers will take advantage of this opportunity to let the rest of us know what we may have missed.

I must say that reflecting on all the fine teachers I have had over the years has been a thoroughly enjoyable activity. I recalled names and faces, expressions on faces, words of encouragement, praise and blame. At different times of my life I have had different needs and interests, and these created different opportunities for teachers to have different kinds of influence upon me. My father died when I was 15 and I think I tended to adopt new fathers from among the male teachers and athletic coaches who crossed my path. I grew up in Cleveland, Ohio and played organized football and ran hurdles from about the ninth grade through university. Most of my coaches and male teachers were veterans of the Second World War, and most of them seem to have had a healthy suspicion about mindless patriotism and a genuine interest in having "their boys" avoid going to war. They were no-nonsense guys,

Michalos, A.C.: 1997. The best teacher I ever had was J. Coert Rylaarsdam. Teaching Business Ethics, 1, pp. 93–95. © 1997 Kluwer Academic Publishers. Printed in the Netherlands.

A.C. Michalos (✉)
University of Northern British Columbia, Prince George, BC, Canada
e-mail: michalos@brandonu.ca

A.C. Michalos, *Philosophical Foundations of Quality of Life*,
DOI 10.1007/978-3-319-50727-9_3

who conveyed a sense of honour, duty and purpose, which was contagious. No wonder, then, that I went to university with the noble aims of playing professional football, running in the Olympics and marrying my high school sweetheart.

By the end of my second year of university (Western Reserve University in Cleveland, now Case-Western Reserve), I discovered that I was not good enough to play professional football, not fast enough to run in the Olympics and my girlfriend found other interests. Fortunately, at just that time I encountered Plato's *Republic* and a brilliant teacher of the history of religions named Horace Abram Rigg. Between the two of them, Plato and Rigg lit an academic fire under me that has continued to burn to this day. Until I met Rylaarsdam in graduate school, Rigg held the crown for the best teacher I ever had. And it is no trick determining what special quality he had that was so good. He was a spectacular lecturer. Without notes he lectured to a class of about 300, three hours a week and kept most of us spellbound with stories from the world's great religions carefully wrapped in his homespun humour. To help us understand religious ritual, for example, he told us about his "research" in the faculty bathroom watching distinguished faculty members who were disciplined enough to run their hands under the faucet but not disciplined enough to make sure that the water actually touched their hands. Above all else, he was in command, in command of his subject matter and in command of his audience. He was a living testament to Jesus Christ's comment that the truth shall make you free, and I was totally convinced that if I could find such truth, I too could be free.

So, as my undergraduate career came to an end, I decided I would go to graduate school to study the history of religions and become a university professor. In a word, I wanted to be like Rigg. I enrolled in the Divinity School of the University of Chicago and it was there that I met J. Coert Rylaarsdam, Professor of the Old Testament, and the best teacher I ever had. What he had was not unlike what Rigg had. He was an absolutely captivating lecturer. But more than that, he had virtually limitless patience and generosity with his time. I remember that he invited me to his office for tea with the remark that he supposed if he did not invite me, I would not get to his office at all. That was true. As approachable as he and other teachers were, I never would have dropped in for a chat. I just assumed that they had better things to do and it was not right for me to bother them.

But with Rylaarsdam things were different. He seemed to want to know what I thought about things as much as I wanted to know what he thought. I went to Divinity School as an atheist and I graduated as an atheist, and I don't recall ever sliding from this position throughout my 3 years in the School, or since, for that matter. But my atheism didn't seem to put anyone off, especially Rylaarsdam, who was some sort of a theist and Christian. We spent hours every week drinking tea and exploring all aspects of theology and philosophy. I was hardly a budding Socrates and must have bored him to tears sometimes, but I never saw it or heard it from him. My memories are of endless hours of serious investigation with a first rate scholar and teacher as my guide and confidant. He was a fearless searcher after truth and a tireless instructor. I think the pursuit of truth was at least as important to me then as it is now, and Rylaarsdam gave it legitimacy. He knew it was worth the effort and he “walked the talk” as we say today by helping me find my own way into the life of scholarship.

I don’t think I am a great teacher but if I am any good at all, I think it is mainly because I had at least one great teacher. Thanks again for everything, Coert.

Chapter 4
The Case for Atheism

Alex C. Michalos

Introductory Comments

Here are some of my basic assumptions

The discussion is about the existence or non-existence of a God that would be a suitable object of worship, including prayer as a form of communication and not just a form of meditation.

As I use the terms,

a *theist* is one who affirms that God exists,

an *agnostic* is one who denies that one can have knowledge one way or the other, and

an *atheist* is one who denies that God exists.

My thesis is that of an *atheist*, i.e., God does not exist.

I suppose that everything we have to say on both sides of this debate has been known and said since at least Saint Augustine and the Council of Nicaea in the fourth century.

Besides denying precisely what a theist affirms, I also deny what an agnostic affirms.

Since I believe and will produce what I take to be good reasons for atheism, I deny that we cannot know one way or the other.

Assuming that one has knowledge insofar as one has good reasons for believing propositions that happen to be true, I believe one can know that God does not exist.

It is possible to be an *agnostic theist* or *agnostic atheist*. An agnostic theist affirms that God exists but denies that one can satisfy the conditions for knowing it

---

Notes for a debate at UNBC September 20, 2005 by Alex C. Michalos.

A.C. Michalos (✉)
University of Northern British Columbia, Prince George, BC, Canada
e-mail: michalos@brandonu.ca

A.C. Michalos, *Philosophical Foundations of Quality of Life*,
DOI 10.1007/978-3-319-50727-9_4

to be true, while an agnostic atheist denies that God exists but also denies that one can satisfy the conditions for knowing it to be true.

Unfortunately, I have never seen an uncontroversial argument for or against God's existence, but that is not surprising given the extremely complicated nature of the subject.

General Problem of all theological discourse according to Thomas Aquinas: One must try to avoid the anthropomorphism of univocal predication on the one hand and the agnosticism of equivocal predication on the other.

In plain English this means that because God is supposed to be an absolutely unique being, one must admit first, that words that mean one thing when applied to people cannot mean exactly the same thing when they are applied to God. Insofar as one assumes they mean exactly the same thing, one is liable to mistakenly turn God into some kind of an extraordinary human being (=the error of anthropomorphism of univocal predication).

Second, however, one must admit that the more one insists that words that mean one thing when applied to people cannot mean exactly the same thing when they are applied to God, the more one is liable to have no idea what one knows or can know about God (=the error of agnosticism of equivocal predication).

My impression is that atheists tend to error on the side of univocal predication and theists tend to error on the side of equivocal predication.

The General Argument

Premise 1. There are two kinds of concepts of God,

(1) those that apparently would designate suitable objects of worship if the objects could exist, and
(2) those that designate objects that do exist but are not suitable objects of worship (e.g., the familiar Biblical craven images and things like nature, energy and love).

Premise 2. Concepts in the first class imply logical contradictions either in world views or in themselves.

Premise 3. It is unreasonable to accept concepts that imply contradictions (because contradictions are literally nonsensical and designate logically impossible states of affairs).

Conclusion 1. So, it is unreasonable to accept concepts of God that apparently would designate suitable objects of worship if those objects could exist.

Final conclusion. Therefore, since neither concept of God is reasonably acceptable, there cannot be an entity designated by a reasonably acceptable concept of God, i.e., God cannot exist.

Essential characteristics of a concept of God that apparently would designate a suitable object of worship if such an object could exist

Traditionally, in much of western theology and philosophy God is supposed to be:

1. *Creator (and sustainer) of the universe*. This is necessary for those who want to answer the cosmological question "Why is there something rather than nothing?", who believe the universe is not simply a chance event. 'Sustainer' is added parenthetically because most people who think there is a need for a creator also seem to think some ever-present force is necessary to keep the universe going.
2. *Transcendent*. This means "wholly other than the universe" and is a logical implication of the assumption of God as creator. God must be other than the universe because God is posited as that which brings the universe into existence.
3. *Eternal*. This means "ever present" or somehow existing all at once rather than living and developing through time. It is also a logical implication of the assumption of God as the creator of time.
4. *Self-sufficient*. Another logical implication of God as the creator of everything. Sometimes it is expressed by saying that God's essence is to exist.
5. *Omniscient*. This means "knows everything knowable" (including future freely chosen human acts) and is another logical implication of God as creator of everything. God can't know what is empirically false (e.g., that Prince George is in China) or self-contradictory (e.g., that $1 + 2 = 4$).
6. *Provident*. This is a direct implication of God's omniscience and creativity. God is supposed to act on people through divine foresight and, in some religions, through grace.
7. *Omnipotent*. This means "more powerful than anything else" or possibly "infinitely powerful". Without this attribute it would be possible for something to overcome God's creative acts and will, which would undermine people's belief that finally whatever happens is dependent on those acts and will.
8. *Perfect*. This means "without defects" or possibly "without limitations that would count as defects", e.g., the fact that God can't find Prince George in China is a kind of limitation but not a defect. Without this attribute, it would be possible for God to believe, choose and do the wrong thing, including creating the universe.
9. *Personal*. This means God has mental characteristics such that people can communicate with God (e.g., through prayer) and God can love or care about and for people. Without this attribute, prayer and worship would be pointless.
10. *All Good*. This means especially, but not necessarily only, "wholly morally good" or "wholly just". This is a logical implication of God's being perfect and personal, because moral perfection is supposed to be the supreme virtue or perfection of persons.
11. *Incorporeal*. This means "immaterial" or "not made of matter" and is a logical implication of God's creativity and perfection, since material things are created, exist in and through time, are changeable and have limitations.

12. *Immutable*. This means "unchangeable" and is a logical implication of God's creativity and perfection, like incorporeality.
13. *Immanent*. This means somehow "inherent in everything" but not as a quality (e.g., as mass or colour) or as the formal essence of things. This is a logical implication of God's being the "creative ground" or "source" of existing things.

Although one would be hard-pressed to give rigorous definitions of most of these characteristics, it would be difficult to abandon any of them. Since many of them are logically implied by others, if the former fail to hold then the latter fail also, e.g., if God is not transcendent then God cannot be the creator either since the former characteristic is logically implied by the latter.

Argument to show that some concepts designate objects that do exist but are not suitable objects of worship (e.g., the familiar Biblical craven images and things like nature, energy and love)

Premise 1. If the familiar Biblical craven images and things like nature, energy and love lack some of the 13 essential characteristics of God then they are not suitable objects of worship.

Premise 2. The familiar Biblical craven images and things like nature, energy and love lack most if not all of the 13 essential characteristics of God.

Conclusion. So, they are not suitable objects of worship and it would, therefore, be unreasonable to accept concepts of God designating such things as suitable objects of worship.

Arguments to show that concepts of God that apparently would designate suitable objects of worship if the objects could exist imply logical contradictions either in world views or in themselves.

Argument 1 showing concept of God implies a contradictory world view (The Inconsistent Triad)

P1. If God is the omnipotent and all good creator of the universe then evil should not exist.

P2. Evil exists.

C1. So, it is not the case that God is the omnipotent and all good creator of the universe.

C2. So, either God is not omnipotent or not all good or not the creator of the universe.

P3. If God lacks any of these attributes then God as a suitable object of worship does not exist.

Fc. Therefore, God as a suitable object of worship does not exist.

Argument 2 showing concept of God implies a contradictory world view: Transcendent object of worship

P1. If God is transcendent (=wholly other than the universe) then all of God's characteristics must be wholly other than anything known to humans.

P2. If all of God's characteristics must be wholly other than anything known to humans then nobody can know what is true to say of God.
P3. If nobody can know what is true to say of God then nobody can know if it is true to say that God is Omnipotent, All Good, and so on.
P4. But religious people claim to know that it is true to say that God is Omnipotent, All Good, and so on.
C1. So, religious people claim that they know what is true about God and that nobody can know what is true about God, which is logically impossible.
P5. If a world view implies logical impossibilities then it is reasonable to reject it.
Fc. So, it is reasonable to reject a world view that affirms God's existence.

Argument 1 showing that the concept of God apparently designating a suitable object of worship is self-contradictory: Personal and Incorporeal

P1. The concept of God is that of a personal and incorporeal being.
P2. To be a person, one must be capable of feeling/experiencing love, care and concern.
P3. Without a corporeal body, one would be literally incapable of feeling or experiencing anything.
C. Therefore, the concept of a personal and incorporeal being is self-contradictory and it is logically impossible for it to designate an existing being, i.e., God cannot exist.

Argument 2 showing that the concept of God apparently designating a suitable object of worship is self-contradictory: Omniscient and Omnipotent

P1. If God is omniscient, then everything that will happen in the future is known to God now.
P2. If everything that will happen in the future is known to God now then God cannot change the future.
P3. If God cannot change the future then God is not omnipotent.
C. Therefore, the concept of an omniscient and omnipotent being is self-contradictory and it is logically impossible for it to designate an existing being, i.e., God cannot exist.

Argument 3 showing that the concept of God apparently designating a suitable object of worship is self-contradictory: Perfect Creator

P1. The creator of the universe must have a purpose for the creation or not.
P2. If God does not have a purpose then the act of creation is frivolous, and God is not perfect.
P3. If God does have a purpose then the act of creation is designed to achieve some goal that requires such an act.
P4. If God has a goal to be achieved then God is not perfect.
C1. So, whether God has a purpose in creating the universe or not, God is not perfect.

P5. But by hypothesis God is perfect.
C2. So, the idea of a perfect creator is that of a being that is and is not perfect, which is logically impossible, i.e., a God with such attributes cannot not exist.

Argument 4 showing that the concept of God apparently designating a suitable object of worship is self-contradictory: Personal and Omniscient

P1. The concept of God is that of a personal and omniscient being.
P2. To be a person, one must be capable of learning, doubt and error.
P3. An omniscient being would be incapable of learning, doubt and error.
C. Therefore, the concept of a personal and omniscient being is self-contradictory and it is logically impossible for it to designate an existing being, i.e., God cannot exist.

A being incapable of learning, doubt and error would be incapable of intending to learn, trying to learn, succeeding or failing to learn, incapable of doubting anything doubtable, incapable of worrying about what is true or false, right or wrong, incapable of knowing by experience how it feels to learn, succeed, fail, worry or doubt. In short, such a being would lack many of the characteristics that make persons personal and that give persons personality.

Argument 5 showing that the concept of God is self-contradictory: Divine Providence and Creativity versus human free will

P1. If God knows exactly what every human will choose before the choice is made and is creatively active in every choice then human choices are determined and not entirely free or autonomous.
P2. If human choices are determined and not entirely free or autonomous then people cannot be held morally praiseworthy or blameworthy, and the institution of morality is pointless.
P3. The institution of morality is a necessary condition of human communities and as such it is supremely important for human existence.
C1. So, human choices must not be determined, but free or autonomous, and God cannot know exactly what every human will choose before the choice is made.
P4. But by hypothesis God has precisely such knowledge.
C2. So, God both knows and does not know exactly what every human will choose before the choice is made, which is logically impossible.
Fc. Therefore, since the concept of God is self-contradictory, it is logically impossible for it to designate an existing being, i.e., God cannot exist.

Argument 6 showing that the concept of God is self-contradictory: Self-sufficiency (=a being whose essence is existence)

P1. Everything that exists is supposed to be characterized by an essence (saying what it is, what features it has) and by existence (saying merely that it is, that it exists).

P2. To say that God's essence is existence is equivalent to saying that God's existence is existence.
P3. The claim that 'existence is existence' is logically true (tautologous) and has no descriptive content.
P4. But people who claim that God's essence is existence offer this as a central description of one of God's characteristics.
C1. So, people who claim that God's essence is existence are asserting that a sentence without descriptive content has descriptive content, which is logically absurd.
Fc. If the concept of God implies logical absurdities, then the concept cannot designate a logically possible entity or state of affairs, i.e., God cannot exist.

Argument 7 showing that the concept of God is self-contradictory: Creativity, Omnipotence and Rationality

P1. If God is a perfectly rational and omnipotent creator then God's creation would not be at war with itself.
P2. But God's creation is at war with itself.
C1. So, it is not the case that God is a perfectly rational and omnipotent creator of the universe.
C2. So, either God is not perfectly rational or not omnipotent or not the creator of the universe.
P3. If God lacks any of these attributes then God as a suitable object of worship does not exist.
Fc. Therefore, God as a suitable object of worship does not exist.

Examples of a Creation at War with Itself

1. Diseases and cures: Why not just create healthy people that grow old gracefully and die peacefully in their sleep?
2. Still-born births: Why not just prevent conception?
3. Famines and humans needing food: Why not create exactly enough food for everyone born?
4. Poverty and idle wealth: Why not provide financial security for everyone instead of too little for some and too much for others?
5. Tortured and murdered innocents: Why not punish only the guilty instead of punishing the guilty and innocent alike?
6. People with different faiths, sacred writings and religious practices all sincerely believing they are right but others are wrong: Why not give one clear message upon which all could easily agree?

Note that although there are some moral issues in these examples, my argument here is not intended as a moral condemnation. Here I am only arguing that an omnipotent and perfectly rational creator would not produce a product that displays such inconsistency of purpose.

Summary of the Last 7 Arguments

P1. If the concept of God is an oxymoron then God cannot exist.
P2. The concept of God is an oxymoron.
C. God cannot exist.

Chapter 5
Logic, Philosophy of Science and the Quality of Life

Alex C. Michalos

Introduction

The *Encyclopedia of Life Support Systems* is based on the assumption that sustainable human development across the whole world is a goal worthy of pursuit by the human community. Unfortunately, it is not a particularly salient or compelling goal for many people, and many of those who do view it as salient and compelling have different ideas about its nature and about the best way to achieve it. Since one's chances of hitting a target tend to improve as one's view of the target is clarified, it is reasonable to expect that the clarification of the goal of sustainable human development will improve our chances of reaching that goal. This essay is a modest contribution to the quest for clarification.

At least since the emergence of philosophy in the fifth century BCE in ancient Greece, some people have appealed to *reason* as the instrument for solving human problems. Growing up in a world in which the differences between supernatural and natural phenomena were far from clear, and in which the ultimate determinants of life and death were probably more readily perceived as the result of poorly understood and unconstrained passions, brute force and dumb luck, ancient philosophers were rare in number and their outlook on life was even more rare. Perhaps the characteristic that most distinguished philosophers from all other people was their assumption that people have the capacity to *reason* or *think critically* about issues, and that it is both possible and worthwhile to train oneself and others in the efficient

Michalos, A.C.: 2006. Logic, philosophy of science and the quality of life. In Philosophy and World Problems, John McMurtry (Ed.) the Encyclopedia of Life Support Systems (EOLSS), Developed under the Auspices of the UNESCO, Eolss Publishers, Paris, France (http://www.eolss.net). © UNESCO-EOLSS 2006.

A.C. Michalos (✉)
University of Northern British Columbia, Prince George, BC, Canada
e-mail: michalos@brandonu.ca

A.C. Michalos, *Philosophical Foundations of Quality of Life*,
DOI 10.1007/978-3-319-50727-9_5

and effective exercise of this capacity. What is perhaps even more remarkable than the fact that such people had such insight was the fact that other people apparently appreciated it. Thus, the initiative of a few and the appreciation of many led to the social construction of principles and systems of logic, and methods of critical thinking about the world and its inhabitants. In fact, since the earliest divisions of philosophy from the fifth century BCE included logic, physics and ethics, the structure of this essay bears a family resemblance to its illustrious ancestors.

In this essay some of the foundational elements of logic, philosophy and science will be explained. Some light will be shed on the philosophers' understanding of good versus bad reasons for believing some things rather than others, or of reasonable versus unreasonable arguments. Once the general foundation of critical thinking is laid, some foundational concepts of all the sciences will be examined with a view to revealing their variety, strengths and limitations. It is not an exaggeration to say that the total corpus of accepted scientific knowledge rests on the foundations to be examined here. As well, our understanding and appreciation of a sort of life or quality of life that is worthy of pursuing, obtaining and sustaining for present and future inhabitants of planet earth rests on the very same foundations.

Logical Foundations

Some claims, assertions, sentences or propositions are *worthy of belief* and some are not. Among those that are worthy of belief, some merit complete certainty relative to some other claims and assumptions, while others merit acceptance short of complete certainty. In both cases, one may be said to have knowledge insofar as one's claims are worthy of belief. The difference between knowing that a claim is true and merely believing that it is true is that knowledge requires a good reason for what one believes. Structurally, a good reason is a good argument, and logic is the study of arguments and things essential to their appraisal as good or bad.

An argument may be defined as a sequence of sentences divided in such a way that some of the sentences are supposed to be the reason, justification, guarantee, warrant or support for some other sentence in the sequence. The sentences that provide the reason or warrant are called 'premises'. The sentence that is supposed to be warranted by the premise(s) is called the 'conclusion'.

An argument whose conclusion is supposed, alleged or claimed to be certain relative to its premises is called 'deductive'. Even if the argument has an error in it and does not do what it is supposed to do, it is called 'deductive.' Calling it 'deductive' does not make it good or bad. It just tells everyone what is to be expected of it. More precisely, it specifies the appropriate rules according to which it should be evaluated.

An argument whose conclusion is supposed, alleged, or claimed to be more or less acceptable relative to its premises is called 'inductive'. Even if the argument has an error in it and does not do what it is supposed to do, it is called 'inductive'. Calling it 'inductive' does not make it good or bad. It just specifies the appropriate rules according to which it should be evaluated.

Notice that the definition of an 'inductive argument' contains the word 'acceptable' rather than the 'probable'. The former is merely more general. Usually the conclusion of an inductive argument is described as more or less probable relative to its premises. But sometimes it is described as more or less likely, well supported, well confirmed, reasonable, useful, sensible and so on. That is, there are many ways to characterize the relation that obtains between the premises and the conclusion of an inductive argument. The somewhat general term 'acceptable' is intended cover this variety.

Good arguments must be truth-preserving in the sense that they never lead from true premises to false conclusions. They must satisfy our intuitive notion of a *proof.* The technical name for such arguments is 'sound.' A sound argument must satisfy three conditions. It must be patterned after a valid form, have only true premises and contain no methodological flaws. Each of these three conditions is necessary for a sound argument and collectively the three conditions are sufficient. Thus, an unsound argument is one that fails to satisfy at least one but possibly every one of the conditions for soundness. The first necessary condition for a sound argument is a matter of logical form while the other two necessary conditions are typically (not always) matters of content. Each condition will be examined in turn.

The notion of a valid logical form is perhaps the most important concept in the study of logic. Every argument has a logical form (structure, pattern or skeleton) and some material content. For example, consider the following deductive arguments:

All cats are animals.
All tigers are cats.
So, all tigers are animals.
All humans are mortal.
All Greeks are human.
So, all Greeks are mortal.

Each of these arguments is about different things. The first is about animals, cats, and tigers; the second, about mortals, humans, and Greeks. Arguments that are about different things are said to have different contents. So, these arguments have different contents. But they have the very same logical form, pattern, or structure. The form of each of these arguments is this:

All ____ are - - -
All … are ____
So, all … are - - -

The only words occurring in this skeleton are logical guides called 'logical operators'.

The word 'so' tells us that what follows is a conclusion. The words 'all' and 'are' tell us that everything following the former is in the same class as everything following the latter. Just as the whole structure is called an 'argument form', each line is called a 'sentence form', e.g., 'All____are - - -' is the form of the sentence 'All humans are mortal'.

An argument form or skeleton is called 'valid' if, and only if, it *must* yield a true conclusion whenever its place markers (e.g., the solid, broken and dotted lines) are replaced in such a way that each of its premises becomes a true sentence. The ordinary argument obtained from a valid argument form by consistently or uniformly replacing its place markers appropriately is called a 'valid argument'. Hence, the two arguments above (about tigers and Greeks) are valid because they are patterned after a valid argument form, and the argument form in those arguments may be recognized as valid because with the appropriate replacements of its place markers it must produce a true conclusion from true premises.

An argument form is called 'invalid' if, and only if, it is *possible* to uniformly or consistently replace its place markers in such a way that each of its premises is true but its conclusion is false. Such an argument is clearly not truth-preserving in the required sense. The ordinary argument obtained from an invalid argument form by uniformly replacing its place markers appropriately is called an 'invalid argument'. Any argument based on an invalid argument form is an unsound argument. It has a formal defect that is sufficient to render it unsound. On the other hand, any argument based on a valid argument form may be a sound argument insofar as it has satisfied the formal necessary condition of soundness.

Having passed the formal test of validity, sound arguments must pass the material tests of having only true premises and no methodological flaws. The phrase 'methodological flaws' is used to designate a variety of defects in arguments that usually result from informal or material features of arguments, with one notable exception. The notable exception concerns circular arguments. Structurally speaking, as the name suggests, circular arguments have the defect of containing one or more premises that are substantially equivalent to the conclusions that are supposed to be established by those arguments. Accordingly, such arguments are formally valid but methodologically flawed because anyone in doubt about the conclusion of such arguments would have the same doubts about the premises. Apart from the case of circular arguments, methodologically flawed arguments include such errors as proving propositions that are entirely irrelevant to a question at issue, presenting premises that are biased for or against a question, presenting an oversimplified set of premises, using defective definitions of key terms, and using threats or emotional appeals that might lead one to assent to unwarranted conclusions.

While much more will be said in the following sections about the pursuit truth in diverse forms, using diverse procedures, based on diverse assumptions and paradigms, a brief review of theories of truth will provide a useful resting place for this overview of topics in the study of logic that have a particularly important role to play in the philosophy of science.

Very early in school students learn that there are four kinds of sentences, namely, questions or interrogatives (e.g., How are you?), commands or prescriptives (e.g., Close the door.), exclamations (e.g., Ouch!) and declaratives or assertions (e.g., Vancouver is in British Columbia). They also learn that by definition, only declarative sentences can be true or false (i.e., can have a truth-value), and only if they are cognitively or descriptively meaningful. Philosophers have refined the preceding sentence by distinguishing ordinary sentences, which have some physical form such as marks on paper or sounds; judgments, which have some mental form such as ideas in people's heads; and propositions, which are supposed to be the meanings of declarative sentences and have their own special form that is regarded as metaphysical by those who draw these distinctions. (See section "Scientific Significance" for an explanation of 'metaphysical'.) Using these distinctions, it is more accurate to say that by definition only propositions can be true or false. Thus, for example, one would say that the two distinct sentences 'John is taller than Bob' and 'Bob is shorter than John' have the same meaning or are used to assert or affirm the same proposition. What's more, it is the meaning or proposition that has a truth-value, rather than any particular sentence. Following this tradition, then, our basic question is: What does it mean to say that a proposition is true? Setting aside propositions that are true by definition (about which more is said in section "Scientific Significance"), four theories have been proposed to answer this question.

According to the 'correspondence theory of truth', where 'p' is used to designate any proposition, 'p is true' means 'p corresponds to some aspect of the world'. Thus, for example, if p is replaced by the simple sentence 'Toronto is a windy city', then the proposition that Toronto is a windy city is true just in case there is such a city and it does have the characteristic of being windy. This theory is consistent with ordinary usage insofar as anyone hearing that Toronto is a windy city would suppose the proposition to be true if it somehow matched the relevant features of that city. The main problem with the theory is that it is not clear exactly what features of propositions must match what features of the world, or exactly what form the matching should take.

According to the 'coherence theory of truth', 'p is true' means 'p is consistent with all other propositions accepted as true'. For example, if it is true that Toronto is a windy city, then it would be reasonable to believe that most people living there would accept the proposition, that residents would take special precautions carrying opened umbrellas, that local news media would carry stories about the effects of winds in the city and so on. This theory is also consistent with ordinary usage insofar as all propositions imply many others that collectively form relatively consistent systems of beliefs or bodies of knowledge that tend to reinforce each other. The main problem with the theory is that it does not have any clear connection to the real world. As a result, two people might have self-consistent systems of beliefs about the world which systems happen to be mutually contradictory, but there would be no means of determining which system was actually true of the world in the sense of the correspondence theory.

According to the 'pragmatic theory of truth', 'p is true' means 'action in accordance with p leads to satisfactory results', where 'satisfactory results' is understood as correspondence with the world *and* consistency with all other propositions accepted as true. That is, the inventors of the pragmatic theory of truth constructed the theory by combining the two basic features of the other two theories. As a result, this theory solves the problem of being able to determine which of two self-consistent but mutually contradictory belief systems is true of the world, but it has nothing special to offer to solve the problem of exactly defining 'correspondence'.

Finally, according to the 'semantic theory of truth', all other theories are defective insofar as they assume that the predicate 'is true' has any descriptive force at all. On the contrary, the semantic theorist says that 'p is true' descriptively means nothing more than 'p' itself. For proponents of the semantic theory, the predicate 'is true' only has expressive or prescriptive force. Thus, for example, 'p is true' has the force of 'Of course p' or perhaps 'Behave as if p', i.e., "'Toronto is a windy city' is true" has the force of 'Of course Toronto is a windy city!' or perhaps 'Behave as if Toronto is a windy city'. According to these theorists, then, all other theorists failed in their attempts to find the descriptive force of the predicate 'is true' because they failed to realize that sentences patterned after the declarative form 'p is true' are functionally exclamations or prescriptions. This is indeed a radical departure from traditional approaches to the theory of truth. While it has the advantage of capturing some of the nondescriptive force of truth claims, it has the disadvantage of offering a theory that is relatively far from ordinary usage. Instead of rejecting all other theories, it seems more reasonable to accept the fact that truth claims perform diverse functions that are articulated more or less accurately by the different theories.

Philosophy of Science

While it has been the logicians' task to explain the differences between good or sound arguments leading to propositions worthy of belief and bad or unsound arguments leading to unwarranted propositions, the task of explaining appropriate methods for discovering true premises (outside of formal logic and mathematics) has been assigned to other specialists. As late as the middle of the twentieth century, one could still find some introductory logic texts with sections called 'scientific methods', although the authors of those texts knew that disciplines as different as chemistry, sociology, physics and psychology employed many different kinds of methods. The task of searching for common features among the diverse methods used in diverse disciplines fell first to philosophers and historians of science. Their explorations took many forms, including careful inspection of the actual practices of scientists working in different fields as well as careful and critical reflection on alleged good practices. Their aim was not merely to discover features of research regarded as good practice by practitioners, but to discover principles of good practice that would reveal or, if necessary, create some coherence or unity in all scientific investigation.

In the following sections, we will review many of the most important *conceptual features* of scientific practice as those features have been explained by philosophers of science over the past 90 years. It will be shown that science and scientific knowledge is socially constructed on the basis of diverse assumptions, possibilities and priorities. Because it is socially constructed, scientists, philosophers of science and to some extent all members of the human community have a responsibility to ensure that science and scientific knowledge serve the long term interests of that community. More will be said about the identification and measurement of those long term interests in the final section of this essay. Let us turn now, to a review of some common conceptual features of science and scientific knowledge.

Scientific Significance

It was a basic tenet of positivist or empiricist philosophers of science in the 1930s that all cognitively meaningful propositions were either logically true or false, or else in principle experimentally testable. Logically true propositions are often referred to as 'analytic' and are characterized as having self-contradictory denials, or as being true in all possible worlds merely in virtue of the meanings of the terms employed in them.

Nonanalytic propositions are often referred to as 'synthetic' or 'empirical', and a lot of philosophical ink has been shed trying to find a precise criterion of meaningfulness for them. One plausible suggestion was the 'requirement of complete verifiability': A sentence is empirically meaningful if and only if it is not analytic and is implied by a finite logically consistent set of observation sentences. 'Observation sentences' are sentences in which observable characteristics are attributed to objects: e.g., 'This chair is green' or 'John is taller than Frank'.

The trouble with the verifiability criterion is that it makes some scientific laws empirically meaningless. Some laws of nature apply to more objects than anyone could ever observe. For example, there will never be a set of observation sentences that will logically imply the unrestricted generalization 'All men are mortal', since the sentence applies in a totally unrestricted way to all men, including those existing in the future who cannot be observed now. This means that some scientific laws (unrestricted generalizations that are commonly believed to be not only empirically meaningful but true) cannot be regarded as empirically meaningful. Since these laws are quite secure, the criterion has to be abandoned.

Another candidate to be the criterion of empirical meaningfulness is the 'requirement of complete falsifiability': A sentence is empirically meaningful if and only if its denial is not analytic and is implied by a finite logically consistent set of observation sentences. Unfortunately, this criterion suffers the same fate as the other. Although it allows some unrestricted generalizations to be empirically meaningful, it makes their denials meaningless. This is certainly anomalous because if a given claim is meaningful and therefore true or false, then anyone who denies it must be making a claim that is equally meaningful only false or true, depending on the status of the former. Still, that is just the sort of sour pickle this criterion breeds. So it too has been abandoned.

Weaker criteria of confirmability and testability were suggested, but they also turned out to be objectionable. The criteria always excluded or included too much.

Apparently meaningful sentences were ruled out and apparently meaningless sentences were ruled in. Thus, it seemed to some philosophers by the late 1940s that the only way to solve this problem was to design an artificial language whose vocabulary and grammar would prohibit all the unwanted and permit all the wanted sentences. Once again in the history of human affairs, what began as a philosophic sanitation problem was transformed into a philosophic capital works project. Instead of a swift clean-up job, a long-drawn-out development project was proposed.

The analytic-synthetic distinction, explained above, allows us to classify all propositions as follows:

Analytic	A priori	A posteriori
	Propositions in formal sciences, such as logic, mathematics	None
Synthetic	Metaphysical propositions	Propositions in empirical sciences, such as physics, sociology, etc.

In this scheme, metaphysical claims are regarded as claims about the world whose truth status may be investigated without experience or observation. Formal scientific claims are not claims about the world; their truth status may also be investigated without experience. Empirical scientific claims are claims about the world whose truth status requires experiential or observational investigation.

Most philosophers of science who have labored over the problem of finding an empirical meaningfulness criterion have been trying to find decisive identifying characteristics for empirical scientific claims, to specify the necessary and sufficient conditions for classifying any proposition as worthy of consideration by techniques and personnel they already regarded as scientific. Some fields of study struck these philosophers as intellectual and practical dead ends, e.g., theology, esthetics, ethics and, worst of all, metaphysics. Some philosophers even claimed that these fields were downright pernicious, that they gave people an unwarranted sense of security and stifled any inclinations toward intellectual progress or social reform. How sweet it would be, they thought, to have an ironclad empirical meaningfulness criterion to bash the brains of the merchants of soporific slush. Even today a scientist may be heard to throw down the gauntlet to the uninitiated: 'That's not scientific!' one may exclaim, as if a knockdown criterion had been found. Alas, it has not been found.

It may be possible not only to waste one's time but to employ it in destructive ways in the interests of worthless fields of study. However, it is doubtful that a principle distinguishing empirical meaningfulness from meaninglessness, empirical science from nonscience, would also serve to separate out worthwhile from worthless fields of study. Insofar as the exclusion of worthless or dangerous investigations was dear to the hearts of those who labored for an empirical meaningfulness criterion, the labor has been in vain. No one has been able to produce such a criterion, and even if anyone had, it would not have been sufficient for the evaluative task.

Theory and Observation

According to the "received view" of 'scientific theories', they may be characterized as axiomatic systems consisting of a set of

1. Formation rules for constructing well-formed formulas in the system
2. Transformation rules (i.e., rules of inference)
3. Three distinct vocabularies for logical, observational, and theoretic axioms
4. Correspondence rules connecting observation and theoretic terms.

There are very few scientific theories that are cast in this form, and there are plenty of other views of the nature of theories. Nevertheless, this view occupied the center of the stage for at least 30 years in the philosophy of science. It is clearly in the positivist formalistic tradition; i.e., the idea is to analyze the structure of theories in syntactic and semantic terms.

As a simple illustration of the received view, one may consider a physical theory of probability. (For more on this theory, see section "Probability".) In particular, consider it as a theory about the relative frequency of the occurrence of events in repetitive sequences, e.g., flips of a coin, rolls of a die, and so on. Then the formation and transformation rules would include the rules of algebra and set theory, supplemented by some special rules related to the use of a probability operator. The usual set of logical and mathematical terms would be included in the logical vocabulary, e.g., logical operators and place holders for variables of various sorts. The observation vocabulary would include terms like 'coin', 'die', and toss'. The basic theoretic term required is 'probability' itself, and that would be defined and measured by the ratio of the number of favorable events to the total number of events in a selected sequence of repetitive events. Insofar as this definition functions as a correspondence rule, the *definiendum* (defined part) should have only theoretic terms and the *definiens* (defining part) should have only observational terms. The axioms of the theory might be the standard three, concerning the addition and multiplication of probabilities and the constraints put on numerical values. Armed with this theory, then, one may crank out new postulates and test them in the real world of actual coin and dice tosses.

Because, as explained below, there is some difficulty in maintaining a distinction between observation terms and theoretical terms, some people have recommended replacing it with a distinction between old and new terms, where what is regarded as old or new depends on the particular problem being investigated.

Some people have rejected the axiomatic view of theories altogether. Some hold, for instance, that although a theory must organize or systematize a body of knowledge, this can be accomplished without rigorous axiomatization. Many good textbooks provide systematic presentations of scientific material without bundling it up in an axiomatic framework. Scientific theories may be thought of as organizing or systematizing material in this looser sense.

Alternatively, some writers seem to regard theories as nothing more than unrestricted universal generalizations to which people are deeply committed. For these people, there would seem to be no difference between theories and laws from a structural point of view. Perhaps, for them, only a difference in attitude separates scientific laws from scientific theories.

Theories have also been regarded as essentially answers to *why questions*, again with structure playing no significant role. Close to this view is the idea that a theory is a collection of sentences that provides intuitive understanding of something for someone.

An 'instrumentalist view of theories' has also been recommended, according to which theories are typically regarded as sets of inference rules, i.e., as collections of prescriptive sentences rather than declaratives.

According to a 'semantic view of theories', the latter are regarded as sets of statements that have the logical status of definitions without empirical significance. That is, they define a particular sort of natural system without asserting that any given system is of that sort. 'Theoretical claims', on the other hand, assert that a given system is of this or that theoretical sort. Thus, theoretical claims can be true or false. For example, the axioms of preference theory may be said to define a coherent set of preferences, while it is a matter of fact whether this or that individual's set of preferences satisfy the axioms.

In spite of this fairly impressive array of alternative views of the nature of theories, much more has been written about particular theories in diverse sciences. Consider, for instance, the vast critical literature devoted to the theories of Karl Marx, Charles Darwin and Sigmund Freud. It would not be an exaggeration to say that the philosophy of any particular science is always dominated by the philosophical problems of the dominant theories of that science. For example, contemporary philosophy of physics is largely devoted to problems related to quantum theory and relativity theory. After winning their wings in defense of the scientific status of the synthetic theory of evolution, philosophers of biology have flown fearlessly into current battles over socio-biological theories. The theory of innate linguistic capacities, behavioral theory and practically all theories of mental illness have been the subjects of severe philosophical criticisms. Theories of rational decision-making abound in the literature. Clearly, a review of the philosophy of science in the twentieth century could be overwhelmed by a review of philosophical discussions of particular features of particular theories of particular sciences.

Advocates of the received view of theories hold that observation terms and theoretical terms should be clearly distinguished. In fact, the latter should be explicitly defined by the former. The impossibility of constructing explicit definitions of all theoretical terms by observation terms is easy to demonstrate. The proof turns on the nature of 'disposition-designating terms' like 'magnetic', 'intelligent', and 'soluble'. It is characteristic of such terms that they refer to properties that are beyond any referred to by any set of observation terms. As long as one insists that observation terms must designate properties that are in principle observable, and that disposition-designating terms must designate properties that are in principle one step beyond any given observation, one has logically blocked the possibility of exhaustively capturing all the fish of the latter in a net designed by the former. The most one can hope for is a new net.

A new net was invented in the late 1920s, namely, 'operational definitions'. Instead of trying to capture the full meaning of disposition-designating terms by a set of terms designating observable properties, one appeals to a set of operations. For example, an operational definition of 'mentally deficient' might run as follows: One is mentally deficient *if and only if,* when one is given a Stanford-Binet IQ test, one scores below 70. The trouble with operational definitions in this form is that, given standard interpretations of the logical connectives involved, everything turns out to have the defined property as long as no tests are ever performed.

The two logical connectives involved are the material conditional (or hypothetical) and the bi-conditional. Material conditionals have the form of 'if p then q', where 'p' and 'q' are place holders (or sentence variables) for any ordinary sentences like 'the city is covered in smog' and 'it is hard to breath'. So, 'if p then q' might be interpreted as the hypothetical claim 'if the city is covered in smog then it is hard to breath'. By convention going back over 2000 years, sentences patterned after 'if p then q' are regarded as false when their antecedent variables (represented by 'p') are replaced by true sentences and their consequent variables (represented by 'q') are replaced by false sentences. In ordinary English or other languages, hypothetical claims with false antecedents might be true or false or simply indeterminate. In the logicians' world of truth-functional logic, where the truth-value of sentences patterned after 'if p then q' is merely a function of the truth-values of the component sentences replacing 'p' and 'q', interpretations of 'if p then q' are true whenever 'p' is replaced by a false sentence or 'q' is replaced by a true one. Sentences patterned after 'p if and only if q' are called bi-conditionals, and they are true whenever the sentences replacing both variables have the same truth-values, i.e., if the sentences replacing 'p' and 'q' are both true or both false, the sentence patterned after 'p if and only if q' is true.

There is, of course, some artificiality in the logic of truth-functional systems, in all logical systems for that matter. Logicians begin with some common sense intuitions about what sentences logically imply others, and then try to construct systems of rules that allow them to justify those intuitions without forcing them to accept any counter-intuitive claims. Success is seldom complete. Even such apparently trivial assumptions as the truth-functional equivalence of 'p and q' and 'q and p' is a distinct departure from ordinary language. In the latter, 'Ed died and was buried' has a significantly different meaning from 'Ed was buried and died'. Anyone who failed to notice that the truth-functionally valid implication of the second of these sentences from the first is inconsistent with ordinary linguistic usage would have a very impoverished sense of ordinary language and logic. So, it is vitally important to make sure that such anomalies are noticed. The artificialities and resultant anomalies require users to be mindful of the limitations of such formal systems. Such systems can be very helpful in elucidating fundamental notions concerning the construction and evaluation of sound arguments, but they must be used with some care.

Returning to the problem of adequately characterizing an operational definition, one must either give up the logicians' conventional definitions of material conditionals and bi-conditionals or give up the proposed view of operational definitions.

The easiest thing to do is to rearrange the various parts of the proposed operational definition so the test comes first. Then we get what is called a 'reduction sentence': If one is given a Stanford-Binet IQ test, then one is mentally deficient, by definition, if one scores below 70. Now whenever anyone fails to be tested, nothing follows with respect to her or his mental deficiency. We know a priori that one is mentally deficient *if* one has a score below 70, but this is useless information in the absence of any tests. In fact, its usefulness is strictly limited to testable cases. That is, the meaning of disposition-designating terms like 'mentally deficient' is specified only partially, for testable cases, by reduction sentences. As other tests are constructed, the meaning of such terms can be extended. But it can never be exhausted by such a procedure because, as intimated above, disposition-designating terms designate properties that are in principle one step beyond anything right here, right now.

Insofar as the distinction between observational and theoretical terms disguised a hankering for certainty concerning empirical matters, it was bound to fail. Corrigibility is logically built into empirical claims, including those involving the simplest of observables. Two thousand years of epistemology should have been sufficient to alert philosophers of science to the total darkness at the end of that tunnel. Some people have tried to maintain the distinction without having any illusions about the certainty of observation claims. These people just wanted to have some neutral facts available now and then, especially when theories had to be tested. Insofar as observation claims or terms were burdened with theoretical overtones, they reasoned, such claims and terms would be biased. After all, a 'theory-laden claim' or 'theory-laden term' is literally a claim or a term whose very meaning is at least partially determined by some theory. Thus, it cannot be regarded as a neutral datum to be used in the appraisal of alternative theories.

In the worst of all possible worlds, every term, and therefore every claim, would be theory-laden. So it would be impossible to administer an unbiased test of any theory. What is worse, people committed to diverse theories would find it difficult, and occasionally even impossible, to communicate with one another. Their official views of the world might be so different that they could be correctly described as living in quite different worlds.

Given the possibility of this undesirable scenario, it is easy to appreciate the motivation of those who insist upon an observation term-theoretical term distinction. They would like to have some assurance that we are not in fact living in the worst of all possible worlds. Fortunately, the world is crawling with such assurances. When psychologists test alternative theories about the behavior of rats in various kinds of experimental setups, there is typically no question about the observable facts. When political scientists test alternative theories accounting for voter turnout, the same statistical facts are usually employed. The whole point of the exercise is to provide a satisfactory account of the facts. If the facts changed to suit every theory, the exercise would effectively lose its point. Similarly, demographers, epidemiologists, criminologists, and geographers typically have to dip into the very same pool of statistical time series, i.e., facts, in order to test, confirm or disconfirm their theories. Moreover, becoming a demographer, and so on, implies learning to interpret such common pools of facts in the proper ways.

All the preceding problems with the observable-theoretical distinction are central to philosophy of science, but they represent the tip of an iceberg of problems in the philosophy of psychology or philosophical psychology. The problems of innate capacities, mental illness, behaviorism, rational action, goal-directed behavior, theories of the unconscious, and deterministic laws of human behavior, might all be mentioned. One might also mention the question of the role of inference in perception; the nature of mental representation; what it is to have a concept; whether mental images exist and, if so, how; the nature of emotion, feelings and cognition, and their relationships; the problem of split brains or, more generally, of personal identity; intentionality; mind-body relationships; consciousness; privacy and the so-called problem of the existence of other minds. Most of these problems are classics of epistemology and metaphysics, and it would be difficult to distinguish contemporary approaches to them from enlightened approaches taken by our predecessors, although there is, of course, a vast difference in the availability of a wide variety of experimental results and theories.

Without a clear distinction between observation claims and theoretical claims, one road to an incorrigible foundation for science is closed. Moreover, if one thinks of the total body of scientific knowledge and beliefs along the lines of the received view of theories, the whole edifice may appear to be jeopardized by the elimination of suitably stable (i.e., incorrigible) axioms. Some people would find that prospect terrifying. Nevertheless, the loss of certainty is not the loss of science.

To some extent the fear of flying with theory-laden terms and claims is also rooted in the quest for certainty of procedures. Without theory-free facts, some people believe, one cannot be sure that one's testing procedures are unbiased. No one imagines that the possession of theory-free facts is sufficient for impartiality but, as illustrated above, it is not obviously necessary either. Furthermore, the practice and growth of science for at least the past couple hundred years must be accepted as evidence that it is not only logically possible, but at least highly probable. Research procedures, like observation claims, do not have to be infallible in order to be useful, good, reliable and/or valid.

Discovery and Growth

Perhaps nothing about science captures the imagination of everyone, scientist and lay person, as much as the idea of a 'scientific discovery'. Ordinary people have opinions, views or hunches about the way the world works, but scientists have discoveries. It would seem that any reasonable initiation into any scientific community would have to pay some attention to the logical structure of discoveries. After all, without discoveries there would be no growth, and without growth, the scientific enterprise would grind to a halt.

To the casual observer it may seem as if scientific discoveries are nothing more than generalizations from particular observations. Indeed, this view has been held by observers who have been considerably more than casual. The theory is called 'induction by enumeration'. One notices, for example, that a particular thief was raised in a one-parent household in which economic, social and personal security were in short supply. As time passes, one encounters, reads or hears about other thieves coming from similar backgrounds. Then the generalization emerges: All thieves are raised in socio-economically deprived households. By examining the backgrounds of many thieves, a scientist (sociologist, criminologist or psychologist, perhaps) discovers a regular relationship between deprivation and theft. He discovers something that looks as if it may be a law of nature.

It is easy to see why one might think that induction by enumeration is practically sufficient to account for the logic of scientific discoveries. Just as one noticed a relation between deprivation and thieves, one might notice a similar relation between deprivation and drug pushers, murderers, kidnappers and rapists. Thus, one moves up a level, conceptually, still working within the pattern of enumerative induction. That is

All thieves are raised in deprived households.
All kidnappers are raised in deprived households.
All counterfeiters are raised in deprived households.
Thieves, kidnappers, counterfeiters and the like are criminals.
So, all criminals are raised in deprived households.

Notice, however, that the higher-level generalization was logically mediated by the conceptual link between thieves and the like and criminals in the fourth premise of the argument. If one did not know that thieves and the like were all species of the genus criminal, then one could not logically have arrived at the higher-level generalization. Moreover, one does not discover that, say, thieves are criminals the way one discovers that thieves come from deprived households. The conceptual link between thieves and criminals is forged while one is learning to speak English. The deprivational link is, on the 'enumerative inductivist view', built up from observations.

Just as one might design a conceptual link between thieves and criminals, one might design hypotheses that link theft not to some kind of deprivation but to rational calculation or illness. Such an approach might be patterned after a method known as 'induction by elimination'. For example, one might reason that theft may be explained by deprivation, illness or rational calculation, and rule out the first two possibilities for some affluent white-collar criminals. Wherever the alternative hypotheses originate, on the 'eliminative inductivist view' truth is discovered by the elimination of falsehood. Furthermore, it is usually the case that such inductivists do not know and do not care about the origin of scientific hypotheses. Their concern is the discovery of a true hypothesis from a set of options, whereas the enumerative inductivist was concerned with the discovery of lawlike generalizations (i.e., generalizations that turn out to be scientific laws) from lower-level generalizations or from particular claims.

A third analysis of the logical structure of discovery proceeds from analogy. Freud argued, for example, that since people often daydream about events they would like to see happen, and night dreams are similar to daydreams, night dreams probably have a similar source, namely, wish fulfillment. Interestingly enough, an analogical argument based on physiological rather than psychological considerations led to a quite different hypothesis concerning the origin of dreams. It has been argued that since a certain amount of muscle tension remains after strenuous exercise, and mental exercise is similar to physical exercise, (night) dreams are probably caused by a delayed shutdown of conscious processes. Instead of having one's mental faculties stop altogether when one falls asleep, some of the machinery continues to operate in a disjointed way, producing more or less coherent dreams. For our purposes it does not matter whether the psychological or physiological hypothesis is nearer to the truth. The point is that occasionally scientific hypotheses are discovered by means of analogical arguments.

It has also been argued that some discoveries consist in seeing familiar things in unfamiliar or new ways. For example, although people were familiar with shadows and with the phenomenon of straight sticks appearing bent when submerged in water, the idea of explaining such things by thinking of light traveling in straight lines was quite novel. In order to conceive of the Principle of the Rectilinear Propagation of Light, one had to begin to think of shadows and optical illusions as the *effects* of something. Once this discovery was made, additional questions concerning the source, direction and speed of light were bound to emerge. If light travels in straight lines, then one would expect to see shadows bend in predictable ways depending on the source of the light, its angle of direction and speed.

A similar view has been advocated by stressing the social aspect of scientific investigation and discovery. In this view discoveries do not usually arise at particular points of time as a result of a single scientist's efforts. Discoveries or innovations are essentially social phenomena with vague spatial and temporal identities. Moreover, and more importantly, they are not usually the result of bold new flights of fantasy. On the contrary, they are supposed to result from extremely constrained, tradition-bound puzzle solving that is concentrated on generally accepted theories and procedures. The paradox of discovery is that a community of severely indoctrinated scientists whose basic aim is to extend their pet theories as far as possible (rather than to seek new ones) finds itself dragged willy nilly to new and incompatible theories.

Just as eliminative inductivists tend to bypass the question of discovering hypotheses and focus on the question of discovering a true hypothesis in a set of plausible alternatives, some philosophers have focused on the question of discovering growth-ensuring hypotheses. They have been quite opposed to the idea of a *logic* of discovery along the lines of enumerative induction and quite content to leave the question of the ultimate source of discoveries to psychologists. Their problem has been to explain the growth of science in the absence of enumerative induction. Their solution is essentially an appeal to trial and error. Scientists make conjectures and submit them to tests. If a conjecture fails to pass its tests, it is rejected. If it passes, it is provisionally accepted.

This trial-and-error procedure, often referred to as the 'hypothetico-deductive method', has been recommended by several philosophers of science. Schematically, the procedure runs like this.

Given hypothesis *H* and initial conditions C, phenomenon *P* should occur.
If *P* occurs, the conjunction '*H* and *C*' is provisionally acceptable.
If *P* does not occur, '*H* and C' is falsified.
If '*H* and *C*' is false, then either H or C is false, or both are false.
So, either H or C, or both are false.

Four points should be emphasized about this procedure. First, it is basically patterned after a valid deductive argument form known as *modus tollendo tollens*, meaning 'the mood which denies by denying'. Schematically, the form is

If p then q
Not q
Therefore, not p.

Second, it is not asserted that the hypothesis is true when it passes its test. Such an assertion would be tantamount to the Fallacy of Affirming the Consequent, i.e., schematically,

If p then q
q
Therefore, p.

It is merely asserted that because it passed its test, we have no good reason to reject it.

Third, strictly speaking, the hypothesis *and* its initial test conditions stand or fall together following a test. Following a passed test, no one is interested in the fact that the initial conditions were as they were supposed to be. However, following a failed test, proponents of the hypothesis may have serious doubts about the conditions. Since a faulty setup may have been the cause of the unsuccessful prediction, the setup must be inspected. If it is clean, then the hypothesis has to bear the brunt of the failure. For the time being at least, it is provisionally rejected or at least regarded as doubtful.

This third point about the hypothetico-deductive method has received an extraordinary amount of attention in the past 90 years. Pierre Duhem's thesis (sometimes called the "D-thesis":) was that since hypotheses can only be tested in combination with some sort of appropriate experimental conditions, and a single test cannot identify which statement (*H* or *C*) in an experiment is false, there can be no crucial experiments of any hypothesis. Proponents of a hypothesis can always insist that there is some defect in the experimental conditions of the test, just as opponents can insist that the hypothesis itself is defective. So, all hypothesis testing must lead to inconclusive results.

As has already been suggested, if one is practically certain that an experimental setup is not defective then a hypothesis can be seriously undermined, if not completely falsified. The facts that the sympathetic theory of gravity, the phlogiston theory of combustion, the pangenetic theory of inheritance and many others have been thoroughly discredited and abandoned leaves no doubt about that point. Although empirical hypotheses are, from a logical point of view, always subject to reappraisal, it is not always rational or wise to do so. Just as one may have very good reasons to believe that a particular prediction has been successful or not, one may have good reasons to believe that a particular initial condition or hypothesis has been faulty. Thus, the D-thesis is unwarranted.

The fourth point to be noticed about the hypothetico-deductive method is that there is nothing in the procedure described so far that ensures the growth of science. What has to be insisted upon in this scenario is the inverse relationship between empirical content and logical improbability. If one wants bold new scientific hypotheses with an abundance of explanatory power, then one's conjectures must be highly improbable from a logical point of view. As explained more fully in section "Probability", from the point of view of the logical interpretation of 'probability', security can be bought only at the price of timidity. Highly probable hypotheses are highly probable only because they depart minimally from already accepted evidence and beliefs. The hypothetico-deductive method, supplemented by the requirement of testing only logically improbable hypotheses (though not hypotheses that are totally discredited or regarded as false), ensures the continued growth of science.

Another contemporary view of discovery and growth in science has roots that are nearly 150 years old. According to this view, in the process of becoming a scientist one is exposed to certain models or exemplars of good practice. One recreates standard experiments in order to develop an appreciation of the scientific enterprise as it is practiced by physicists, anthropologists or whatever. Little by little one is brought to the frontiers of one's discipline and one develops an appreciation of one's ignorance. In short, one is socialized into a scientific community that may be roughly characterized as a set of individuals committed to what is called a 'paradigm'. A 'scientific paradigm' consists of a set of accepted models of good practice, hypotheses, laws, theories and rules of behavior or regulative principles.

Scientific discoveries and growth, in this view, may be looked at in two ways. Normal or evolutionary discoveries are essentially mopping-up exercises undertaken without any threatened assault on a paradigm. They have the effect of enriching a paradigm by adding to its' stock of models, laws and so on. Revolutionary discoveries are paradigm-testing and, hence, threatening. Such discoveries are supposed to be brought about by a steady accumulation of anomalies within an accepted paradigm. So, new ones are sought. For example, the abandonment of the Ptolemaic geocentric view of the universe in favor of the less cumbersome Copernican heliocentric view was a revolutionary change, a change in scientific paradigms. On the other hand, within the geocentric paradigm, the addition or subtraction of epicycles to the constructed orbits of planets would be regarded as evolutionary changes.

Induction by enumeration has enjoyed enormous popularity as a rough (but very serious) account of what many textbook authors have described as 'the scientific method'. A scientist is supposed to observe, form a generalization, test, observe again, and so on. Whether or not such sequences ever occurred in science as it is actually practiced, a lot of students have been taught that they ought to occur. Thus, this particular view of the path to scientific discoveries has served as a model or exemplar for budding scientists. It has provided the uninitiated with an alleged behavior pattern that is proper, reasonable and accepted by the scientific community. It has given visible form to a scientist's way of pursuing the truth. In a world where appearance, form and style are often as important as reality, the possession of codified institutions cannot be underestimated. Scientists do not proceed by consulting a holy book, by going to court, by a public election, by breaking bread, rolling dice, dealing cards or reading the stars. They have their own method (so the story has gone) the scientific method.

If this approach sounds plausible, then it ought to be easy to appreciate the resistance one encounters from scientists when someone tries to introduce new methods into science. For more than a hundred years, those who have recommended the hypothetico-deductive method or defended induction by enumeration have been engaged in a struggle over scientific credentials. Although the players and procedures have changed today, the principle is the same. To a significant extent, science is a set of accepted procedures. To be a good scientist is, in the first place, to master these procedures. Moreover, since a good scientist is a person with high status in the social hierarchy of the scientific community, and since high status is generally preferable to low status, from a purely personal or ego-enhancing point of view, most scientists would like to be regarded as good scientists. Hence, scientists have personal as well as professional motives for trying to articulate proper procedures.

Explanation

Just as some procedures leading to scientific discoveries and growth are supposed to have a privileged status within the scientific community, some patterns of explanation are supposed to be similarly regarded. The pattern that has occupied the center of the academic stage for at least seventy years is called the 'covering law model'.

Every explanation may be divided into two parts, an explaining part (*explanans*) and a part to be explained (*explanandum*). In the 'deductive nomological form' of the covering law model, the explanans consists of a set of premises that imply the explanandum. Ideally these premises would be true and would contain some general scientific laws. In other words, the model or exemplar for this form of the covering law model is a sound argument. From a logical or structural point of view, explaining something scientifically in this view means providing a sound argument whose conclusion is whatever needed explaining.

To illustrate this type of explanation, we can consider a scientific explanation of the bursting of a water pipe in the winter:

C_1 Last winter the temperature fell below 32 °F.
C_2 An outdoor water pipe contained water.
C_3 If water expands sufficiently in a pipe then it bursts.
L_1 Water freezes at temperatures below 32 °F.
L2 Water expands when it freezes.
E Hence, the pipe burst.

All the conditions for a deductive nomological explanation are satisfied. The argument form is deductive and valid. The premises are true. Three of the premises state initial conditions (C_1–C_3) and two state general laws (L_1 and L_2). Both laws, as is typically the case in explanations of this sort, are causal, i.e., in L_1 freezing water is supposed to be the effect of the temperature's falling below 32 °F, and in L_2 expanding water is supposed to be the effect of its freezing. Hence, the whole account may be regarded as a 'causal explanation' of the bursting of a water pipe.

When the model was first proposed, it was claimed that the only difference between an explanation and a prediction is where one begins. If one has only the premises, they may be used to predict the bursting of the pipe. If one has only the concluding statement of fact, it may be explained by producing the premises. Logically or structurally, explanations and predictions were supposed to be symmetric. The trouble is that it is easy to think of premises that would be excellent for predictive but worthless for explanatory purposes. For example, if we had known nothing about water pipes except that one bursts every winter, then we would have been able to predict the bursting of the pipe last winter. However, once the pipe burst, it would have explained nothing to point out that it bursts every winter. The fact that it bursts every winter is merely a summary of precisely the sort of fact that requires explanation, namely, that it burst last winter.

For reasons of this sort, the symmetry thesis was abandoned early, but that was only the beginning. Regardless of anyone's commitment to scientific laws, it remains logically possible that as empirical propositions any of them will be false. Besides, some laws are accepted not because they are believed to be true, but just because they have a lot of support or, perhaps, merely more support than any alternative. So, there was some sympathy for the idea of requiring premises of acceptable scientific explanations to be merely well supported instead of true. This was the thin end of the wedge.

Once one begins to think of the role of inductive logic in relation to scientific explanations, the attraction of an inductive analogue of deductive nomological explanation becomes irresistible. This is especially true when one considers the fact that so-called 'statistical laws' are inescapable in science. Thus, in the 'inductive-statistical form' of the covering law model, statistical laws are substituted for universal generalizations, inductive validity is substituted for deductive validity, and inductive support of some sort is substituted for the truth of premises. An example of this form of explanation might run as follows.

L_1 All plants have a pair of factors controlling their height.

L_2 The offspring of sexual parents receive one factor from each parent in a random fashion.
C Jones planted seeds that were the offspring of plants having an equal share of both factors.
E Hence, Jones probably had a crop of plants with 3/4 displaying the effects of one of these factors and ¼ displaying the effects of the other.

Here we have an explanation with two laws (L_1 and L_2) and one statement of initial conditions (C). The first law (L_1) is an unrestricted generalization. The second (L_2) is a version of Mendel's First Law. Since it refers to a random distribution of factors in plants, it is essentially statistical. Hence, this feature of the *explanans* is transmitted to the *explanandum*. Thus, if one knew that Jones had produced a crop described as in the conclusion (E), then one could use the premises of this argument as a probabilistic explanation of that crop. On the other hand, if one had only the premises of this argument, then one could use them to make a probabilistic prediction of the crop distribution described in the conclusion.

The 3:1 ratio mentioned in the conclusion arises from several unstated assumptions, namely, that the seeds Jones planted carried genes from each of its parents, that each parent carried a pure line of some sort, say, tall and short, and that the tall sort would be dominant while the short sort would be recessive. Thus, three of the four options in the offsprings' inheritance would be biased in favour of tallness. That is, a tall parent combines with a short parent to produce an offspring with genes for tallness and shortness. When these offspring combine at random with each other, there are four possible results.

Offspring 1 Offspring 2 Jones' crop
Tall Tall Tall
Tall Short Tall
Short Tall Tall
Short Short Short

The second form of the covering law model seems perfectly plausible to most philosophers of science, but some people with special interests in social sciences still think it is too rigid. Since there is still no general agreement about the criteria that must be satisfied for a proposition to count as a scientific law and there is a tendency for contemporary scientists to avoid the term altogether, little would be lost by abandoning the requirement that one of the premises should be a law. Then arguments like the following could be regarded as acceptable scientific explanations.

Political views are normally distributed (i.e., in bell-shaped distribution curves) in any large population.
Politicians try to maximize votes.
Most people are favorably inclined toward people they perceive to be like themselves.
Most people will vote for people toward whom they are favorably inclined.

Hence, most politicians will try to appear as middle-of-the-roaders whether or not they are.

This is a fairly standard explanation of the usual bland or ambiguous type of speech that often flows out of politicians in western democracies. All the premises are well supported by empirical evidence, but none of them has been honored by the title of 'law'. The normal distribution of views mentioned in the first premise implies that about 68% of voters have political views that may be described as centrist rather than extremist. Bland-speaking politicians are aiming to identify with and capture the support of that central core of voters. Moreover, this example from political science of an explanation involving premises citing statistical distributions but no laws is typical of explanatory accounts in the social sciences. Thus, again one either has to weaken one's criteria to accommodate widespread practice or to justify one's criteria on a priori grounds. No one doubts that such explanations are logically weaker than the original deductive nomological type, but some people regard them as acceptable models of scientific explanations while others regard them as mere 'sketches' or truncated versions of acceptable models.

Explanations in the biological sciences have also raised special problems. These sciences are supposed to employ 'teleological explanations' that in one way or another are supposed to account for phenomena in terms of purposes or functions. Teleological explanations may be conveniently divided into two types, namely, goal-directed and functional explanations. In 'goal-directed explanations' the *explanandum* is some sort of goal-directed behavior, e.g., the pecking of woodpeckers is explained by reference to the aim of the activity, namely, finding larvae of insects. In a 'rational action' species of this sort of explanation, human action is explained by reference to the aim of maximizing estimated utility. In 'functional explanations' the *explanandum* is some feature of a physical system that is explained in terms of its function in the system, e.g., the presence of gills in fish is explained in terms of their respiratory function.

Alternative accounts of both types of teleological explanations may be found in the literature, but there seems to be general agreement that goal-directed explanations are easily interpreted as special sorts of causal explanations. Functional explanations, however, seem to be a distinct type. So a fuller analysis of these explanations is warranted. Consider the following example of a functional explanation.

Cows are well adapted (i.e., they have a good chance of surviving and reproducing).
Cows are well adapted only if they have the means to feed their very young.
Cows can feed their very young only if they have udders.
Therefore, cows have udders.

In this example, the presence of udders on cows is explained in terms of their function of supplying food for the very young. Although the presence of udders is in a sense the cause of cows being able to feed their young, it is the presence of udders that is explained in this explanation. Typically, however, it is some effect that is explained in a causal explanation. For example, the bursting of a water pipe was the effect of the water freezing and the other phenomena mentioned in the *explanans* of our first illustration. Thus, insofar as the roles of cause and effect are structurally reversed in functional explanations, they are logically distinguishable from causal explanations.

For all the types of explanations reviewed so far it is assumed that an explanation is essentially an argument. This assumption is explicitly rejected in the 'statistical relevance model'. According to this view, a statistical explanation of an event is a probability claim or assertion concerning that event, rather than an argument with a statement of the event as its conclusion. Perhaps the easiest way to appreciate the idea behind this model is to compare it with that of the inductive-statistical form of the covering law model. According to the latter, we were able to argue to the conclusion (explain the *explanandum*) with some probability that Jones would have a crop displaying a particular distribution of effects. According to the statistical relevance model, we would be able to assert that the *explanandum* was probable to a certain degree relative to the *explanans.* The formal methods used in both models could be identical. The difference is in the way one describes what one is doing when one explains an event, namely, arguing or making a probability claim. The statistical relevance model effectively eliminates the possibility of misunderstanding, although the rejection of the idea of an inductive explanation as a kind of reasoned argument seems to be a high price to pay for such instruction.

Some philosophers think that the attempt to specify syntactic and semantic conditions of adequacy for scientific explanations is fundamentally misguided. The crucial feature of any explanation, they claim, is its capacity to convey understanding. Indeed, some philosophers have held that the fundamental difference between social and physical sciences is that the former aim at an empathic understanding (*Verstehen*) of human action while the latter aim at causal explanations. For *Verstehen* theorists, the syntactic and semantic structures of the sentences that serve as the vehicle for empathic understanding are beside the point. According to these people, an explanation that does not enlighten anyone is as worthless as an argument that does not convince anyone, and social science without *Verstehen* is as worthless as physical science without causal explanations.

What has been presented in the preceding paragraph may be regarded as an extreme softline view of explanation in stark form, in contrast to the relatively extreme hardline view of deductive-nomological explanation. The summary makes it easier to appreciate the relevance of these issues to value questions in science. It is clear that rigorous codification of the structure of scientific explanations would serve the same social purposes as rigorous codification of the logic of scientific discovery. The more the community is able to articulate its accepted models or exemplars, the easier it is to distinguish good science and scientists from everything else, and to distribute rewards and punishments accordingly. Insofar as the view of the extreme softliners can be sustained, the line between the scientific approach toward human understanding and any other approach tends to turn extremely blurred.

Discussions of the structure of explanation have been regarded as having fundamental significance for the ethical neutrality of science. Insofar as human behavior may be explained in accordance with the deductive nomological form of the covering law model, it would appear that such behavior is completely determined. That is, insofar as the model is satisfiable in its strong form, human freedom of choice is supposed to be eliminated. Furthermore, since such freedom (i.e., personal autonomy) is a necessary condition of the ability to hold anyone responsible for his or her actions, it is a necessary condition of morality. Thus, the satisfiability of the strong form of the covering law model with respect to the explanation of human behavior has been regarded as having devastating consequences for morality. Those who assume, or merely hypothesize and try to prove, that human behavior can be explained in a deductive nomological form are engaged in the devil's own work. If they succeed, the argument runs, the moral fabric of all societies will be irreparably torn. Thus, at the very least, no one who adopts the hardline position should assume that his or her research is morally neutral.

It is perhaps also worth mentioning here that one has a moral obligation to pursue the truth and avoid falsehood. Without it, the obligation to speak the truth is at best silly and at worst virtually impossible to satisfy. Honesty requires a reasonable attempt to find out just what sort of world one lives in (i.e., due diligence in the pursuit of truth). If one happens to be engaged in research as a more or less primary activity, then the obligation is even clearer. Thus, no matter what position one adopts with respect to the structure of explanations, one's scientific research is not morally neutral.

Finally, some philosophers have argued that the irreducibility of teleological explanations to causal explanations tends to make biological organisms unique sorts of physical entities. However, as indicated above, there now seems to be general agreement that goal-directed explanations, including rational action explanations as an important special case, can be analyzed as causal explanations. Even if it is granted that functional explanations do not admit of such analysis, it is not clear what sort of uniqueness that confers on living things. More precisely, it is not clear what evaluative or ethical implications would follow from the fact that, say, some features of planaria, pigs, people and potted plants all require functional explanations. This is not the place to undertake a discussion of the moral relevance of various attributes of distinct species. However, as technology advances and it becomes possible to sustain life forms in diverse qualitative states for various lengths of time, the need for clearer lines of demarcation among species and greater appreciation of the moral obligations of humans to their own kind (including borderline cases) as well as other kinds becomes more pressing.

Induction

The concepts of induction and deduction were introduced in section "Introduction". After problems of explanation, problems of induction are the most popular subjects for university courses in the philosophy of science. The fundamental problem of induction is known as 'Hume's Problem', named after the eighteenth century

Scottish philosopher David Hume. It arises as follows. The premises of valid deductive arguments imply their conclusion. That is, one is guilty of self-contradiction to accept the premises but not the conclusion. On the other hand, valid inductive arguments do not provide such a warrant. There is no self-contradiction in accepting the premises while rejecting the conclusion. But we do accept the conclusions of inductive arguments. So, what is our warrant for doing so? This is Hume's problem.

There are several ways to attack the problem. First, it may be said that the warrants for accepting the conclusions of valid inductive and deductive arguments are exactly the same. There are rules of inference that warrant conclusions either certainly or with a certain degree of probability, confirmation, etc. To use these rules and then turn around and reject either the certain conclusions or the conclusions with some degree of probability is equally inappropriate. Warranted inferences are inferences made in accordance with accepted rules. Whether the rules permit inductive or deductive inferences, the warranting game is the same.

Some philosophers have objected to this view on the ground that there are really two ways to warrant an inference, namely, by showing that it is permitted by an accepted rule (as above), and by showing that it is at least as good as any other in an appropriate sense of 'good'. Moreover, formally correct inductive inferences may be shown to be at least as good as any others. This is a good warrant for inductive procedures generally and, although it is significantly different from the preceding solution to Hume's problem, it is certainly compatible with that solution. Neither precludes the other logically. This 'pragmatic approach' has been recommended by several authors.

There are three other proposed solutions that merit some attention. Some people have thought that the way to solve Hume's problem is to add an appropriate universal premise to all inductive arguments. Examples might be 'Nature is everywhere uniform', 'The unobserved is like the observed', or 'The future is like the past'. But the addition of such premises to inductive arguments transforms them into deductive arguments. So, this solution is more drastic than it may seem. It really amounts to the elimination of inductive in favor of deductive arguments, which would not be a solution to the problem of finding a satisfactory warrant for inductive inferences.

Another way to tackle Hume's problem by rejecting inductive inference altogether is to employ the method of 'conjectures and refutations'. Instead of trying to justify claims that go beyond one's evidence, one should merely try to falsify them. The idea is that if one seriously tests one's claims, whether they are generalizations or not, one need not worry about providing a warrant for accepting them. Until they are falsified, one has no good reason to reject them. However, and this is the crucial point, one need not accept them as anything but testable hypotheses. One certainly does not have to judge the degree to which they are supported by any accumulated evidence. On the contrary, one merely accepts a commitment to continue to apply the most severe tests one can find to the boldest hypotheses one can find. So the body of scientific knowledge will grow on the corpses of discarded hypotheses.

Finally, it has been suggested that the way to solve Hume's problem is to codify current inductive practices. Those who hold this view believe quite simply that acceptable rules of inductive inference are just those that are consistent with the kinds of inductive inferences that are presently routinely accepted. Warranted inferences are inferences that are generally allowed. In fact, the more they are allowed, the more secure their warrants become. In other words, inductive procedures and patterns of inductive inference feed upon themselves. The more they are used, the more they are regarded as useable and, therefore, the more they are used, and so on.

Just as Hume found himself embroiled in the problem of induction while attempting to put the institution of morality on a sound evidential basis, philosophers of science have suffered the same fate trying to perform the same task for science. Some philosophers have regarded the failure to solve this problem as "the scandal of philosophy," while others have found it equally scandalous that so many mountains have been made out of such a molehill. If one assumes that in one way or another the scientific enterprise is based on inductive procedures, then the whole edifice would be jeopardized by the failure to provide a rational warrant for such procedures. That is precisely the assumption many people have made, with fear for the life of science being an immediate consequence. As indicated above, however, such fears seem unnecessary.

Probability

Most of the philosophers of science who have tried to codify patterns of warranted inductive inferences have appealed to the 'theory of probability'. Although rigorous axiomatizations of probability theory were not available until the early part of the twentieth century, the basic principles were well known for over a hundred years before that. Most philosophical work related to probability theory did not center on the principles. That was left to mathematicians and, later, to statisticians. Philosophers focused on three fundamental questions. (1) What is the meaning of the term 'probability'? (2) How should one obtain numerical probability values? (3) How should the various interpretations, principles and values be applied to the problem of warranting inductive inferences? We will consider each question in turn.

What is the meaning of 'probability'? Alternatively, one may ask: How should probability claims or statements be interpreted? Examining the possible sources, grounds or origins of such claims or statements, a threefold genetic classification of possible answers to this question may be obtained. Probability claims may arise out of and be based upon physical, psychological or logical considerations. If the claims are generated from an analysis of certain physical properties of the world, probability is given a 'physical interpretation'. If the statements are generated from an analysis of certain psychological properties of someone (e.g., a decision maker), probability has a 'psychological interpretation'. If the statements are generated from an analysis of certain logical properties of a set of statements in some language, probability has a 'logical interpretation'.

Several classifications of interpretations of probability and probability statements have been used in the literature, usually with no criterion of demarcation being systematically employed. The most popular division is the dyadic one consisting of so-called 'objective' and 'subjective probability'. The interpretation referred to here as 'physical' is generally classified as objective. The psychological interpretation is always regarded as subjective, while the logical interpretation is sometimes regarded as objective and sometimes as subjective. People who adopt the logical interpretation often use the term 'confirmation' instead of 'probability'.

For those who believe that probability statements are about logical relations holding among statements in some language, one measurement theory merits special attention. According to the 'classical theory of probability', one measures the initial probability of an event by determining the ratio of the number of cases that are favorable (for some purpose) to the total number of equally possible events of a certain kind. Since the entire analysis is carried out a priori, it is clear that the sort of possibility referred to in the phrase 'equally possible' must be logical and that, strictly speaking, what the classical theorist is basing initial probability appraisals on is not the relations among certain events but the logical relations among claims or statements describing those events.

For those who believe that probability statements are about the physical attributes of certain features of the world, two measurement theories merit attention. According to the 'finite frequency theory of probability', one measures the initial probability of an event regarded as favorable by determining the ratio of the number of such cases to the total number of events in an observed sequence of repetitive events of a certain kind. There are three fundamental differences between this theory and the classical theory. In the first place, the analysis is carried out a posteriori on the basis of observations. Second, the kinds of events involved are necessarily repetitive. An event is said to be 'repetitive' if it is repeatable an unlimited number of times, e.g., drawing a card from a deck with replacement, rolling a six with a fair die and kicking a football. In such cases, strictly speaking, it is the kind, sort or type that is repeated, not any particular event; e.g., one may enjoy as many kicks as one pleases, but one cannot repeat, say, the first kick. In contrast to kicking a football as a kind of repetitive event, the first kick is unique. 'Unique events', by definition, are not repeatable. Finally, this theory differs from the classical theory because it requires sequences of repetitive events.

According to the 'propensity theory of probability', one measures the initial probability of an event regarded as favorable by determining, on the basis of one's experimental setup and scientific theories, the expected relative frequency of such cases in a sequence of events of a certain kind. The basic difference between this theory and the frequency theory just cited is that here probability statements are not reports about observed sequences, but reports about the tendencies of experimental setups to generate certain kinds of sequences. While the frequentist focuses merely on the outputs of experimental setups, the propensity theorist focuses on the setups themselves in combination with whatever scientific theories are available to account for their outputs.

Finally, for those who believe that probability statements are about the psychological properties (attitudes, beliefs and the like) of someone, two measurement theories merit attention. According to what may be called a 'simple judgment theory of probability' one measures the initial probability of an event by simply assigning it a numerical value on the interval between zero and one, inclusive, in accordance with one's intuitive judgment concerning its occurrence or nonoccurrence. Alternatively, one may employ a 'personal odds theory of probability' according to which, if one is willing to give odds of *m to n* in favor of some event, then the probability of that event is $m/m + n$.

Until around the middle of the last century, philosophers haggled about the proper interpretation of probability, as if there could be only one. Since then, it is more usual to find people simply explaining their preference for a particular view, rather than explaining the alleged inadmissibility of alternatives. Although contemporary writers may be inclined to put constraints on probability functions that earlier writers were not aware of, most people seem willing to admit that it may be impossible to obtain initial values in one way only and especially useful to obtain them in several ways. The lesson here is familiar. The richer one's stock of alternative theories, the greater one's chances for success. Insofar as philosophical analyses of probability have contributed to the enrichment of our stock of warranted inductive procedures, such analyses have increased our chances of articulating and, hence, critically evaluating inductive procedures in science and daily affairs.

Utility

Anyone who has an ordered set of preferences that may be exhaustively measured on an interval scale is said to have a 'utility function'. Interval scales are such that their basic units of measurement are of equal size, allowing one to say, for example, not only that one item is larger than another but exactly how much larger in terms of a standard unit of measurement. For some limited areas, provided that they do not contain more than half a dozen items, one may be expected to have such a utility function. However, given the wide variety of things that people value, it would be a rare person indeed who could neatly order her or his total set of preferences. Most people do not have, and probably do not miss, utility functions for all their preferences.

Since preferences are, by anyone's reckoning, closely related to values, it is often assumed that insofar as one has a utility function, one's values are measured on an interval scale. Moreover, by combining utility and probability values, it is possible to increase substantially the variety of one's inductive procedures. The method of combination is straightforward, involving a 'Maximization of Expected Utility Rule', but not necessary to explain here. It has been suggested that the idea of utility considered here is too general to serve the specific interests of science.

After all, the argument runs, the values that are of particular concern to scientists represent only a subset of all the values that people hold. Moral, political, aesthetic, religious, economic and social values, for example, are supposed to be irrelevant to the scientific enterprise. Hence, if one is going to use the Maximization of Expected Utility Rule to determine the acceptability of scientific hypotheses, one is going to have to put some constraints on one's utility function. More precisely, one must distinguish epistemic from pragmatic utility, and employ only the former in science. 'Pragmatic utility' may be identified with the broader concept. Epistemic utility requires a bit more explanation.

The 'epistemic utility' or 'epistemic value' of a hypothesis is its utility or value from the point of view of the aims of pure or basic science. Without getting bogged down in a debate about the difference between pure and applied (or mission-oriented) science, one may safely assume that truth is near the top of the list of aims of pure science. Besides truth, defenders of this position claim, there are other epistemic values e.g., self-consistency and precision. So far as the expected utility of a scientific hypothesis is concerned, then, these are the only kinds of values that should be taken into account.

As one might expect, there is some dispute about the matter. Some people believe that pragmatic values must be considered in the determination of the acceptance of scientific hypotheses. According to these people, the decision to accept or reject a hypothesis is always based, for instance and among other things, on the seriousness of making a mistake. One must take into account the expected utility of accepting a hypothesis that may turn out to be false, and the utility must be as pragmatic as the actions one is likely to perform under the influence of a false belief. That is, because one's scientific beliefs influence one's actions beyond the realm of science, one's assessment of the consequences of holding those beliefs must include an appraisal of the consequences beyond this realm. Hence, the evaluation of the expected utility of scientific hypotheses must be based on pragmatic as well as epistemic utility.

The idea of pragmatic utility has also been used to address the problem of determining the adequacy of rules of inference as well as courses of action. Particular inferences and courses of action may be justified by showing that they are warranted by more general rules, while the latter may be justified by showing that action in accordance with such rules is well-suited to achieve some specified end at a reasonable cost. The former sort of justification is sometimes called 'validation', and the latter 'vindication'.

Social Responsibility

The preceding section has taken us slightly beyond the threshold of a discussion of the social responsibilities of scientists *as* scientists. Although some evaluative issues in science have been discussed to which fundamental problems in the philosophy of science are relevant, the social responsibilities question has not been faced head-on.

As scientists, what, if any, special social responsibilities do scientists have? Since no one has been able to provide precise necessary and sufficient conditions for distinguishing the scientific enterprise from everything else, one should not expect a logically tidy answer to this question. Still, several, worthwhile points may be made.

In the first place, it must be appreciated that scientists are not immune to the buck-passing syndrome. Most of them will almost certainly be inclined to narrow the range of activities for which they are prepared to accept responsibility and, at the same time, widen the range of activities for which they are prepared to accept authority. Notwithstanding the psychological theory of cognitive dissonance, most human beings seem to manage this particular pair of incompatible inclinations.

Although people in business seem to be the only group blessed with the analytic aphorism, 'The business of business is business', others certainly try to have their way in the same fashion, namely, by fiat. In the case of science, the inclination is to come down very hard on the *as scientist* part of our question, thereby paving the way for the narrowest possible purview. Scientists, after all, are not moralists, politicians or social workers. So, the argument runs, they need not have the concerns of moralists, politicians and so on. So, according to those holding this view, the answer to our question is a flat *no*. Scientists *as scientists* have scientific responsibilities and nothing more.

The trouble with this argument is that it assumes that all concerns or problems can be uniquely sorted into mutually exclusive pigeonholes. On the contrary, most concerns or problems can be regarded as species of several genera. For example, unemployment is an economic, moral, political and scientific, as well as a social problem. The task of correctly measuring the number of unemployed people in a country or region continues to haunt official and unofficial researchers around the world. In fact, about this problem there remains a considerable disparity of views from one country to the next. Officially unemployed people may be eligible for compensation. Hidden unemployed people are surely unemployed but not officially unemployed and not eligible for compensation. To be counted as a member of the hidden unemployed is to be counted as a person without hope at best and as a slacker at worst. In either case, because they are no longer trying to find work, they are not officially regarded as unemployed. Their official status thus depends on their desires and the activities in which they engage in the interest of satisfying those desires. Or rather, it depends on some interviewer's perception of those desires and activities. Needless to say, the self-images of the hidden unemployed are affected by their employment classification. Indeed, it is unlikely that the self-image of anyone in a work-oriented society is unaffected by her or his employment status. Clearly, then, the question, 'Who ought to be regarded as unemployed?' is as much moral, political, economic and social as it is scientific. Hence, anyone who sets out to measure unemployment scientifically must be aware of, and must make decisions concerning, the propriety and consequences of a number of alternatives. Anyone attempting to measure unemployment without regard for the presumably nonscientific facts of unemployment would be a poor scientist. A good scientist *as* a scientist would address the problem in all its richness. He or she may not be able to manage the problem in that form and may have to introduce arbitrary restrictions in order to manage it at all. But that is not the same as refusing to grapple with its richness on the grounds of its unscientific character, whatever that may be.

Apart from the fact that more or less scientific and unscientific aspects of problems are inextricably woven together, there are independent arguments for attributing special social responsibilities or obligations to scientists *as* scientists.

First, since the results of scientific investigation may be used intentionally to influence or control human action, investigators should at least be required to share some of the responsibility for aberrant uses. Although one may balk at the suggestion that Pavlov should be condemned for all the immoral uses to which operant conditioning has been put, one should not be oblivious to the unseemly side of the social impact of his discovery. Undesirable consequences unleashed by scientific discoveries may be as real as desirable consequences.

Second, if allegedly scientific claims are used to legitimize socioeconomic policies, then the scientists making those claims in behalf of those policies should be held partly responsible for the consequences of the policies if they are put into effect. Whenever social programs are initiated on the strength of the recommendations of scientists, whose recommendations would not be heeded at all if they were not made *as* scientific, the scientists must share the responsibility for the consequences of the programs. If scientists are not held accountable for the consequences of their scientific pronouncements then they will be encouraged to be irresponsible, and they will enjoy an unwarranted social privilege that most people cannot and should not enjoy.

Finally, because scientists draw from the same limited resource pool from which the rest of the human race draws, they have an obligation to make their demands reasonable from the point of view of the public interest. The assumption behind this argument is that there is no invisible hand operating to allocate the world's resources equitably or even efficiently. Moreover, it is demonstrably certain that if everyone attends only to what he or she perceives as his or her own interests, a socially self-destructive result may occur. It is also the message of two children in a playpen who finally tear the toys apart rather than share them. Scientists *as* scientists must look beyond their own interests in order to preserve those interests. They must try to assess the total demands on the resource pool that they are tapping in order to avoid what one author has called "the tragedy of the commons." Here, as on our roadways, one must drive defensively. To assume that the 'other guy', an elected representative, civil servant or kind-hearted citizen is going to be wise enough or morally good enough to balance all interests equitably and efficiently is to reject the lessons of history. The public good is the business of everybody, scientists and nonscientists alike.

Quality of Life

At various points in this essay on logic and the philosophy of science references have been made to the importance of our topics for sustaining particular views about rational or reasonable beliefs and behaviour. The fundamental assumption of the essay is that the concepts of such beliefs and behaviour, including the quite magnificent bodies of scientific knowledge and practice, are socially constructed by human beings. Consequently, these beliefs and behaviour proceed from human perceptions, interests and choices, and are subject to moral appraisal. The question is, then: What contribution do logic and the philosophy of science make to defining, building and sustaining a morally good life? Although all of the complicated and subtle issues relevant to this basic question cannot be considered here, some essential aspects of an answer can be sketched.

Broadly speaking, moral philosophers may be divided into two groups, depending on which of the following two principles they regard as the fundamental basis of morality.

1. **Principle of Beneficence**: One ought to act so that one's actions tend to impartially improve the quality of life.
2. **No Harm Principle**: One ought to act so that one's actions tend not to harm anyone.

There is no uncontroversial argument for either position. People operating on the Principle of Beneficence will try to produce as much good as possible, for as many people as possible. People operating on the No Harm Principle will try to produce as little harm as possible. If the production of good includes the reduction of harm, then the requirements of the second principle are included within those of the first principle. Those who believe that moral goodness ought to require more of people than a life of anxious inactivity mixed with pious hopes for our common future will prefer the more inclusive principle. Insofar as one has a choice about what sort of moral ideal one ought to be guided by, what sort one ought to recommend to family, friends and the rest of the human race, it is wise to aim high rather than low. So, from this point of view, the more inclusive Principle of Beneficence is a more reasonable basis for morality, and morally right actions may be defined (with some qualifications noted below) as those performed in the interest of satisfying that Principle.

If one's fundamental moral obligation is to act in accordance with the Principle of Beneficence as articulated above, one's understanding of the concept of the quality of life has paramount importance. A few sentences beyond the famous definition of 'sustainable development' in the report of the Brundtland Commission one finds the following, less famous but more relevant sentence for our purposes. "The essential needs of vast numbers of people in developing countries—for food, clothing, shelter, jobs—are not being met, and beyond their basic needs these people have legitimate aspirations for an improved quality of life."

From ancient Greece to today, and around the globe, most people's understanding of a good life or a good quality of life is very similar. It is a life lived in good health, with loving friends and family, an attractive and safe built and natural environment, good government, financial security, and freedom to pursue one's own dreams in peace.

More precisely, the quality of life of a person or a nation (or a community, city or region) is a function of two variables, the actual living conditions of the person or people in a community, and what that person or those people make of those conditions. What a person or community makes of those conditions is in turn a function of how the conditions are perceived, what the person or community thinks and feels about those conditions, and finally, what a person or community does.

Taking the two main variables together (conditions of life and what people make of them), one can construct four scenarios which, with some exaggeration and over-simplification, may be described as different kinds of Paradise and Hell.

1. If one's living conditions are good, and one accurately perceives and thinks about them, feels good and acts appropriately in those conditions, we may describe that as 'Real Paradise'.
2. If one's living conditions are bad, and one accurately perceives and thinks about them, feels bad and acts appropriately in those conditions, we may describe that as 'Real Hell'.
3. If one's living conditions are bad, and one inaccurately perceives and thinks about them, feels good and acts inappropriately, we may describe that as the classical 'Fool's Paradise'.
4. If one's living conditions are good, and one inaccurately perceives and thinks about them, feels bad and acts inappropriately, we may describe that as a 'Fool's Hell'.

In each of these scenarios, the evaluative terms 'good' and 'bad' are used in two senses. In both senses, 'good' and 'bad' have the usual positive and negative connotations, respectively. Regarding living conditions, 'good' may be understood as 'life sustaining' in a broad and descriptive sense. Regarding people's feelings, 'good' may be understood as experientially pleasant in a descriptive sense. Besides these two relatively descriptive senses of 'good' (life sustaining and experientially pleasant), there is an evaluative sense recognizable insofar as one grants that some lives are not only longer and pleasant but richly or poorly endowed with mental and physical advantages and disadvantages of various kinds, with relatively vast or meager opportunities to put endowments to work in the pursuit of noble or base purposes, courageously or cowardly, and wisely or foolishly. Just as there are individuals with developed characters displaying a propensity to choose morally right or just actions, for the right reason and with the right attitude (as Aristotle might have said), there are communities or societies with developed cultures that provide socio-economic and political environments conducive to nourishing such individuals. Clearly, then, when we speak of a good quality of life for individuals or societies, we are speaking about life in both descriptive and evaluative terms.

In the best of all possible worlds, Real Paradise, people would have perceptions, thoughts, feelings and actions consistent with each other and appropriate to their living conditions, given the fundamental moral obligation to act in accordance with the Principle of Beneficence. Given the great variety of living conditions, perceptions, thoughts, feelings and actions, it is impossible to make the crucial evaluative term in the previous sentence, 'appropriate' precise. In different particular circumstances, the specification of what is appropriate to perceive, think, feel and do in the interest of satisfying the requirements of the Principle of Beneficence may be different, as well as constructed as different by different people or even the same people in different circumstances. Although this is not particularly satisfying, it is an accurate description of the human condition. Aristotle addressed the problem by recommending consultations with the best people, in the sense of the most virtuous or excellent people. (Somewhat analogously and at least as dissatisfying, some epistemologists suggest the need for "ideal observers" to provide the foundations of knowledge.) Unless one believes (contrary to the assumption of this essay) that there is, finally, a naturalistic basis and solution to moral problems, it may not be possible to go father than Aristotle at this point. In any case, this is not the place to attempt a final resolution of the problem of the ultimate basis of morality. Let us return, therefore, to the four scenarios.

While the first two cases are uncontroversial (notwithstanding the foundational issues in the previous paragraph), the second two are not. In fact, what is most interesting about the second two cases is that some people seem very supportive of one or the other as *ideal.* This is revealed most clearly by the numbers of publications around the world in which the quality of people's lives is measured on scales consisting only of 'objective indicators' (e.g., counting things like crime rates, mortality and morbidity rates, education achievement rates, per capita income) or only of 'subjective indicators' (e.g., people's reported satisfaction with their jobs, health, government services, life as a whole or overall happiness). While there are many researchers who recommend the use of both kinds of indicators and there are some mixed indicator sets, there are many more in which one or the other sort of indicator is simply omitted from consideration. Because it is impossible to make sense of the classical notion of a Fool's Paradise unless both sorts of indicators are considered, a reasonable set of quality of life indicators should include both sorts. The good life that we should want and achieve for all people is not just a life in which people feel good, no matter how terrible their real life conditions are, but one in which they feel good with the best of all reasons, because the objectively measurable conditions of their lives are worthy of a positive assessment.

The identification and measurement of a good life meeting the conditions just specified requires understanding and appreciation of the elements of logic and philosophy of science reviewed above as well as a vast accumulation of other theoretical knowledge and practical expertise in the natural, human and social sciences, humanities and arts. At a minimum, it requires communities of people to reach agreement on acceptable answers to the following critical questions and then to follow through with appropriate collective action. The questions are not categorized or presented in any particular order of priority or importance because no single principle or set of principles seems sufficient to provide a single rank order of the total set. Some are clearly logically prior to others in the sense that answers to some must be obtained before others, e.g., one cannot select measures of causal interaction (#12) or benefits and costs (#8) without knowing what sorts of things (#5) have been selected for possible interaction or evaluation. Other ordering principles would lead to different orders, e.g., one might suppose that the most important question in the lot is who gets to assess the adequacy of answers to all other questions (#18), or perhaps, who is entitled to any consideration at all (#1). As well, it is unlikely that this set of questions or their answers are mutually exclusive and exhaustive. Nevertheless, for all their limitations, in order to identify and measure *a life worthy of pursuit*, an individual or community must decide (most likely among other things):

1. *Recipient population*: Who should be included as a recipient of benefits and/or burdened with costs?
2. *Spatial coordinates*: Across what amount of space should one look, from the actors' own homes and backyards to the whole world?
3. *Temporal coordinates*: Across what length of time should one look, from now into the future?
4. *Population composition*: How should the affected individuals be characterized, if at all, in terms of sex, age, education, ethnic background, income and so on?
5. *Domains of life composition*: What domains of life should be examined?
6. *Objective versus subjective indicators*: Should one ask recipients how they feel or what they think (subjective indicators) about how they or others are affected by actors' action, or is it enough to merely observe their behaviour or other things that may be affected (objective indicators), e.g., what people think or feel about being unemployed versus unemployment rates?
7. *Input versus output indicators*: Should one measure only what one invests in actions, what comes out of the investments, or both?
8. *Benefits and costs*: What particular kinds of benefits and costs should be counted?
9. *Discount rates*: How much should one discount costs and benefits delivered some time in the future, compared to those delivered today?
10. *Measurement scales*: How should one choose the best sort of scale or measuring devices for the diverse measurements to be taken?
11. *Distributions*: How should central tendencies and variations be measured in diverse fields?
12. *Interaction effects*: How should one measure causal interactions in any particular array of phenomena?
13. *Probabilities*: What interpretations of 'probability' should be employed and how?
14. *Confidence levels*: What level of confidence should one require to accept any particular claim?
15. *Research procedures*: What adequacy criteria should be used to assess the acceptability of any procedures employed?

16. *Research personnel*: How should one choose one's experts, if indeed experts are to be chosen at all?
17. *Aggregation function*: How should all the diverse elements of the assessment be aggregated?
18. *Assessment assessor*: Who should decide (audit) if any assessments are adequate or appropriate?
19. *Assessment criteria*: What criteria should be used to assess (audit) the adequacy of assessments, the adequacy of the procedures used for the audit, indeed, the adequacy of the answers to all the previous 18 questions?

The last question reveals the threat of either an infinite regress, a circular argument or an arbitrary end to analysis. Clearly, none of these options is very attractive, but it is in the very nature of foundational work that such a point must be reached. In any event, long before individuals or communities reach their most basic assumptions, considerable progress can be made in the interests of improving the quality of people's lives. Accepting the fact that our capacity is practically always limited in matters of public policy-making to improve the quality of life, the most one can hope for from any review of critical issues or questions is that it will serve as a good heuristic device for calling attention to such issues. If such devices turn out to be inadequate, which is highly probable, our clear duty is to replace them with those that are more adequate. As we search for better instruments to build a better world for our own and future generations, we will share the accumulated wisdom of previous generations who pursued the same goals and, like them, we will hope that reason aided by compassion and hard work will bring all the earth's inhabitants nearer to a good life.

Glossary

Analytic sentence A sentence with a self-contradictory negation.

Analogy Things are analogous insofar as they are similar. Arguments from analogy and scientific discoveries from analogies are therefore arguments and discoveries based on similarities.

Antecedent Sentences following "if" and preceding "then" in conditional claims.

Argument Sequence of sentences such that some of the sentences (premises) are offered as reasons for accepting another part (conclusion).

Argument form Logical structure, pattern or skeleton of an argument.

Calculus of sentences	System of logic containing variables representing whole sentences and logical operators applying to such variables.
Categorical sentence	Sentences used in the theory of syllogism and patterned after All S is P, No S is P, Some S is P and Some S is not P.
Classical theory of probability	Theory designed to obtain numerical values for probability based on logical relations among sentences.
Coherence theory of truth	'p is true' means 'p is consistent with all other propositions accepted as true'.
Conjunction	A truth-functional sentence formed by connecting two sentences by 'and' such sentences are true if and only if all their component conjuncts are true.
Contradictory sentence	The negation of a tautologous sentence.
Correspondence theory of truth	'p is true' means 'p corresponds to some aspect of the (natural or even supernatural) world'.
Covering law model of scientific explanation	A model which assumes scientific explanations are sound arguments containing at least one premise that is a scientific law.
Deduction	An argument whose premise(s) are supposed to logically imply its conclusion.
Deductive nomological explanation	Type of covering law model which assumes the argument form required is a deductively valid one.
Disjunction	A truth-functional sentence formed by connecting two sentences by 'or' such sentences are true if and only if at least one of their component disjuncts is true.
Disposition terms	Terms designating entities with tendencies or propensities to behave in certain ways, e.g., magnetic, intelligent.
Epistemic utility	The value of scientific hypotheses (including laws and theories) insofar as they are for example, true, consistent with other claims believed to be true and precise.
Falsifiability theory	Proposed criterion of empirical meaningfulness for sentences, based on their falsifiability by observation sentences.

Formally fallacious argument	An invalid argument.
Hypothetico-deductive method	A method of scientific discovery based on positing hypotheses, deriving predictions, and testing the latter to obtain confirmation or disconfirmation.
Induction	An argument whose premise(s) are supposed to make its conclusion more or less acceptable or probable.
Induction by elimination	A method of discovering true scientific hypotheses (including laws and theories) based on the elimination of false hypotheses from a set of relevant alternatives.
Induction by enumeration	A method of scientific discovery of universal generalizations (e.g., All S are P) based on the enumeration of particular claims (e.g., Some observed S are P).
Inductive statistical explanation	Type of covering law model which assumes the argument form required is an inductively valid one.
Informally fallacious argument	An argument with a false premise or methodological flaw. Circular arguments are informally defective but formally valid.
Instrumentalism	(Theoretical) The theory asserting that scientific laws and theories are rules of inference rather than truth claims or sets of truth claims.
Interpretation	Interpretations of sentence and argument forms are ordinary sentences and arguments patterned after the forms interpretations of the term 'probability' are views about the meaning of probability claims.
Invalid argument schema	An argument form or skeleton such that if its variables are appropriately replaced making all its premises true, then it is still possible that its conclusion may be false (assuming no methodological flaws in the argument).
Hume's problem	Because it is self-contradictory to accept the premises of a deductively valid argument but not the conclusion, and it is not self-contradictory to accept the premises of an inductively valid argument but not the conclusion, some other reason must be found for accepting the conclusion of an inductively valid argument.

Logic	The study of arguments and things essential to their appraisal as good or bad.
Logical operator	Expressions that connect terms, sentences and variables of various sorts in logical systems.
Material biconditional	A truth-functional sentence formed by connecting two sentences by 'if and only if'; such sentences are true if and only if the two sentences connected have the same truth value.
Material conditional	A truth-functional sentence formed by connecting two sentences by 'if' and 'then'; such sentences are false if and only if they have true antecedents and false consequents.
Negation	The denial of a sentence.
No harm principle	One ought to act so that one's actions tend not to harm anyone.
Observation sentence	A sentence without theoretical content designating an observable phenomenon.
Operational definition	A type of definition such that words are defined by describing some operations designed to produce observable results.
Pragmatic theory of truth	'p is true' means 'action in accordance with p leads to satisfactory results'.
Pragmatic utility	The value of scientific hypotheses (including laws and theories), all things considered, including the moral, political and economic consequences of anticipated action based on those hypotheses.
Principle of beneficence	One ought to act so that one's actions tend to impartially improve the quality of life.
Proposition	The meaning of declarative sentences or assertions which must have a truth-value of truth or falsity.
Quality of life	The objectively measurable and subjectively experienced aspects of life. What philosophers traditionally have called a good life would be a life with a good quality.
Self-contradictory sentence	The negation of an analytic sentence.
Semantic theory of truth	'p is true' descriptively means nothing more than 'p' itself.

Scientific method Traditional name used to describe procedures for obtaining empirical knowledge by means of careful observation of the world versus a priori speculation.

Scientific paradigm A set of accepted models of good practice, hypotheses, laws, theories and rules of behavior or regulative principles.

Scientific theory Several alternative definitions have been proposed, but most people would define a scientific theory as an organized set of propositions designed to describe some aspect of the natural world, including aspects and behaviour of individuals and social groups.

Sentence form The logical structure or pattern of an ordinary sentence.

Sentence variable A letter representing any ordinary sentences.

Sound argument An argument with all true premises, a valid logical schema and no methodological flaws.

Syllogism An argument formed by some combination of categorical sentences, containing two premises and three distinct terms, with one term (middle term) occurring in both premises but not in the conclusion.

Tautologous schema A sentence schema such that it necessarily becomes a true sentence (tautology) when its variables are appropriately replaced.

Theoretical sentence A sentence essentially containing a term whose meaning is embedded in a particular scientific theory.

Theory of probability A theory designed to interpret the term 'probability' and to obtain initial probability values for probability claims.

Truth-functional argument schema An argument schema whose validity may be determined by converting it to a conditional sentence schema and testing the latter for tautologousness.

Truth-functional sentence Any sentence whose truth-value is a function of the values of its component sentences.

Truth-table definition A type of definition for logical operators based on an exhaustive listing of the truth-value of sentences formed by those operators.

Truth-table test A type of test for tautologousness of truth-functional sentences.

Unsound argument An argument with at least one false premise, an invalid logical schema, a methodological flaw, or any combination of these defects.

Valid argument An interpretation of a valid argument schema.

Valid argument schema An argument form or skeleton such that if its variables are appropriately replaced making all its premises true, then its conclusion must be true (assuming no methodological flaws in the argument).

Validation of particular rules Showing that the rules are warranted by more general rules.

Verifiability theory Proposed criterion of empirical meaningfulness for sentences, based on their complete verifiability by observation sentences.

Vindication of general rules Showing that action in accordance with such rules is well-suited to achieve some specified end at a reasonable cost, i.e., that the rules have pragmatic utility.

Bibliography

Brown, J. R. (2001). *Who rules in science? An opinionated guide to the wars* (236 pp.). Cambridge: Harvard University Press. (This contains several analyses of basic disputes in science and philosophy of science over such notions as instrumentalism, realism, objectivity and reason.)

Enderton, H. B. (2000). *A mathematical introduction to logic* (2nd ed., 317 pp.). San Diego: Harcourt Academic Press. (This is an introduction to mathematical or symbolic logic.)

Friedman, M. (2001). *Dynamics of reason: The 1999 Kant lectures at Stanford University* (141 pp.). Stanford: CSLI Publications. (This presents a thorough examination of two points of view in the philosophy of science, namely, the naturalistic pragmatism of W. Quine and the historical relativism of T. Kuhn.)

Hodgson, B. (2001). *Economics as moral science* (320 pp.). Berlin: Springer. (This is a close examination of the philosophical and ethical foundations of the discipline of economics.)

Hughes, W. H. (2004). *Critical thinking: An introduction to the basic skills* (403 pp.). Peterborough: Broadview Press. (This is a very readable introduction to elementary logic.)

Jaynes, E. T. (2003). *Probability theory: The logic of science* (727 pp.). Cambridge: Cambridge University Press. (This is a rather advanced text covering a wide variety of theoretical and applied issues related to probability theory.)

Johnson, R. H., & Blair J. A. (Eds.). (1994). *New essays in informal logic* (164 pp.). Windsor: Informal Logic. (This is a collection of essays reviewing the state of the art of informal logic.)

Kincaid, H. (1996). *Philosophical foundations of the social sciences: Analyzing controversies in social research* (283 pp.). Cambridge: Cambridge University Press. (This is a defence of naturalism and holism in the social sciences.)

Leary, C. C. (2000). *A friendly introduction to mathematical logic* (218 pp.). Upper Saddle River: Prentice-Hall. (This provides a readable introduction to the basic concepts of symbolic logic.)

Michalos, A. C. (1969). *Principles of logic* (443 pp.). Englewood Cliffs: Prentice-Hall. (This provides introductions to calculus of sentences, calculus of terms, predicate calculus, calculus of probability, standard fallacies and modes of definition.)

Michalos, A. C. (1970). *Improving your reasoning* (129 pp.). Englewood Cliffs: Prentice-Hall. (This has a thorough review of nearly 100 types of informal fallacies with many examples.)

Michalos, A. C. (1971). *The Popper Carnap controversy* (124 pp.) The Hague: Martinus Nijhoff. (This has thorough discussions of issues related to the logic of discovery and confirmation theory.)

Michalos, A. C. (Ed.) (1974). *Philosophic problems of science and technology* (624 pp.). Boston: Allyn and Bacon. (This has a fine array of papers covering alternative views of scientific meaning, explanation, laws, theories and interpretations of probability.)

Michalos, A. C. (1978). *Foundations of decision making* (290 pp.). Ottawa: Canadian Library of Philosophy. (This book provides detailed analyses of all concepts relevant to decision making, including needing, wanting, choosing, deciding, rational decisions, rational decision processes, benefits and costs, and values.)

Michalos, A. C. (2003). *Essays on the quality of life* (492 pp.). Dordrecht: Kluwer Academic Publishers. (This collection of essays has a variety of essays explaining concepts of the quality of life, relating those concepts to ethics and public policy-making, and to specific issues like health and health care, public services, sustainable human well-being, crime and victimization, ethnic relations, social capital, modern prejudice and gender equity.)

Nelson, L. H., & Nelson, J. (Eds.). (1996). *Feminism, science and the philosophy of science* (311 pp.). Dordrecht: Kluwer Academic Publishers. (This is a collection of essays explaining several feminist points of view regarding fundamental concepts in the philosophy of science.)

Roeper, P. (1999). *Probability theory and probability logic* (240 pp.). Toronto: University of Toronto Press. (This has a good combined introduction to both formal logic and the calculus of probability.)

Chapter 6
Philosophy of Social Science

Alex C. Michalos

Introduction

The aim of this essay is to briefly review the past 20 years of work in the philosophy of social science and to suggest-worthwhile areas for further research. Since others have been assigned the task of reviewing psychology, linguistics and statistics, I have tried to keep my remarks on these disciplines to a minimum. For reasons that will be made clear later, psychology got more attention than originally planned.

In the next section some of the general problems of the task are described. This is followed by three sections covering recent dissertations, articles and books. In the sixth section some caveats are offered concerning the suggestions for future research. Following that there is a section on the future as an image of the past and finally a section on the future beyond the recent main stream.

Aspects of the Problem

In this week's issue of *Science* (23 September 1977) W.W. Lowrance (1977) has a nice review on "The NAS Surveys of Fundamental Research 1962–1974, in Retrospect." He claims that the $2 million spent on these surveys was well spent. I will not review that review here, but it's worthwhile to put the efforts of the

Michalos, A.C.: 1979. Philosophy of Social Science. In P.D. Asquith & H. Kyburg (Eds.) Current Research in Philosophy of Science (pp. 463–502). Baltimore: Philosophy of Science Association. © 1979 by the Philosophy of Science Association.

A.C. Michalos (✉)
University of Northern British Columbia, Prince George, BC, Canada
e-mail: michalos@brandonu.ca

A.C. Michalos, *Philosophical Foundations of Quality of Life*,
DOI 10.1007/978-3-319-50727-9_6

participants of this conference (and the size of our grant) into the wider context of the NAS efforts. It's also worthwhile to repeat the following relevant remark from that article. "A good survey reestablishes bench marks, legitimates boundary shifts, exposes claims that otherwise would be disputed only in private, and commits to easily examined record a combination history, inventory, census, and projection" (Lowrance 1977, p. 1256).

Part of the problem of reviewing the recent history of the philosophy of social science is that we don't seem to have any classics. We don't have a *Logical Foundations of Probability* (Carnap 1950) or a *Logic of Scientific Discovery* (Popper 1961) to point to as absolutely essential reading for new students. One could point to well-known books, but none of them seem to be in the same class as Carnap's and Popper's classics.

Another part of the problem is the impossibility of distinguishing philosophy of social science from social science and social philosophy. Interestingly enough, Lowrance claims that "one of the surest signs that a discipline has fulfilled its purpose is that it pervades the other fields so thoroughly that it loses its own identity and thereby passes on, as many venerated disciplines have, into the history of science" (Lowrance 1977, p. 1256). For me, rightly or wrongly, sharp distinctions among disciplines have never seemed worth the effort. I have always focused on problems and solutions, never on disciplinary proprieties. For example, when I was working full time on group decision-making, on problems related to making good decisions in various senses of 'good', I began with the literature of formal voting theory and multi-attribute decision-making associated with the names Arrow (1951), Black (1963), Harsanyi (1976), Rothenberg (1961), Farquharson (1969), Alker (1965) and Fishburn (1973). There were no people trained as professional philosophers at the frontiers on this work, although the normative side of group decision-making was always apparent. Arrow's famous Impossibility Theorem, for example, rested on a set of normatively loaded axioms involving assumptions about the rationality of individuals and groups, the connectedness and transitivity of preference sets, the nonimposition of alternatives, Pareto's principle and the infamous principle of the independence of irrelevant alternatives. While segments of the literature of econometrics and political science shook with excitement for many years following *Social Choice and Individual Values*, not much happened in the world of philosophy in this area. Even though questions of the formal structure of multi-attribute decision-making are fundamental for an analysis of the acceptability of scientific theories (a main stream problem in the philosophy of science), no major efforts were made by philosophers to pioneer in this area.

In the 60s the Public Choice Society was born to carry on the discussion of group decision-making across disciplines. New names like Tullock and Buchanan (1962), Downs (1957), Olson (1965) and Riker (1962) came into prominence. We got our own journal, *Public Choice*. The group is still largely made of economists, but the mix is much more varied than it was. Occasionally a philosopher will turn up at the meetings, Tom Schwartz or me. Out of this literature has come some explanatory principles of great power related to the size of groups, the rationality of political participation and the significance of the public-private goods distinction.

To some extent Rawls's *Theory of Justice* (Rawls 1971) belongs in this literature, which is no mean contribution. But Rawls is a good case in point. Is that book political philosophy, philosophy of social science, social philosophy, political science or something else? Does much hang on a "correct" answer to the question?

From the point of view of reviewing the philosophy of social science literature, these questions are important. But from the point of view of the importance of the work itself as a treatise on justice, these questions are unimportant. When a philosopher of physical science reviews recent work on space and time, he should look at the psychology literature on perceptions of space and time as well as at the literature from physics and philosophy. Similarly, when a philosopher of social science reviews recent work on, say, systems of criminal or civil justice, he should look at the literature from political science, sociology, criminology, psychology, economics and social-political philosophy. I find no sharp principles of demarcation that could legitimately restrict one's review to the literature produced by professionals in any of these academic disciplines.

Psychologists and sociologists have also contributed to our stock of literature on decision-making. There were, for example, the string of experiments by Edwards and Tversky (1967) and his followers demonstrating probability preferences. And there were Rapaport's (1965) experiments on prisoners' dilemmas. Coalition theory, the answer to problems created by prisoners' dilemmas, is as much sociology as political science. The point is, again, that solutions to the problem of designing good decision procedures for groups drove me into many allegedly distinct social scientific disciplines. So when I am asked to review the philosophy of social science, if I draw upon my own experience then I am practically obliged to write a review of social science in the past 20 years. Hopefully, the preceding paragraphs illustrate my problem. If not, the following quotation from the *Encyclopedia of Philosophy* (v. 6, p. 370) may be instructive.

> The Encyclopedia features two detailed survey articles, POLITICAL PHILOSOPHY, HISTORY OF and POLITICAL PHILOSOPHY, NATURE OF. It also includes the following articles on political or social concepts and doctrines and on methodological problems of the social sciences: ANARCHISM; AUTHORITY; COMMUNISM; CONSERVATISM; CULTURE AND CIVILIZATION; CUSTOM; DEMOCRACY; ECONOMICS AND ETHICAL NEUTRALITY; ECONOMICS AND RATIONAL CHOICE; EQUALITY, MORAL AND SOCIAL; FASCISM; FREEDOM; FUNCTIONALISM IN SOCIOLOGY; GEISTESWISSENSCHAFTEN; GENERAL WILL, THE; GERMAN PHILOSOPHY AND NATIONAL SOCIALISM; HISTORICAL MATERIALISM; HISTORICISM; HOLISM AND INDIVIDUALISM IN HISTORY AND SOCIAL SCIENCE; IDEOLOGY; JUSTICE; LIBERALISM; LOYALTY; MYTH; NATIONALISM; NATURAL LAW; PHILOSOPHER-KINGS; POWER; PROGRESS, THE IDEA OF; PROPERTY; PUNISHMENT; RACISM; RIGHTS; SOCIAL CONTRACT; SOCIALISM; SOCIETY; SOCIOLOGY OF KNOWLEDGE; SOCIOLOGY OF LAW; SOVEREIGNTY; STATE; TOLERATION; TRADITIONALISM; and UTOPIAS AND UTOPIANISM.

Obviously each of these terms 'anarchism', 'authority', etc. represents a vast literature most of which is unfamiliar to me. While I could certainly read the *Encyclopedia* articles and review our progress up to nearly 1967 that way, that doesn't seem possible in the space and time available to me, nor does it seem worthwhile. After all, the reviews have already been written.

There is another very interesting side to this question of scope. When I tried to find careful conceptual analyses of such key ideas as wants, needs, preferences, values, good and so on, you can guess where I ended up. I spent a lot of time with *Mind, Philosophical Review, APQ*, and so on. But I found that philosophers of science don't. Most philosophers of science seem to regard action theorists, epistemologists in the traditional sense and philosophers of mind as empirically, scientifically uninformed speculators. Maybe they are, but I still find it remarkable that we seem to be able to draw so little from the professional philosopher tradition.

A third part of the problem of reviewing the recent history of the philosophy of social science is that it is indistinguishable from the philosophy of physical science. That is, there is a common literature concerned with explanation, laws, theories, acceptance, etc., in science *simpliciter*, not physical or social science. Since I have recently written a long review of this common literature for *A Guide to the Culture of Science, Technology and Medicine* (still in preparation). I will not repeat that story here.

Part One of the Solution: Dissertations

So much for problems. In the best of all possible worlds one would do a thorough analysis of three kinds of publications, namely, articles, books and dissertations related to the philosophy of social science. I will review recent work in all three areas but, given the resources at my command, the reviews will not be thorough. I suppose, however, that they are better than anything else available and better than nothing.

I have reviewed all dissertation abstracts in philosophy from 1961 to 1977, paying special attention to philosophy of social science. Excluding those explicitly related to psychology and those that I could not understand, there were 111 relevant dissertations. (See Appendices 1 and 2.)

In Appendix 1, I have tried to single out the central theme of each dissertation so far as this was discernible from the abstract. I don't know if the authors really proved what they said they proved. It is logically impossible for all of them to have proved everything they claimed to have proved because some of the claims contradicted others. Some of the dissertations seemed to be literary or historical works in which nothing was proved. Some of the dissertations seemed to be proving propositions that were silly, trivially true, false or nonsensical. While some

Table 6.1 Dissertation frequencies by

(a) Issue		(b) Discipline		(c) Person	
Explanation	12	Sociology	34	Marx	11
Political obligation	10	Politics	24	Dewey	9
Values	8	Economics	19	Perry	2
Human nature	7	Law	6	Hobbes	
Community	6	Education	5	Mead	
Objectivity		History	4	Schutz	
Social Change				Oakeshott	
Justice	3				
Theory					
Decision making					
Rationality					
Property	2				
Historicism	1				
Holism					

Source See Appendix 1

participants at our Conference were appalled by the collection of themes listed in Appendix 1, I suspect that any fair sample of dissertations in any discipline would produce a similar abundance of apparently appalling treatises.

I was not able to find a classificatory scheme to collect every dissertation under a significant rubric. Table 6.1a–c represent three sorts of aggregation. In Table 6.1b, 92 dissertations are aggregated by disciplines. Most dissertations (34) seemed to be concerned with issues in sociology broadly conceived. *Everything is broadly conceived here*! Politics was next (24) and then economics (19).

In Table 6.1a, 71 dissertations are aggregated by issues. Most dissertations (12) seemed to be concerned with issues related to covering-law explanations of human action. Most of those opted for such explanations. Ten dissertations were on political obligation. I noticed only one on holism-individualism.

In Table 6.1c, 30 dissertations are aggregated by persons dealt with. Marx is the favourite, with 11 dissertations related to his work. Dewey is second with 9. Actually, the works of both of these people figure in more dissertations in a more or less minor way. After these two people, a wide variety of names appear.

This brief dissertation survey provides a rough idea of what has been happening in North American graduate philosophy programs related to philosophy of social science. If I had enough time or money to hire someone to review all social science disciplines with an eye out for dissertations involving "philosophical analysis" (supposing I knew what that is), we could get a much better view of what is going on.

Part Two of the Solution: Articles

My request for a computer-search of relevant abstracts stored in the Philosophy Documentation Center (Bowling Green State University, Ohio) turned up over 600 titles. They came from 287 journals for the years from 1966 to 1977. As every copy of *The Philosopher's Index* informs us, "All major philosophy journals in English, French, German, Spanish, and Italian are indexed, along with selected journals in other languages and related interdisciplinary publications." I'm sure several hundred more journals publish relevant material, since few social science journals (few *people* for that matter) would be able or interested in distinguishing good conceptual analysis related to some science from good science.

I requested a computer search by more key words than the Center could conveniently handle. So unfortunately the dissertation search doesn't match the article search. The latter was keyed to social sciences, social-sciences, behavioural science, sociology and, contrary to my mandate, psychology. It captured law, education, history, economics, action, social philosophy and politics to some extent, but not completely. I am sure that if I were to initiate a new search on the basis of these other words, I would get at least another 600 titles with many overlaps from the first search. There still would be no efficient way to know if the key words selected by the Documentation Center to identify an article were the same key words most people or even I would use. That's just an inescapable fudge-factor in this approach. All things considered, I think it is best to work with the data-set that I have, and warn you of its limitations and peculiarities.

A lot of good articles in the philosophy of social science do not appear in any journals. They originate in colloquia and conferences, and are printed in proceedings volumes. I examined several of such volumes and found 235 relevant titles in 42 volumes. Again, there was nothing very systematic about my search. As you can see from Appendix 3, I tapped the most obvious sources.

Table 6.2 summarizes the results of the journal and proceedings volume search. More work was put on decision making than on anything else. Forty nine articles were devoted to this subject. Moreover, since most of the articles on values (46), rationality (25) and utility (21) are related to decision making, this subject easily dominates the literature in the philosophy of social science (Table 6.2a). The fact that there is a journal, *Theory and Decision*, and a book series, *Theory and Decision Library*, devoted to just these issues is both a cause and an effect of the flurry of activity.

Most of the decision making literature was related to individual rather than group decision making. Most of it tended to be formal, rather than informal, and most of it was concerned with some notion of good decision making. Usually 'rational' substituted for 'good' and the questions at issue were how to characterize and make rational decisions. Answers to these questions turn on a handful of basic moves. One may focus on processes leading to decisions or on the decisions themselves. The alleged rationality of a decision may be attributed to the process or the product. It may be regarded as essentially measurable or not, and a single sort of thing or not.

Table 6.2 Article frequencies by

(a) Issue		(b) Discipline		(c) Person	
Decision making	49	Psychology	268	Marx	35
Values	46	Sociology	118	Popper	12
Behaviourism	45	Social science	68	Skinner	11
Explanation	41	Education	24	Freud	
Observation	31	Politics	14	Husserl	10
Rationality	25	Economics	12	James	9
Causality	24	History	10	Weber	8
Utility theory	21	Law	4	Habermas	7
Information	20			Mannheim	5
Objectivity	17			Dewey	
Theory	16			Merleau-Ponty	
Brain/Mind	14			Aristotle	
Language				Jung	4
Functionalism	12			Chomsky	
Reduction				Wittgenstein	
Motivation				Durkheim	
Verstehen	6			Mead	3
Laws				Thomas	
Measurement				Levi-Strauss	
Historicism				Piaget	
Mental illness				Mill	
Intentions	5			Hegel	
Creativity				Marcuse	
Prediction				Schutz	
Memory				Brentano	
Heritability				Winch	
Models					
Control	4				
Negation					
Rules	3				
Culture					
Innate ideas					

Source Review of 571 abstracts computer-searched by social sciences, social-sciences, behavioural sciences, sociology, psychology, October 4, 1977, Philosophy Documentation Center (Bowling Green State University, Ohio), and 235 titles from proceedings volumes of special conferences and colloquia

If the rationality of decision making is regarded as measurable then some account of what it is that must be measured is required. This typically leads to an analysis of value or utility of some sort. The measurable things required in the measurement of rationality may be regarded as demanding maximization or not, in the long, short or some specifiable run. A thorough review of the literature concerning all these alternative basic moves may be found in my *Foundations of Decision Making* (Michalos 1978).

Behaviourism (45), explanation (41) and causality (24) were also near the top of the list of issues considered by philosophers of social science. Again, many of the articles that dealt primarily with one of these subjects touched upon the other. Most of the authors of the papers on behaviourism were trying to show that it failed to capture some essential aspects of human nature. Many people attacked Skinner on this ground, usually ignoring a distinction between methodological and ontological behaviourism. Clearly, however, there is an important difference between restricting one's research to behavioural analysis and asserting that there are no psychological correlates to behaviour. It has been some years since I met any ontological behaviourists, but one of the Conference participants assured me that there are plenty of them where he comes from, the University of Illinois.

Most of the papers on explanation were written by people trying to show that some sort of covering law model was applicable to human action. Typically then, the question of causal laws of human action figured centrally in these discussions.

Other very popular topics were the nature of observation in the social sciences or, more generally, the nature of perception. Thirty one papers were devoted to one or the other of these closely related issues.

Collectively these eight most popular topics accounted for about 60% of the papers reviewed, while the other 40% were involved with 24 or three times as many different issues. So within the main stream of recent work in the philosophy of social science (at least as much of that work as I have been able to classify after reviewing over 800 abstracts and titles), there is a clearly visible main current that is roughly characterizable as concerned with decision and action theory. Interestingly enough, while philosophers seem to have a (probably deserved) reputation for inactivity, they have spent a lot of time thinking about activity. In their hearts and minds, they are a very active group!

So far as the work of particular people is concerned, the work of Karl Marx got more attention than that of anyone else. There were papers on Marx on determinism, motivation, values, theory, objectivity, revolution and so on (Table 6.2c). Considering the fact that the computer did not search for material on economics or politics, the triumph of Marx is remarkable. It would seem to be a safe bet that if all disciplines were searched, Marx would be the most popular historical figure studied by philosophers of social science. Moreover, most of the authors who wrote on Marx seemed to be sympathetic to his views.

After Marx came Popper (12), Skinner (11) and Freud (11). Popper's views on critical rationalism and historicism seemed to draw the most attention. Skinner's views or alleged views bore the brunt of most of the attacks on behaviourism, while Freud's work played a similar role for psycho-analysis. This was tantamount to fighting the behaviourists at their strongest point and the psycho-analysts at their weakest. Freud, after all, has been dead for many years and an enormous psychoanalytic literature has developed since his time. Those who are interested in finding the truth or virtue of psycho-analysis or psycho-analytic theory should look at contemporary work.

Finally, as I suggested above, nothing much can be made of Table 6.2b on disciplines. A different key word computer search would have generated a different output mix. It is probably fair to say that psychology dominates the disciplines in the subset of disciplines examined, but the subset may or may not represent the total set of titles in the data bank that are relevant to the philosophy of social science.

I suppose the real moral of this brief discipline count is that we are well beyond the point where one can hope to review recent work in the philosophy of social science. There's just too much material to examine. I suspect one would be hard-pressed to review a single discipline. Just because philosophy of social science tends to be parasitic on the social sciences, it tends to be as widespread as its hosts. We have sent an army to study the philosophy of science. We apparently need an army to study the philosophy of social science too, and I am not an army.

Part Three of the Solution: Books

Perhaps the place to begin a brief review of some basic books in the philosophy of social science is with those that are or easily lend themselves to use as textbooks. Kaplan (1964) would have to head the list of this sort of book. Indeed, one participant at the Conference suggested that this book might qualify as a classic in this field. It has excellent scope and is widely accepted as sound by most philosophers and many social scientists. Rudner (1966) is also widely accepted, but its range is severely restricted (by design). The most recently published text is Nowak (1977) which, in spite of its title, covers a wide range of philosophic issues in social science.

If one prefers a formalistic approach to philosophic problems, then Ackoff (1962), Ackoff and Emery (1972) or Blalock (1969) might be used. A student would not get an introduction to main stream philosophy of social science from these books, but he or she would get a good introduction to a hardheaded approach to social science.

Leaving psychology aside, philosophers seem to have written more on the philosophy of history than on any other social science, and history, of course, is very much a borderline case for many people. That is, many people regard it as more of an art than a science. In any case, there are a variety of positions represented.

In Dray (1957) one finds his famous assault on the covering law model of historical explanation and his defence of "good reason assays". His intention was to emphasize the pragmatic aspect of explanations and to insist that causal laws are, apparently paradoxically, irrelevant to causal explanations. Danto (1965) defends the covering law model. In his view there are historical laws, but they tend to be truisms or nearly truisms. Moreover, he insists that the particularism typical of historical narratives is essential to history, unlike other sciences.

White (1965) also accepted covering law historical explanations and the essential role of historical narratives. On the question of historical laws, he argued that there are laws about individuals as well as types and that causal sentences don't presuppose corresponding causal laws. The last point has particular relevance for some inductive systems (e.g., Hintikka-Hilpinen) which seem to demand precisely the opposite.

In Meiland (1965) it is argued that historical knowledge is impossible and that therefore historians have to create the past rather than merely report it. The first part of his thesis is put forward on the grounds of the fallibility of memory, the impossibility of verifying historical reports and other fairly well-worn, arguments. So, as one might expect, the work is mainly epistemological. In this respect it contrasted with Todd (1972). Todd examined and classified a dozen sorts of historical work, and arrived at two generalizations. First, historians construct explanations that employ contrary-to-fact conditionals and presuppose causal laws, and second, such explanations tend to involve evaluations.

Besides Nowak's text mentioned above, there are a couple philosophical treatises on sociology that might be mentioned. Abel (1970) analyzes some of the work of Durkheim, Weber and Simmel, and shows how work after 1920 is continuous with these early foundations. Isajiw (1968) reviews a lot of sociological literature related to the issues in its title, and defends an anti-reductionist view of "telecausality".

There is no doubt at all that Merton (1949) has plenty of philosophy in it and should not be neglected by philosophers of sociology. Gouldner is also philosophical, but a bit more sociology of sociology than philosophy of sociology.

I have already mentioned some treatises on group decision making that have philosophical significance although they were written by economists. I believe Rosenberg (1976) represents the first fairly general philosophy of economics book produced by a philosopher. It's a carefully reasoned and worthwhile beginning.

There are a number of interesting books by philosophers on specific issues or clusters of issues in the philosophy of social science. For example, Diesing (1971) is an attempt to elucidate the logic of discovery and growth in social science by a careful analysis of diverse practices. It is, therefore, in the tradition of Hanson, Kuhn and Feyerabend. Runciman (1972) tries to support the notion of the unity of science by arguing that methods in natural science may be extended to social science. That pretty well commits him to causal explanations of social behaviour.

Cunningham (1973) tries to show the unsoundness of all major arguments purporting to show the impossibility of objectivity in social science. Scheffler (1967) deals with a closely related problem, namely, that of explaining how observation can be conditioned without being biased. These books are arguing roughly the reverse of Winch (Winch 1958). Winch claims that there are severe limits to objectivity in social science, and that one must in any case live by rules in order to thoroughly understand them. In Ganz (1971) the idea of a rule and what it means to follow rules are examined.

There are several books in the general area of rational decision and action, including value theory. One of the most useful happens to be the oldest, namely, Simon (1945). Like Churchman (1961) it doesn't have the sensitivity to linguistic nuance that is characteristic of a lot of philosophy of the past 30 years. But both books are thought-provoking and worth careful scrutiny.

Shackle (1973) argues for the impossibility of rational choice on grounds similar to those of Simon. The difference is that Simon rejected the synoptic model of rationality while Shackle accepts it along with its alleged disastrous consequences for economics. Diesing (1962) tries to outline five models of rationality and to review their advantages and disadvantages. Kurtz (1965) tends to be broad in scope like Diesing's book, but the theses are not as carefully defended.

There are a pair of books by Handy (1969, 1970) in which a naturalistic theory of value is defended. In both books values are defined by needs, an exercise that is apparently circular. In the first (Handy 1969) Handy reviews the work of his predecessors, Perry, Dewey and Pepper. In the second (Handy 1970) he considers the work of psychologists on value measurement.

Rescher's four books (Rescher 1966, 1969, 1972, 1973) all deal with basic issues of rational decision making. The first (Rescher 1972) reviews issues related to definitions of poverty and measurement of the quality of life. The second (Rescher 1969) reviews alternative approaches to value theory, and individual and group decision making. In the third (Rescher 1973) Rescher argues for a two-level justification of truth claims in which acceptance of the latter is warranted by some criterion and acceptance of the criterion is warranted by successful practice. In the fourth book (Rescher 1966) alternative divisions and ways of making divisions of outputs are examined.

Caws (1967) presents a theory of value based on human freedom and decision making. It's a peculiar view in that values are alleged to be essentially futuristic. Margenau (1964) does not have a theory of values or ethics, but he tries to show how a scientific theory of either might be structurally similar to ordinary scientific theories.

Suchman (1967) deals with a set of issues not found in any of the other books mentioned here. He is concerned with techniques of evaluating social programs and with ways of guaranteeing that fair evaluations are made.

Mitroff (1974) also represents a significant departure from standard methods. He did a sociological study of scientists working on the Apollo moon shots and, on the basis of results from this study, proposed some distinct normative principles. It is philosophy of science based on sociology and psychology, rather than on history.

Finally, I should mention Radnitzky (1968) as a special case. The sort of analysis recommended in his book is similar to Dray's, but it is proposed not on cognitive but on normative grounds. The aim is to increase freedom and communication among proponents of different schools of philosophy, not merely to increase our understanding of science. I'm sure Gary Gutting will have more to say about this general approach in his essay in this volume.

Suggestions for the Future

A couple nights ago I watched a TV movie in which the hero was a 30 year old stockbroker who suddenly got hooked on jogging. Then the jogging turned into racing. As the show progressed, bit by bit the stockbroker's world began to flake away. His job, his marriage, his normal routines were shed in various degrees as he became consumed by his desire to run and win a one mile race. As I watched that show it occurred to me that this was symbolic of a lot of human activity, or inhuman activity maybe. We tend to mount our hobbyhorses and gallop away for all we're worth as the rest of the living room passes into oblivion.

All of this is relevant to the task immediately before me. I want to address the question of future priorities for philosophers of social science. I haven't taken a survey to find out what most people or the best people or even my closest pals think we ought to do next. It's by no means clear in this business that there is a "next", since that suggests that we have just finished something. I'm sure some of you have heard the story about theories dying with theorists. What we do next may be largely a matter of what we're tired of doing now, rather than what God in his infinite wisdom would propose. Obviously I can't speak for God. For all I know, I can't even speak to God. And I don't have a marvelous theory that would allow me to generate proposals for our future. Of course, if we assume that we're confronted by a set of mutually exclusive and exhaustive possible courses of action and possible states of affairs, that we have a utility function and an objective measure of probability, then all our problems are solved. Unfortunately, I don't know where one might begin to find all those assumptions. There's a moral there!

In the presence of all these limitations then, perhaps it is understandable that I'm a bit suspicious of my own recommendations. You will be suspicious too when you hear the recommendations. Without further ado, I will mount my trusty wooden steed, throw caution to the wind and "sin bravely that grace may all the more abound."

The Future Following Past Performance

If future work in the philosophy of social sciences is patterned after past work in the philosophy of physical sciences, then several familiar lines of attack become evident. One might begin by analyzing alternative theories in different sciences. In the field of criminology, for example, there are theories accounting for criminal behaviour in terms of physiology, social environment, personality and combinations of these. The theories exist in diverse stages of development, with a wide variety of precision, explanatory power, coherence and so on.

Criminology is only one exciting field of sociology. There are theories in the sociology of the family, religion, work, law, politics, education, medicine, and the community. There are theories of rural and urban sociology, kinship systems, migration, population, social change, social welfare, social stratification and social psychiatry. Philosophers of social science have not even scratched the surface of sociology and sociological theories yet.

All the subfields of social sciences tend to generate their own jargon. So there are ample opportunities for conceptual analysis. In the field of criminology, for example, such key notions as 'crime', 'delinquency' and 'white collar crime' still do not have generally accepted definitions. Rural sociologists haggle about notions of 'solidarity', 'differentiation' and 'linkages'. Definitions of 'urban environment' differ from country to country. Definitions of minority groups and races admit of many variations. In Canada, for example, we have one count of Native People originating from Statistics Canada and another originating from the Department of Indian and Northern Affairs. In the United States there are at least three different official counts of deaths resulting from railroad accidents. One comes from the Metropolitan Life Insurance Company, one from the U.S. Federal Railroad Administration and one from the U.S. National Center for Health Statistics. These agencies are aware that the different numbers are the result of different definitions, but there is no single generally accepted definition of "death resulting from a railroad accident".

There are some conceptual issues that arise in all social sciences. For example, all social scientists worry and write about alternative concepts of validity and reliability. Philosophers might more naturally use the terms 'accuracy' and 'consistency' to designate the same concepts. Philosophically familiar disputes between teleological and deontic approaches to reliable and valid measurement arise. The question of the need for and possibility of operationalizing basic concepts is also ubiquitous in social sciences. The search for crisp explications of rule-following, law, role, social structure, explanation and a host of other more or less familiar ideas is bound to go on for some time.

In short, if philosophers of social science want to remain within the main stream of work that has characterized our discipline for the past 20 years or so, there is plenty to be done. Some people have referred to this sort of philosophy of science as cognitive and contrast it with the more normative type of philosophy to be considered next. I would like to emphasize two points with respect to the search for problems in cognitive philosophy of social science. First, one should not needlessly restrict one's view of any given discipline. For example, criminology, industrial relations and family studies are extremely rich subdisciplines of sociology which should not be neglected by students or mature scholars in the philosophy of social science. And second, one should not become fixated on historical figures or issues. Just as it would be silly to identify the philosophy of physics with the study of Newton or Galileo, it would be silly to identify the philosophy of sociology with the study of Durkheim or Spencer. What happened yesterday is often important and interesting, but what is happening today or tomorrow is often just as important and interesting. No one should harbour the suspicion that to be a philosopher one must be a historian as well.

The Future Beyond the Present Main Stream

I would like to see philosophers of science make a major effort toward the development of a national socio-economic accounting system. Essentially this would be an annual assessment of the socio-economic costs and benefits of living in some country. Just as firms prepare an annual report indicating their assets, liabilities, profits and losses, I would like to see countries prepare annual reports accounting for all our social assets, liabilities and so on. That is what the social indicators movement is about. It is an attempt to quantify the quality of human existence, to measure it in order to sharpen our understanding and appreciation of the sort of world in which we are living and the direction in which we are moving. It is thoroughly normative (esthetic, evaluative, etc.) and scientific. Or, to put it another way, it is science and philosophy combined in the interests of a particular set of normative concerns. If I briefly review some of the kinds of problems involved in social accounting, it will be easier to see why I think philosophers of science generally, but especially philosophers of social science, should branch out into this area.

First, one would like to have an inventory of the most important kinds of assets and liabilities to be counted in an annual report. For example, we will want some information on health, education, employment, politics, crime and science. There are lots of alternatives to consider, lots of ways to cut our socio-economic world. But we want to talk about "most important aspects" of that world. So, for openers, social accounting requires some systematic view of what there is to be studied, then some setting of priorities. No one is training anyone to try to get a view of our social world as a whole and to select priorities. Philosophers of social science, because they are trained to look at metascientific issues or transdisciplinary issues, are at least slightly trained to take the broader views required in this field. I say *slightly* because I believe most of us are still disciplinarians talking to the properly initiated and few others. You remember Carnap said he was greatly disappointed to discover that both physicists and philosophers had no use for "bridge people" like him. I'm afraid that what began as a bridge building exercise years ago has become today another discipline, philosophy of science. Nevertheless, I think we are a little better prepared than most people to look across disciplines. If not, my first reason for proposing social indicators research for philosophers is a bad one.

Suppose one picks a particular area of concern to work in, say, crime and justice. One wants to know how to measure the quality of a criminal justice system. What should a good law enforcement agency be like? What criteria should a good judicial system satisfy? Note: The question is not "What is justice?" again, though it requires some answer to that. How should one compare the seriousness of various kinds of crime? How should one measure white collar crime?

Questions like these are philosophically loaded in the sense that they involve issues that are part of the basic training of philosophy students. People with that kind of training plus training in social science should be better prepared to deal with such issues than people without any philosophical training. If not, then we ought to take a close look at our philosophy undergraduate programmes.

The same argument can be made in any area of concern for social accounting. If one looks at the health care system, technology, arts, religion, housing, transportation or whatever, the picture is substantially the same. Philosophers are trained to address normative questions in a way that others are not trained. If they will take the time to learn the essentials of, say, transportation systems then they can make a novel contribution to problems of measuring the quality of such systems. This is not the place to defend the development of social indicators and social accounting. Many of us have done that elsewhere. (See, for example, Michalos 1974, 1976.) Here I only want to insist that philosophers of social science can find a wide open field of study in this area and that they should get into it. It allows one to mix science and philosophy in a way that will be beneficial to each field and, more importantly, to the improvement of human existence. That's more than you can say for grue and bleeding bleen!

As a second area of major endeavour for philosophers of social science, I suggest science policy. (See, for example, Speigel-Rosing and de Solla Price 1977.) The issues here involve national support for science in the form of resource investment of various sorts. There are, of course, common themes shared by science policy studies and social indicators research. A view of our socioeconomic system as a whole would be useful. Normative considerations are essential. The payoffs for work well done clearly press beyond the congratulations of other philosophers. They may include a more reasonable allocation of the earth's resources.

A third area ripe to be picked is that of policy sciences or policy studies. Whatever these rubrics denote, they generally include social science designed to influence social policies. I believe that social scientific information is pressed into service for social policies all the time. For example, school boards, city planners, businessmen of all sorts and politicians make frequent use of demographic data. People don't build homes, schools, shopping plazas, etc., without trying to determine local population flows and stocks. Nevertheless, policy scientists try to provide information specifically for social policy. Put in another way, policy scientists try to make policy-making scientific- whatever that means to them. Here again is a mix of normative concerns and science that can be profitably exploited by philosophers of science. The two journals, *Policy Sciences* and *Policy Studies Journal* would be excellent places to begin one's investigation.

Finally, a fourth area, or perhaps a subarea of either science policy or policy sciences, is that of the science court. The science court is a misleadingly named procedure recommended to help decision-makers arrive at a timely and authoritative agreement about issues broadly classifiable as scientific. It is roughly a hybrid procedure consisting of elements of adversary, mediation and Delphi tactics. It was designed and has been studied and advocated by Arthur Kantrowitz and the U.S. Task Force of the Presidential Advisory Group on Anticipated Advances in Science and Technology.

Although the idea of the court is loaded with philosophical assumptions, no philosophers of science had any input into the Task Force. However, when I did my homework on the court and sent Kantrowitz a copy of my views about the idea and criticisms of it, he was delighted. He duplicated my paper and circulated it among his friends and Task Force members. One might wonder if I would have had such a reception if I had not come down on his side, but that is beside the points of my story. The points are that (1) people trained in philosophy of science *can* make a contribution to ideas like that of the science court, and (2) communication between philosophers of science and some influential scientists is still very poor.

These four areas then, social indicators, science policy, policy sciences and the science court seem to me to be perfect areas for philosophers of social science to move into. But, of course, my biases are hanging out all over. I believe some people go into the philosophy of science with roughly the same motivation that people go into monasteries, i.e., to avoid the world of ordinary affairs and contemplate the good instead of doing any good. I don't expect to make any converts. Besides, there are still plenty of main stream issues to examine. My recommendations are analogous to the recommendations of earlier philosophers of science to established philosophers. I want to push back the shores of the main stream, but main streams have fantastic momentum and resilience. They tend to just keep rollin' along. So let me just conclude by saying that there are vast uncharted frontiers for philosophers of social science to explore and I hope they will move into them. Most importantly, I hope that we will all follow Carnap's lead and help build bridges across the channels of self-interest and special privilege that separate academic disciplines.

Appendix 1: Issues Discussed or Theses Defended in Recent Dissertations in Philosophy of Social Science

[1] Dewey held a view of category continuity in physical, biological and social science 1977.
[2] Utilitarian theory cannot justify capitalism 1977.
[3] Hobbes' analysis of corporate state clarified 1974.
[4] Government is unacceptable because non-coercive means are available for its ends 1974.
[5] Madisonian and Rousseauian democracy are equivalent 1977.
[6] Perry's theory of value is objectivist and not substantiated 1976.
[7] Human action is explainable on covering-law model 1976.

[8] Question of political obligation is not a philosophical problem 1976.
[9] Moral education for Aristotle began with paradigms 1975.
[10] A new principle of methodological individualism is formulated 1976.
[11] Weber's arguments for values in cultural inquiry are challenged 1976.
[12] Marx changed from an idealist to a materialist theory of history 1976.
[13] Mill's and Oakeshott's philosophy influenced their social policy views in similar ways 1976.
[14] Negative and positive freedom are complementary 1976.
[15] Needs and wants should be coextensive, and society should fulfill members 1976.
[16] Marx's view of human nature is incoherent 1976.
[17] Ethical relativism defended as empirical generalization on anthropological evidence 1976.
[18] Political obligation based on utilities 1975.
[19] Fundamental problem of political life is the care of the soul 1975.
[20] Theory of society rather than of social action is a better ground for social change theory 1976.
[21] Rawls's theory of justice as fairness can't accommodate communitarian values 1975.
[22] Concepts of quantity and quality are necessary to understand surplus value in Marx 1976.
[23] Marx's theory of value and his views on alienation are connected 1975.
[24] Human action is amenable to causal explanation 1975.
[25] Scientists must make ethical value judgments 1975.
[26] Human action is amenable to causal prediction 1976.
[27] Political consequences of accepting social theory should play a role in deciding how acceptable it is 1974.
[28] Axiomatic social choice theory has semantic difficulties 1975.
[29] Socialist theory of property is preferable to a liberal theory 1975.
[30] Explanation of human action is limited by normative sense of rationality and by mental states 1975.
[31] We should have an androgynous world 1975.
[32] Mead's theory of social acts and knowledge are elucidated 1975.
[33] There are three senses of 'social philosophy' 1975.
[34] Marx's theory of distribution is defended 1975.
[35] Linguistic analysis is used in political theory 1975.
[36] Demonstration of originality of A. Schutz's phenomenological approach to social theory 1975.
[37] Solves the crisis of historicism 1975.
[38] Socialist rights are necessary for liberal's civil rights 1975.
[39] Dewey misunderstood Marx 1975.
[40] Marxism's relation to phenomenological and structuralist philosophies of human science 1974.

[41] Political philosophy should not be expected to justify obedience to law 1974.
[42] Ortega y Gasset's view of society is analyzed 1975.
[43] Schutz's category of relevance is analyzed 1975.
[44] Non-exploitive community rather than objectivity is at the basis of rationality 1974.
[45] Winch's view of social science is basically sound 1974.
[46] Sartre helps explain Marx 1973.
[47] Social science should be behaviouristic but avoid survey research 1973.
[48] Justice and equality are linked by relevance 1973.
[49] Moderate forms of the Duhemian argument are sustained in pluralist-elitist dispute 1972.
[50] Revolutionary consciousness develops in societies characterized by master-slave relations 1972.
[51] Concepts of prudence and ethics can be developed without a concept of empirical value-quality 1973.
[52] Ethics is culturally relative and subjective 1973.
[53] Marx's analysis of social structures is scientific rather than ideological 1973.
[54] Nonviolent political activity is justified 1972.
[55] An axiomatic theory of organizational development is constructed 1972.
[56] Civil disobedience can be based on moral or political concerns 1972.
[57] Fact-value bifurcation is not well-founded 1972.
[58] A theory of society is developed 1972.
[59] Individuals are related by similarity and difference in community 1971.
[60] Military conscription should be abolished 1973.
[61] An analysis of the explication of unclear theories in social science 1973.
[62] Ethical idealism can be applied in an industrial world 1971.
[63] Economic laws are causal conjoining reasons and actions 1971.
[64] Integration of themes of community and quality 1971.
[65] A process social paradigm is used to explain social order 1971.
[66] Social philosophy of Justice W.O. Douglas is criticized 1971.
[67] Explanations of behaviour don't require general laws 1971.
[68] Dewey's philosophy of education is defended 1971.
[69] Notion of objectivity in social science is unclear 1971.
[70] Analysis of legal and moral obligation 1970.
[71] Morality is not essentially social 1971.
[72] All systems of approaching decision making are limited but complementary 1971.
[73] Collective is superior to individual in Levi-Strauss 1970.
[74] Insanity defense is analyzed 1970.
[75] Concepts of ideology are explicated 1970.
[76] Oakeshott's view of rational conduct is criticized 1970.

[77] Analysis of moral objectivity is given with a theory of moral education 1970.
[78] A satisfactory preference-aggregation rule is designed 1969.
[79] Social science can't be value-free 1969.
[80] Dewey was a practical Idealist 1969.
[81] Perry's socio-moral theory is inadequate 1969.
[82] Marxian unified materialist theory of culture is developed 1969.
[83] Hobbes' *Leviathan* represents a coherent moral and political view 1968.
[84] US Military represents American disposition to violence and moral crusades 1968.
[85] Covering law model of explanation is not necessary for explaining human behaviour 1968.
[86] Analysis of mental disorder and criminal responsibility. 1968.
[87] Historical roots of concepts of alienation are examined 1968.
[88] Dichotomy between moral and self-interested reasoning is illusory 1967.
[89] Heidegger's work lays a foundation for a social philosophy 1967.
[90] Idea of 'good moral character' in US citizenship law is useless 1967.
[91] Royce's social philosophy is analyzed 1967.
[92] Brightman's educational theory is analyzed 1967.
[93] Analysis of functional statements in anthropology 1964.
[94] Shows how to decide if a revolutionary act is right 1966.
[95] Covering-law-type historical explanation is defended 1966.
[96] Human action can be explained without offending materialists or vitalists 1966.
[97] Marx's theory of democracy is defended 1966.
[98] Social philosophies of Dewey and Bosanquet are compared 1966.
[99] Covering-law-type historical explanation is defended 1965.
[100] Mead's metaphysics of sociality is explained 1965.
[101] Profit maximization in economic theory is analyzed 1965.
[102] Analysis of idea of fundamental change in law and society 1964.
[103] Scheler's philosophy is consistent 1964.
[104] Dewey has a doctrine of political rights 1964.
[105] Ricoeur's philosophical anthropology is analyzed 1964.
[106] Analysis of social thought of R. Niebuhr and H.R. Niebuhr 1963,
[107] Analysis of ethical foundations of the labour movement 1963.
[108] Educational philosophy of Dewey and Thomas are compared 1961.
[109] Dewey's approach to social philosophy-is analyzed 1962.
[110] Dewey's theory of value is valuable 1962.

Appendix 2: Dissertation Bibliography. Philosophy of Social Science 1961–1977

[1] Abbate, P.J. *Politics and Principles: A Critique of Michael Oakeshott's Conception of Rational Conduct*. Columbia U., 1970.
[2] Ackley, C.W. *The Modern Military in American Society; An Ethical and Theological Critique*. Claremont Graduate School and U. Center, 1968.
[3] Aichele, R.G. *John Dewey's Democracy and Education: From a Logical Point of View*. U. of Missouri, Columbia, 1971.
[4] Akinpelu, J.A. *Moral Education and Moral Objectivity*. Columbia U., 1970.
[5] Bardi, J.F. *Philosophy and the Phenomenon of Political Obligation*. U. of Missouri, Columbia, 1974.
[6] Beebe, W.A. Rev. *Value and Society: A Study of the Socio-Moral Thought of Ralph Barton Perry. Catholic U. of America, 1969.*
[7] Bennett, W.J. *Societal Obligation*. U. of Texas at Austin, 1970.
[8] Berleant, A. *Logic and Social Doctrine: Dewey's Methodological Approach to Social Philosophy*. U. of Buffalo, 1962.
[9] Bhattacharya, D. *"Relevance" in the Concept of Justice and its Application to the Question of the Distribution of Education*. Columbia U., 1973.
[10] Bordeau, E.J. *The Practical Idealism of John Dewey's Political Philosophy: An Answer to Some Critics*. Fordham U., 1969.
[11] Bramann, J.K.R. *The Problem of Objectivity and Ideology in the Social Sciences*. U. of Oregon, 1971.
[12] Brandon, W.P., Jr. *Linguistic Analysis, Political Science and Political Theory: Some Applications of Contemporary Anglo-American Philosophy to the Study of Politics and Political Theory*. Duke U., 1975.
[13] Cell, H.R. *Rousseau's Theory of Community*. Temple U., 1977.
[14] Creer, L.M. *A Defense- of the Covering Law Theory of Historical Explanation*. U. of Utah, 1966.
[15] Damhorst, D.E. Rev. *Social Norms and Protestant Ethics; The Ethical Views of Reinhold Miebuhr and H. Richard Niebuhr*. St. Louis U., 1963.
[16] D'Amico, R. *Consciousness and History; Phenomenological and Structuralist Philosophies of the Human Sciences*. State U. of New York at Buffalo, 1974.
[17] Diorio, J.A. *Ethics, Actions and Things: A Cross-Cultural Analysis of the Ontological Foundations of Moral Deliberation*. Columbia U., 1973.
[18] Dusek, R.V. *The Implications of the Duhemian Argument for the Social Sciences*. U. of Texas at Austin, 1972.
[19] Dyke, C.E. *Political Duties and Their Limits*. Brown U., 1966.
[20] Ellard, G. *Science and Ideology in Karl Marx*. Yale U., 1973.
[21] Enteman, W.F. *A Philosophic Critique of the Economic Concept of Profit Maximization*. Boston U. Graduate School, 1965.

[22] Fagot, Anne M. *Causal vs. Teleological Explanation of Behavior*. Stanford U., 1971.

[23] Feinberg, W. *Comparative Study of the Social Philosophies of John Dewey and Bernard Bosanquet*. Boston U. Graduate School, 1966.

[24] Ferguson, E.E. *Ralph Barton Perry's Value Theory: Its Relation ship to His Epistemology*. Saint Louis U., 1976.

[25] Fischer, N.A. *Alienation, Reification, and the Labor Theory of Value: The Philosophical Basis of Marx[1]s Economics*. U. of Washington, 1975.

[26] Fleck, L.M. *G.H. Mead's Pragmatic Theory of Knowledge*. Saint Louis U., 1975.

[27] Clyde, James. *On the Moral Autonomy of Science*. Washington U., 1975.

[28] Gambino, Richard. *Concepts of Mental Disorder and Criminal Responsibility in Law*. New York U., 1968.

[29] Gay, W.C. *Action Versus Society: An Analysis of Weber and Marx*. Boston Col., 1976.

[30] Gibson, Mary B. *Behind the Veil of Ignorance: A Dim View. A Critical Study of Rawls's Theory of Justice*. Princeton U., 1975.

[31] Gordon, P.M. *The Development of Marx's Conception of Human Mature*. U. of California, San Diego, 1976.

[32] Grassian, V.D. *Criminal Responsibility and the Mentally, 111 Offender*. U. of California, Los Angeles, 1970.

[33] Greenstein, H. *Philosophy, Science and Human Behavior*, New York U., 1968.

[34] Grim, P.N. *Ethical Relativism in the Context of the Social Sciences*. Boston U. Graduate School, 1976.

[35] Gross, Richard. *Quality and Quantity; An Analysis of the Influence of Hegel's Logic on Marx's Capital*. Boston Col., 1976.

[36] Hackler, Chris. *Political Obligation*. U. of North Carolina at Chapel Hill, 1975.

[37] Hare, P.H. *G.H. Mead's Metaphysics of Sociality*. Columbia U., 1965.

[38] Helm, *C.J. Causality and Explanation in the Social Sciences*; *The Case of the SRC*. U. of North Carolina at Chapel Hill, 1973.

[39] Hines, J.N. III. *A Theory of Society*. Emory U., 1972.

[40] Hunt, T.J. *Is Morality Essentially Social?* Vanderbilt U., 1971.

[41] Lavely, J.H. *Paul Ricoeur's Phenomenological Methodology and Philosophical Anthropology*. Boston U. Graduate School, 1964.

[42] Joly, R.P. *The Human Person in a Philosophy of Education*, Catholic U. of America, 1961.

[43] Ketchum, Sara Ann. *Needs, the Good Life and the Good Society*: *Toward a Philosophical Foundation for Radical Humanism*. U. of Michigan, 1976.

[44] Kim, Hong-woo. *Phenomenology and Political Philosophy: A Study of the Political Implications of Husserl's Account of the Life-World*. U. of Georgia, 1975.

[45] Korn, F.F. *Dissolving the Problem of Political Obligation*. U. of Michigan.
[46] Kraus, R.J. *Free Individual in a Free Society: The Philosophy of Justice William O. Douglas*. Fordham U., 1971.
[47] Lambert, Garth R., *A Study of Aristotle's Concepts of Moral and Intellectual Education in the Context of Modern Educational Theory*. U. of Toronto, 1975.
[48] Landesman, B.M. *The Obligation to Obey the Law: An Essay on Law, Social Institutions, and Morality*. U. of Michigan, 1971.
[49] Leach, J.J. *Historical Explanation and Value-Neutrality*. Michigan State U., 1965.
[50] LiBrize, J.A. *A Study in the Philosophy of Labor*. State U. of New York at Buffalo, 1963.
[51] Lindemann, Kathryn M. *A Clarification of the Meaning of 'Social Philosophy' Through an Examination and Clarification of the Extension of the Domain of Social Philosophy*. Michigan State U., 1975.
[52] Lithown, R.J.M. *Actions: Their Identification and Explanation. An Essay in the Philosophy of Action and the Epistemology of the Social Sciences*. U. of Western Ontario, 1976.
[53] Lcmbardi, J.L., *The Ethics of Distribution: Three Methods of Appraisal*. New York U., 1975.
[54] Long, J.B. *Dewey and Pragmatism: Towards a True Conception of Values in Process*. Fordham U., 1962.
[55] Luban, D.J. *The Misuse of Objectivity in the Foundations of Politics, Language, and Knowledge*. Yale U., 1974.
[56] Malinovich, Stanley. *Morality as Reasoning About the Concept of Man*. New York U., 1967.
[57] Mannolini, C.A. *Toward a Philosophy of Feminism: A Matter of Androgyny*. Southern Illinois U., 1975.
[58] McBride, W.L. *The Concept of Fundamental Change in Law and Society*. Yale U., 1964.
[59] McKim, V.R. *Human Action and a Scientific Image of Man*. Yale U., 1966.
[60] McNabb, J.R., Jr. *C.I. Lewis and the Foundations of Practical Reason*. State U. of New York at Buffalo, 1973.
[61] Megill, K.A. *The Community as a Democratic Principle in Marx's Philosophy*. Yale U., 1966.
[62] Murchland, B.G. *Alienation: The Problem and Some Philosophical* Antecedents. State U. of New York at Buffalo, 1968.
[63] Nissen, B.A. *Moral Means and Ends in Social Change: Dewey and Marxism*. Columbia U., 1975.
[64] O'Connor, R.F. *The Social Philosophy of Ortega y Gasset*. U. of Texas at Austin, 1975.
[65] Odoni, E.M. *Sartre's Contribution to the Phenomenology of Marxism*. Boston U. Graduate School, 1973.

[66] Onwuanibe, R.C. *An Ethical Inquiry on Franz Fanon's Revolutionary Humanism: A Critique of the Use of Violence*. Georgetown U., 1975.
[67] Overholt, W.H. *Organization, Revolution and Democracy: Toward a Sociology of Politics*. Yale U., 1972.
[68] Panichas, G.E. *The Liberal Theory of Property*. U. of Arizona, 1975.
[69] Park, Dong Huan. *Organization and Conflict: Value Theory and the Policy Sciences*. Southern Illinois U.
[70] Perkins, Lisa Haenlein. *The Concept of "Good Moral Character" in Naturalization Proceedings*. Columbia U., 1967.
[71] Perry, Clifton B. *Methods and Explanations in Social Science*. U. of California, Santa Barbara, 1976.
[72] Philip, Edward Parkinson. *Scientific Method, Behavioral Science, and Rationality*. Columbia U., 1975.
[73] Phillips, C. *John Stuart Mill and Michael Oakeshott: A Case Study of Some Differences in Social Policy and Philosophical Theory*. City U. of New York, 1976.
[74] Piggush, J.R. *Peter Winch and the Philosophy of the Social Sciences: A Critical Analysis*. U. of Notre Dame, 1974.
[75] Power, R.J. *The Bases of Political Rights in the Philosophy of John Dewey*. Emory U., 1964.
[76] Preuss, P.S. *The Individual in Community*. U. of Toronto, 1971.
[77] Radest, H.B. *Toward a Philosophy of Culture (A Study of Felix Adler's View of Education)*. Columbia U., 1971.
[78] Ramsdell, R.D. *Brightman's View of the Person and Educational Theory*. Boston U. Graduate School, 1967.
[79] Ranly, E.W. *Scheler's Phenomenology of Community*, St. Louis U., 1964.
[80] Robertson, A. A. *Alienation and Political Economy*. State U. of New York at Buffalo, 1976.
[81] Rogers, C.T. *A Critique of Axicmatic Social Choice Theory*: *Certain Difficulties in the Semantics of Social Choice*. Indiana U., 1975.
[82] Rosenberg, A. *Microeconomic General Statements: A Philosophical Analysis*. John Hopkins U., 1971.
[83] Sanders, John T. *The Ethical Argument Against Government*. Boston U. Graduate School, 1977.
[84] Sargeant, B.A. *Corporate Theory in Them as Hobbes*. U. of Toronto, 1974.
[85] Schatz, M.S. *Application of an Ethical Theory to the Problem of Military Conscription*. Boston U. Graduate School, 1973.
[86] Schwartz, A.T. *The Collective Interest*. U. of Pittsburgh, 1969.
[87] Schweickart, Charles D. *Capitalism: A Utilitarian Analysis*. Ohio State U., 1977.

[88] Senter, N.W. *Civil Disobedience and Moral Autonomy*. U. of Virginia, 1972.
[89] Sessions, R.A. *Positive Freedom and Autonomy*. U. of Michigan, 1976.
[90] Shalvey, T.J, *The Philosophical Foundations of the Role of the Collective in the Work of Lévi-Strauss*. Georgetown U., 1970.
[91] Shapiro, V.M. *The Philosophy and Social Thought of Josiah Royce*. Brandeis U., 1967.
[92] Sharkey, P.J. *Human Rights: The Relationship Among Civil, Socio-Economic and Political Rights*. New York U., 1975.
[93] Shier, J.D. *Scientific Objectivity and Moral Values*. U. of Wisconsin, 1972.
[94] Smith, Joanmarie. *John Dewey and the Ideal Community*. Fordham U., 1971.
[95] Stern, H.S. *The Question of a Value-Free Social Science*. New York U., 1969.
[96] Stevens, C.T. *Interconnections Among Philosophy, Science, and Social Practice: B.F. Skinner and Carl Rogers, A Case Study*. U. of Missouri, Kansas City, 1974.
[97] Sullivan, R.J. *The Formation of Alfred Schütz's Category of Relevance: The Fundamental Category of the Sociology of Knowledge*. Boston Col., 1975.
[98] Sullivan, W.M. *The Process Social Paradigm and the Problem of Social Order*. Fordham U., 1971.
[99] Tice, T.N. *Ideology Old and New: Historical-Analytical Back ground for Use of the Concept "Ideology" in Scholarly Discourse, with Systematic. Bibliography*. U of Michigan, 1970.
[100] Truitt, W.H. *Social Theory and the Foundations of Aesthetic Culture: A Critique of and Contribution to the Marxian Theory of Art*. Boston U. Graduate School, 1969.
[101] Uffelmann, H.W. *Towards an Ontology of Social Relations*. North western U., 1967
[102] Valone, J.J. *The Phenomenology of Alfred Schütz: Toward a Philosophy of the Social Sciences*. Boston Col. 1975.
[103] Van Dohlen, R.F. *A Case Study in the Explication of Unclear Theories in the Social Sciences: The Relationship of Values to Freedom in the Social Theory of Talcott Parsons*. Boston U. Graduate School, 1973.
[104] Vetterling, M.K. *Social Science Prediction*. Boston U. Graduate School, 1976.
[105] Wicclair, M.R. *Max Weber and the Logic of Cultural Inquiry*. Columbia U., 1976.
[106] Widomlansky, D. *"Category Continuity" as a Key to Understanding the Foundation of Dewey's Social Psychology*. City U. of New York, 1977.
[107] Wilmot, P.F. *Student Revolt, Decolonization and the Master-Slave Relation*. Vanderbilt U., 1972.

[108] Wood, Sanford Watts. *Christian Politics and Civil Philosophy: An Interpretation of Hobbes's Leviathan.* Vanderbilt U., 1968.
[109] Woodward, B.A. *Commitment to Nonviolence: A Theory of Action and Politics.* New School for Social Research, 1972.
[110] Wu, L.C.-F. *Prediction and Explanation in the Behavioral Sciences.* U. of Texas at Austin, 1975.
[111] Zanardi, W.J. Transcendental Method and the crises of Historicism. Loyola U. of Chicago, 1975.

Appendix 3: Proceedings and Colloquia Volumes

[1] Achinstein, P. and Barker, S.F. (eds.). *The Legacy of Logical Positivism.* Baltimore: The Johns Hopkins Press, 1969.
[2] Blalock, H.M. (ed.). *Causal Models in the Social Sciences.* Chicago: Aldine Atherton, Inc., 1971.
[3] Borger, R. and Cioffi, F. (eds.). *Explanation in the Behavioural Sciences.* Cambridge: Cambridge University Press, 1970.
[4] Buck, R.C. and Cohen, R.S. (eds.). *PSA 1970: In Memory of Rudolf Carnap* (*Boston Studies in the Philosophy of Science,* volume VIII") Dordrecht: D. Reidel, 1971.
[5] Bunge, M. (ed.). *The Critical Approach to Science and Philosophy.* New York: The Free Press of Glencoe, 1964.
[6] Bunge, M. (ed.). *The Methodological Unity of Science.* Dordrecht: Reidel, 1974.
[7] Cherry, C. (ed.) *Pragmatic Aspects of Human Communication.* Dordrecht: D. Reidel, 1974.
[8] Cohen, R.S., Hooker, C.A., Michalos, A.C. and Van Evra, J. (eds.). *PSA 1974: (Boston Studies in the Philosophy of Science,* Volume XXXII) Dordrecht: D. Reidel, 1976.
[10] Cohen, R.S. and Wartofsky, M.W. (eds.). *In Honor of Philipp Frank, Proceedings of the Boston Colloquium for the Philosophy of Science, 1962/1964 (Boston Studies in the Philosophy of Science,* volume II) Dordrecht: D. Reidel, 1965.
[11] Cohen, R.S. and Wartofsky, M.W. (eds.). *In Memory of Norwood Russell Hanson, Proceedings of the Boston Colloquium for the Philosophy of Science, 1964/1966 (Boston Studies in the Philosophy of Science,* volume III) Dordrecht: D. Reidel, 1967
[12] Cohen, R.S. and Wartofsky, M.W. (eds.). *Proceedings of the Boston Colloquium for the Philosophy of Science, 1966/1968 (Boston Studies in the Philosophy of Science,* volume IV) Dordrecht: D. Reidel, 1969

[13] Cohen, R.S. and Wartofsky, M.W. (eds.). *Proceedings of the Boston Colloquium for the Philosophy of Science, 1966/1968 (Boston Studies in the Philosophy of Science,* volume V) Dordrecht: D. Reidel, 1969
[14] Cohen, R.S. and Wartofsky, M.W. (eds.). *Logical and Epistemological Studies in Contemporary Physics* (*Boston Studies in the Philosophy of Science*, volume XIII) Dordrecht: D. Reidel, 1974.
[15] Cohen, R.S. and Wartofsky, M.W. (eds.). *Methodological and Historical Essays in the Natural and Social Sciences* (*Boston Studies in the Philosophy of Science*, volume XXV) Dordrecht: D. Reidel, 1974.
[16] Colodny, R.G. (ed.). *Frontiers of Science and Philosophy* (volume 1, *The University of Pittsburgh Series in the Philosophy of Science*) Pittsburgh: University of Pittsburgh Press, 1962.
[17] Colodny, R.G. (ed.). *Mind and Cosmos* (Volume 3, *The University of Pittsburgh Series in the Philosophy of Science*) Pittsburgh: University of Pittsburgh Press, 1966.
[18] Feigl, H. and Maxwell, G. (eds.). *Current Issues in the Philosophy of Science.* New York: Holt, Rinehart and Winston, 1961.
[19] Feigl, H. and Maxwell, G. and Scriven, M. (eds.). *The Foundations of Science and the Concepts of Psychology and Psychoanalysis* (*Minnesota Studies in the Philosophy of Science*, volume I) Minneapolis: University of Minnesota Press, 1956.
[20] Feigl, H. and Maxwell, G. and Maxwell, G. (eds.). *Concepts, Theories, and the Mind-Body Problem* (*Minnesota Studies in the Philosophy of Science.* Volume II) Minneapolis: University of Minnesota Press, 1958.
[21] Hintikka, J. and Suppes, P. (eds.). *Information and Inference*. Dordrecht: D. Reidel, 1970.
[22] Hook, S. (ed.). *Psychoanalysis, Scientific Method and Philosophy.* Washington Square: New York University Press, 1959.
[23] Hook, S. (ed.). *Human Values and Economic Policy*. Washington Square: New York University Press, 1967.
[24] King-Farlow, J. and Shea, W.R. (eds.). *Values and the Quality of Life* ("Canadian Contemporary Philosophy Series") New York: Science History Publications, 1976.
[25] Knorr, K.D., Strasser, H. and Zilian, H.G. (eds.). *Determinants and Controls of Scientific Development*. Dordrecht: D. Reidel, 1975
[26] Lakatos, I. and Musgrave, A (eds.). *Problems in the philosophy of Science.* Amsterdam: North-Holland Pub. Co., 1968
[27] Leach, J., Butts, R., Pearce, G. (eds.). *Science, Decision and Value* (*The University of Western Ontario Series in Philosophy of Science*, Volume I). Dordrecht: D. Reidel, 1973.
[28] Leinfellner, W. and Kohler, E. (eds.). *Developments in the Methodology of Social Science*. Dordrecht: D. Reidel, 1974.
[29] Lerner, D. (ed.). *Cause and Effect*. New York: The Free Press, 1965.

[30] Menges, G. (ed.) *Information, Inference and Decision*. Dordrecht: D. Reidel, 1974.
[31] Morgenbesser, S., Suppes, P. and White, M. (eds.). *Philosophy, Science and Method*. New York: St. Martin's Press, 1969.
[32] Rapoport, A. (ed.). *Game Theory as a Theory of Conflict Resolution*. Dordrecht: D. Reidel, 1974.
[33] Rescher, N. (ed.). *The Logic of Decision and Action*. Pittsburgh: University of Pittsburgh Press, 1967.
[34] Schaffner, K. and Cohen, R.S. (eds.). *PSA 1972*. (*Boston Studies in the Philosophy of Science*, volume XX) Dordrecht: D. Reidel, 1974.
[35] Seeger, R.J. and Cohen, R.S. (eds.). *Philosophical Foundations of Science* (*Boston Studies in the Philosophy of Science*, volume XI) Dordrecht: D. Reidel, 1974.
[36] Shea, W.R. (ed.). *Basic Issues in the Philosophy of Science* ("Canadian Contemporary Philosophy Series") New York: Science History Publications, 1976.
[37] Skala, H.J. *Non-Archimedean Utility Theory*. Dordrecht: D. Reidel, 1975.
[38] F. Suppe and Asquith, P.D. (eds.). *PSA 1976:* Volume One. East Lansing: Philosophy of Science Association, 1976.
[39] F. Suppe and Asquith, P.D. (eds.). *PSA 1976:* Volume Two. East Lansing: Philosophy of Science Association, 1977.
[40] Wartofsky, M.Q. (ed.). *Proceedings of the Boston Colloquium for the Philosophy of Science, 1961/1962* (*Boston Studies in the Philosophy of Science*, volume I) Dordrecht: D. Reidel, 1963.
[41] Wendt, D. and Vlek, C. (eds.). *Utility, Probability, and Human Decision Making*. Dordrecht: D. Reidel, 1975.
[42] Wilson, B.R. (ed.). *Rationality*. Oxford: Basil Blackwell, 1970.

References

Abel, T. (1970). *The foundation of sociological theory*. New York: Random House Inc.
Ackoff, R. L. (1962). *Scientific method: Optimizing applied research decisions*. New York: Wiley.
Ackoff, R. L., & Emery, F. E. (1972). *On purposeful systems*. Chicago: Aldine-Atherton Pub. Co.
Alker, H. R. (1965). *Mathematics and politics*. New York: Macmillan Co.
Arrow, K. (1951). *Social choice and individual values*. New York: Wiley.
Black, D. (1963). *The theory of committees and elections*. Cambridge: Cambridge University Press.
Blalock, H. M. (1969). *Theory construction: From verbal to mathematical formulations*. Englewood Cliffs: Prentice-Hall Inc.
Carnap, R. (1950). *The logical foundations of probability*. Chicago: University of Chicago Press.
Caws, P. (1967). *Science and the theory of value*. New York: Random House.
Churchman, C. W. (1961). *Prediction and optimal decision*. Englewood Cliffs: Prentice Hall, Inc.
Cunningham, F. (1973). *Objectivity in social science*. Toronto: University of Toronto Press.
Danto, A. C. (1965). *Analytical philosophy of history*. Cambridge: Cambridge University Press.
Diesing, P. (1962). *Reason in society*. Urbana: University of Illinois Press.

Diesing, P. (1971). *Patterns of discovery in the social sciences*. Chicago: Aldine-Atherton Pub. Co.
Downs, A. (1957). *An economic theory of democracy*. New York: Harper and Row Pub.
Dray, W. (1957). *Laws and explanation in history*. London: Oxford University Press.
Edwards, W., & Tversky, A. (Eds.). (1967). *Decision making*. Middlesex: Penguin Books.
Farquharson, R. (1969). *Theory of voting*. New Haven: Yale University Press.
Fishburn, P. C. (1973). *The theory of social choice*. Princeton: Princeton University Press.
Ganz, J. S. (1971). *Rules: A systematic study*. The Hague: Mouton.
Handy, R. (1969). *Value theory and the behavioral sciences*. Springfield: Charles C. Thomas.
Handy, R. (1970). *The measurement of values*. St. Louis: Warren H. Green, Inc.
Harsanyi, J. (1976). *Essays on ethics, social behavior, and scientific explanation*. Dordrecht: D. Reidel Pub. Co.
Isajiw, W. W. (1968). *Causation and functionalism in sociology*. London: Routledge and Kegan Paul.
Kaplan, A. (1964). *The conduct of inquiry*. San Francisco: Chandler Pub. Co.
Kurtz, P. (1965). *Decision and the condition of man*. Seattle: University of Washington Press.
Lowrance, W. W. (1977). The NAS surveys of fundamental research 1962–1974, in retrospect. *Science, 197,* 1254–1260.
Margenau, H. (1964). *Ethics and science*. Princeton: D. van Nostrand Co., Inc.
Meiland, J. W. (1965). *Skepticism and historical knowledge*. New York: Random House.
Merton, R. K. (1949). *Social theory and social structure*. New York: The Free Press.
Michalos, A. C. (1974). Strategies for reducing information overload in social reports. *Social Indicators Research, 1,* 131–107.
Michalos, A. C. (1976). Measuring the quality of life. In J. King-Farlow & W. R. Shea (Eds.), *Values and the quality of life* (pp. 24–37). New York: Science History Pub.
Michalos, A. C. (1978). *Foundations of decision making*. Ottawa: Canadian Association for Publishing in Philosophy.
Mitroff, I. I. (1974). *The subjective side of science*. New York: American Elsevier Pub. Co.
Nowak, S. (1977). *Methodology of sociological research*. Dordrecht: D. Reidel Pub. Co.
Olson, M. (1965). *The logic of collective action*. New York: Schoken Books.
Popper, K. R. (1961). *The logic of scientific discovery*. New York: Science Editions, Inc. (Originally published as *Logik der Forschung*. Vienna: Springer, 1933).
Radnitzky, G. (1968). *Continental schools of metascience*. Goteborg: Akademiforlaget.
Rapoport, A. (1965). Laboratory studies of conflict and cooperation. In J. R. Lawrence (Ed.), *Operational research and the social sciences* (pp. 396–398). London: Tavistock Pub.
Rawls, J. (1971). *A theory of justice*. Cambridge: Harvard University Press.
Rescher, N. (1966). *Distributive justice*. Indianapolis: Bobbs-Merrill Co., Inc.
Rescher, N. (1969). *Introduction to value theory*. Englewood Cliffs: Prentice Hall Inc.
Rescher, N. (1972). *Welfare*. Pittsburgh: University of Pittsburgh Press.
Rescher, N. (1973). *The primacy of practice*. Oxford: Basil Blackwell.
Riker, W. H. (1962). *The theory of political coalitions*. New Haven: Yale University Press.
Rosenberg, A. (1976). *Microeconomic laws: A philosophical analysis*. Pittsburgh: University of Pittsburgh Press.
Rothenberg, J. (1961). *The measurement of social welfare*. Englewood Cliffs: Prentice-Hall, Inc.
Rudner, R. S. (1966). *Philosophy of Social Science*. Englewood Cliffs: Prentice-Hall Inc.
Runciman, W. G. (1972). *A critique of Max Weber's philosophy of social science*. Cambridge: Cambridge University Press.
Scheffler, I. (1967). *Science and subjectivity*. New York: The Bobbs-Merrill Co.
Shackle, G. L. S. (1973). *Epistemics and economics: A critique of economic doctrines*. Cambridge: Cambridge University Press.
Simon, H. A. (1945). *Administrative behavior*. New York: The Free Press.
Speigel-Rosing, I., & de Solla Price, D. (1977). *Science technology and society*. London: Sage Pub. Ltd.
Suchman, E. A. (1967). *Evaluative research*. New York: Russell Sage Foundation.

Todd, W. (1972). *History as applied science: A philosophical study*. Detroit: Wayne State University Press.
Tullock, G., & Buchanan, J. M. (1962). *The calculus of consent*. Ann Arbor: University of Michigan Press.
White, M. (1965). *Foundations of' historical knowledge*. New York: Harper and Row.
Winch, P. (1958). *The idea of a social science*. New York: Humanities Press.

Chapter 7
Postulates of Rational Preference

Alex C. Michalos

The postulates of rational preference suggested by Von Neumann and Morgenstern have been defended as descriptive or empirical generalizations and as normative principles. It is argued that the postulates are inaccurate empirical generalizations and unacceptable normative principles.

The postulates of rational preference suggested by John Von Neumann and Oskar Morgenstern in (1947) have been recommended as descriptive or empirical generalizations and as normative principles.[1] That is, according to some writers, people's "systems of preferences" *do* as a matter of fact have the following properties, and according to others, people's "systems of preferences" *ought* to have these properties.

1. The system is complete and consistent; that is, an individual can tell which of two objects he prefers or whether he is indifferent between them, and if he does not prefer C to B and does not prefer B to A, then he does not prefer C to A. (In this context, the word "object" includes combinations of objects with stated probabilities; for example, if A and B are objects, a 40–60 chance of A or B is also an object).
2. If the object A is preferred to the object B, then a combination of A and any object C with stated probabilities is preferred to a combination of B and C with the same probabilities, provided that the probability attached to C is less than unity. Conversely, if a combination of A and C with stated probabilities is preferred to a combination of B and C with the same probabilities, then, A is preferred to B.

Michalos, A.C.: 1967. Postulates of rational preference. Philosophy of Science, 34, pp. 18–22.

---

[1]Examples of the former view may be found in (Luce and Raiffa 1964), p. 32 and (Friedman and Savage 1952a); examples of the latter view may be found in Anscombe (1964), p. 162 and (Savage 1954), p. 20.

A.C. Michalos (✉)
University of Northern British Columbia, Prince George, BC, Canada
e-mail: michalos@brandonu.ca

A.C. Michalos, *Philosophical Foundations of Quality of Life*,
DOI 10.1007/978-3-319-50727-9_7

3. If the object A is preferred to the object B and B to the object C, there will be some probability combination of A and C such that the individual is indifferent between it and B. (Friedman and Savage 1952b, p. 71).

Von Neumann and Morgenstern show that these postulates entail the following decision or preference rule: Given a choice of one among any number of mutually exclusive courses of action, choose that one which maximizes estimated utility. Since, broadly speaking, a course of action might be the choice or preference of a particular hypothesis (including a scientific law or theory), the postulates apparently lead to either a descriptive or a normative claim about preferable, and hence, in some sense acceptable hypotheses. In Levi (1963), Michalos (1965, 1966) the merits of this claim as a normative principle are compared with those of an alternative principle recommended by Karl Popper. The present discussion may be regarded as a supplement to the defense of the view adopted in Michalos (1966). To be more specific, it is shown first that the first two postulates substantiating the rule of maximizing estimated utility are false if taken as empirical generalizations. That is to say, there is abundant evidence that people whose preferences or behavior would ordinarily be considered rational very often have preferences which violate these postulates. In the second place, it is argued that the postulates are unacceptable normative principles because there are cases in which preferences *ought* to be ordered contrary to the order prescribed by the postulates.[2] Let us consider each of these two objections more carefully.

In an experiment designed to test the descriptive adequacy of the Von Neumann and Morgenstern postulates, Mosteller and Nogee found, contrary to the "completeness" assumption, that an individual can *not* always tell whether he prefers one alternative to another or is indifferent between them. "For example," they write,

> if one were offered one chance in five of winning $5.00 against four chances in five of losing 5 cents, one would almost certainly take the bet If one were offered the same chance of losing 5 cents, one would almost certainly not take the bet. However, as the offer increases from 1 cent towards $5.00, vacillation sets in, the bet is taken occasionally, then more and more often, until, finally, the bet is taken nearly all the time. There is not a sudden jump from no acceptances to all acceptances at a particular offer, just as in a hearing experiment there is not a critical loudness below which nothing is heard and above which all loudnesses are heard. (Mosteller and Nogee 1951, p. 374).

In view of this result, it seems that the claim that "completeness" is a necessary characteristic of "rational systems, of preferences" is as unwarranted as the claim that "completeness" is a necessary characteristic of "normal" auditory systems.

The "consistency" assumption is equally gratuitous, for both indifference and preference are *neither* transitive *nor* intransitive. In general, if a person does not

[2]It should be mentioned that Anatol Rapoport has defended roughly the same position for a different reason in Rapoport (1964, 1965), pp. 19 ff. Rapoport claims that the Von Neumann and Morgenstem postulates lead to a "useless" normative utility theory because the theory "assumes as given what, according to the theory of decision under risk, is supposed to be calculated from other givens." (Rapoport 1964, p. 21). In short, the "completeness" assumption renders the resulting utility theory "useless" according to Rapoport.

prefer C to B and does not prefer B to A, then he may or may not prefer C to A. That *indifference* is not intransitive is obvious. For example, many people would be indifferent between any pair of the following triples [going to, a movie, a ball game, a play], [coffee, tea, milk], [carrots, peas, corn], [Ford, Plymouth, Chevrolet], etc. To show that indifference may just as well be non-transitive, we suggest the following sequence of alternatives: holding one's breath for one second, for two seconds, for three, etc. If this sequence were made long enough, say, to holding one's breath for an hour, few people would remain indifferent between the first and last alternatives. Similarly, one might consider the sequences: losing one cent, losing two cents, etc.; forgetting one thing, forgetting two things, etc.; solving one problem, solving two problems, etc.

That *preferences* are not intransitive may be granted. However, there is no doubt that preferences are just as likely to be non-transitive. Consider, for example, the following suggestions by Kenneth O. May.

> Among observed non-transitive relations linked with preferences (choices) may be mentioned the dominance concept in game theory, numerous examples of combat superiority (battleship sinks destroyer sinks submarine sinks battleship; mongoose kills cobra kills cat kills mongoose; tank beats machine gunner beats bazookaman beats tank, etc.,) and winning ability in such games as "rock breaks scissors cuts paper wraps rock." (May, K. O. 1954, p. 6).

Considering any one of these "circular triples" say, [battleship, destroyer, sub-marine], it is apparent that a "rational" better would be committed to a non-transitive set of preferences. That is, given the information we have about the fighting capabilities of these vessels (and assuming that only *even* bets may be made), one would have to bet on the battleship over the destroyer, the destroyer over the submarine, and the submarine over the battleship.

Again, consider the famous "paradox of voting." Suppose a three-membered committee is selecting a chairman from three candidates, A, B and C. The first member prefers A to B to C; the second prefers B to C to A; and the third prefers C to A to B. Evidently then, the majority prefers A to B, B to C, and C to A. But, suppose a fourth member is put on the committee and his preferences are in complete agreement with the majority, If follows that his "system of preferences" is non-transitive.

The second postulate of Von Neumann and Morgenstern, namely, that of the additivity of preferences, is obviously not empirically justifiable. A carpenter might prefer glue to nails, but a hammer and nails to a hammer and glue. Many people would prefer coffee to tea, but tea with lemon to coffee with lemon. Robert Aumann has noted that

> Four tires may be preferred to a Cadillac without tires (at least tubes can be used for swimming), but *many* would prefer a Cadillac with tires to eight tires; so we have reversed preferences simply by adding four tires. Other examples in which the additivity assumption does not hold are those governed by a law of diminishing returns, or personnel assignment problems in which compatibility considerations play an important part. (Aumann 1964, p. 227).

This completes the presentation of our objections to the first two postulates of Von Neumann and Morgenstern taken as descriptions or empirical generalizations about rational preferences. We turn now to an objection to these postulates taken as normative principles used to derive and justify the (normative) rule of maximizing estimated utility.

Our objection to the Von Neumann and Morgenstern postulates as normative principles of rational preference is just this: Strict adherence to the postulates could force one to order his preferences in a plainly *irrational* fashion. To put it in a *slightly* different way, there are cases in which one *ought* not to order his preferences according to these postulates. Although it would, perhaps, be naive to suppose one could formulate a conclusive argument for such a claim, the remarks that follow may strike some philosophic consciences as persuasive.

We assume that a person's behavior is rational so far as it is likely to *satisfy* the person's needs, goals or purposes.[3] Hence, the Von Neumann and Morgenstern postulates may be used as normative principles of rational behavior if, and only if, action in accordance with these postulates is likely to satisfy certain selected needs or purposes. That action in accordance with these postulates is *not* likely to satisfy certain specified needs or purposes may be illustrated by reconsidering two of the situations introduced earlier.

Case 1 It is known that battleships in combat are superior to destroyers, destroyers are superior to submarines, and submarines are superior to battleships. According to the transitivity postulate, if X chooses or prefers to bet on the battleship Over the destroyer and the destroyer over the submarine, then X *should* prefer the battleship over the submarine. But if X wants to win his bet, he *should* prefer the submarine over the battleship, because he knows submarines are superior to battleships. Thus if X is going to behave rationally, in the sense that he is going to choose that action which is most likely to satisfy his desire, (i.e., win the bet), then X *should not* act in accordance with the transitivity postulate.

Case 2 X wants to join two pieces of wood in the most secure manner available. His neighbor offers to lend him either some glue or some nails. Since the nails without a hammer are useless, he prefers the glue. But then his neighbor offers him a hammer and, following the additivity postulate, claims that unless X prefers the hammer and glue to the hammer and nails, X is behaving irrationally. He *ought* to prefer the hammer and glue. Obviously, if X chooses the hammer and glue over the hammer and nails then he is behaving irrationally, in the sense that he is *not* choosing the alternative that is most likely to satisfy his desire (i.e., join the two pieces of wood). Thus X *should not* act in accordance with the additivity postulate.

Such examples could easily be multiplied. Whether or not they are sufficient to reject the Von Neumann and Morgenstern postulates depends, as we suggested, on the reader's philosophic conscience.

---

[3]This more or less pragmatic definition of rational behavior is, of course, not novel. See, for example, Feigl (1961), p. 213 and Simon (1961), Chap. 4.

Before concluding this discussion, one other claim should be noticed. It is sometimes asserted that whether or not the Von Neumann and Morgenstern postulates are postulates of "rational" preferences, they are certainly postulates of "consistent" preferences. Alternative postulates or alternatively ordered sets of preferences then, are supposed to be "inconsistent." What should be clear by now is that, in a perfectly straightforward sense of the term, the Von Neumann and Morgenstern postulates may, with equal justification, be considered postulates of "inconsistent" preferences (and *some* alternatives, postulates or systems of "consistent" preferences). That is to say, for example, that if X (in the two cases just considered) were a rational agent and chose alternatives according to the Von Neumann and Morgenstern postulates, X would have to affirm such inconsistent pairs of propositions as the following: 'I always choose that alternative which I believe is most likely to satisfy my needs' and 'I am now choosing an alternative which I believe is *not* most likely to satisfy my needs.'[4]

References

Anscombe, F. J. (1964). Some remarks on Bayesian statistics. In M. W. Shelly & G. L. Bryan (Eds.), *Human judgments and optimality*. New York: Wiley.

Aumann, R. J. (1964). Subjective programming. In M. W. Shelly & G. L. Bryan (Eds.), *Human judgments and optimality*. New York: Wiley.

Feigl, H. (1961, April). On the vindication of induction. *Philosophy of Science*.

Friedman, M. & Savage, L. J. (1952a, December). The expected utility hypothesis and the measurability of utility. *The Journal of Political Economy*.

Friedman, M. & Savage, L. J. (1952b). The utility analysis of choices involving risk. In Irwin *Readings in Price Theory*. Chicago: Irwin, American-Economic Association.

Levi, I. (1963, February). Corroboration and rules of acceptance. *The British Journal for the Philosophy of Science*.

Luce, R. D. & Raiffa, H. (1964). *Games and decisions*. New York: Wiley.

May, K. O. (1954, January). Intransitivity, utility, and the aggregation of preference patterns. *Econometrica*.

Michalos, A. C. (1965, December). Two theorems of degree of confirmation. *Ratio*.

Michalos, A. C. (1966, February). Estimated utility and corroboration. *The British Journal for the Philosophy of Science*.

Mosteller, F. & Nogee, P. (1951, October). An-experimental measurement of utility. *The* journal *of Political Economy*.

Rapoport, A. (1964). *Strategy and Conscience*. New York.

Rapoport, A. (1965). Game theory and human conflict. In E. B. McNeil (Ed.), *The nature of human conflict*. Englewood Cliffs.

Savage, L. J. (1954). *The Foundations of Statistics*. New York: Wiley.

Simon, H. A. (1961). *Administrative behavior*. New York: Macmillan.

Von Neumann, J. & Morgenstem, O. (1947). *Theory of games and economic behavior*. Princeton: University Press.

[4]I wish to thank the referees for their helpful suggestions.

Chapter 8
Decision-Making in Committees

Alex C. Michalos

Introduction

This paper has two aims, one fairly general and the other fairly specific. The general aim is to provide a basis for logical and empirical investigations of a particular type of group-decision procedure. The type is distinguished by the fact that inequalities in the "weight" of individual voters *and* their votes are permitted. For reasons which will become clear shortly, if such procedures are practicable at all, they would seem to be so only for small groups, say, of two to fifteen people. Since most committees contain less than fifteen members, if such procedures are practicable at all, they should be practicable for committees. Hence, our discussion is oriented toward decision-making in committees.

The more specific aim of this paper is to introduce and critically evaluate certain *prima facie* plausible solutions to the problem of selecting an acceptable group-decision procedure. We begin with a precise statement of the problem in section "The Problem". In section "Criteria of Adequacy" five informal necessary conditions of adequacy for proposed solutions are introduced. Section "Weighting Voters" introduces the notion of "weights of influence" and defines seven fundamental types of distributions. This is followed by a presentation of six more or less plausible "voting schemes" that involve the application of various "weights of influence." In sections "Objections and Replies: Weighting Voters" and "Objections and Replies: Weighted Voting" the constructive work of sections

Michalos, A.C.: 1970. Decision making in committees. American Philosophical Quarterly, 7, pp. 91–106. © University of Illinois Press 1970.

A.C. Michalos (✉)
University of Northern British Columbia, Prince George, BC, Canada
e-mail: michalos@brandonu.ca

A.C. Michalos, *Philosophical Foundations of Quality of Life*,
DOI 10.1007/978-3-319-50727-9_8

"Weighting Voters" and "Weighted Voting" is examined in the light of our adequacy conditions. The upshot of this examination is, unfortunately, that none of the six schemes appears extraordinarily attractive.

The Problem

Very often individuals are called upon to share their decision-making capacities with others. They are asked to serve on committees. There are many reasons for establishing a committee, e.g., to keep people busy (Idle hands get into trouble!), to give them a sense of "belonging," to keep them interested, to fix responsibility, to separate problems and solutions (divide and conquer), and so on. Some committees are supposed to solve problems or make decisions. They frequently plan conventions, parties, and dances, i.e., they *choose* locations, entertainment, refreshments. They *select* textbooks, candidates for new positions, visiting professors, office furniture, etc.

To avoid difficult epistemological problems which for present purposes need not be solved, we shall assume that *a decision is made* if and only if a person or group of people come to accept a certain sentence. The sentence would normally be in the imperative or in the indicative mode. Since committees are social organizations with their own rules, norms, procedures, etc., ordinarily *a committee makes a decision* if and only if there is a sentence which is accepted by the committee according to its operating rules. The operating rules of many committees are such that when there are conflicts of interest, the decision of the committee might not be similar to those of any of its members, e.g., a "compromise candidate" may become the first choice of a committee in which no member ranked him first.

Given the sense of "a committee decision" explained in the last paragraph, the primary question we shall attempt to answer in this paper is: How *should* the various decisions (with respect to some issue) of the members of a committee be amalgamated for the committee decision to be determined in the most acceptable fashion?[1] Three points must be made immediately about this question. In the first place, although it is a normative sort of question, it cannot be answered by logical analysis and intuition alone. What we ought to do to reach more (rather than less) acceptable committee decisions depends, among other things, on the *composition* of and the *issues* considered by this or that committee. That is to say, proposals for optimal group decision-making must be guided by some knowledge of the behavior, skills, resources, preferences, ambitions, etc., of human beings in fairly well-defined circumstances. Such knowledge is not only usually meager, it is also usually difficult to obtain. In the second place, it should be noted that in this paper the term "acceptable" will be used in a very broad sense to designate characteristics or dispositions frequently referred to by such (equally vague) terms as "competent,"

[1]The best introductory survey of recent work on amalgamation procedures is R. Duncan Luce and Howard Raiffa, *Games and Decisions* (New York, John Wiley and Sons, Inc., 1964), pp. 327–371.

"wise," "good," "skillful," "enlightened," "rational," and so on. For the purposes at hand this usage is innocuous and convenient. Finally, it should be emphasized that we are primarily concerned with the procedures, methods, or means used to arrive at committee decisions, *not* with the products, ends, or committee decisions themselves.[2] Although in practice a peculiar committee decision often leads us to question the procedure used to obtain it (just as we might have suspicions about an argument schema which yielded a bizarre conclusion from ostensibly true premisses), it is important to distinguish the former from the latter, the *decision* from the *decision procedure*.

Criteria of Adequacy

Lest we become dizzy chasing our own tails, something should be said about the *necessary* conditions of adequacy that might be applied to the amalgamation procedures offered as solutions to our problem. The following five are consistent (jointly satisfiable) and seem fairly plausible, although I suspect that they are neither independent nor in any technical sense complete.[3] As we shall see later, they are considerably stronger than they appear.

(3.1) The procedures must be *free from coercion* in the sense that committeemen are not forced to cast their votes contrary to their preferences. This is to guarantee each voter the opportunity to use his influence (the "weight" of his vote) exactly as he sees fit.

(3.2) The procedures must be self-consistent or *logically coherent*. This is merely a formal requirement excluding inconsistent procedures from which contradictory decisions could be obtained.

(3.3) The procedures must be *practicable* or/manageable. Practicability is bound to be relative to people and issues, so this is bound to be a pretty unstable

---

[2]In Karl Mannheim's terms, our concern is with "means rationality" rather than "substantail rationality". *Man and Society in Age of Reconstruction* (London, Routledge and Kcgan Paul, 1940), pp. 51–53.

[3]Readers who are familiar with the literature on "social-welfare functions" which arose out of Kenneth J. Arrow's classic *Social Choice and Individual Values* (New York, John Wiley and Sons, Inc., 1963) will notice that the five conditions introduced below differ from Arrow's. In part this merely a result of the fact that Arrow's problem and primary concerns differ from mine. However, it is also partially the result of my rejection of some of his basic assumptions, Roughly speaking, the two sets of conditions are related as follows. My condition (3.1) implies his conditions of nondictatorship and nonimposition. Conditions (3.2)–(3.5) are logically independent of his conditions of collective rationality, pair-wise comparisons, and Pareto optimality. Collective rationality and pair-wise comparisons are explicitly rejected in section "Objections and Replies: Weighted Voting" (below) and I have nothing to say about Pareto optimality. Similarly, so far as I know, Arrow has been silent regarding conditions analogous to (3.3)–(3.4), would probably reject (3.5), and accept (3.2). The most through discussion of Arrow's conditions in Jerome Rothenberg, *The Measurement of Social Welfare* (Englewood Cliffs, N.J., Prentice-Hall, Inc., 1961).

criterion. But if a procedure is so complicated that for every group of people and every sort of issue some *other* procedure is simpler and equally effective, then our procedure would have to be regarded as relatively (relative to the other procedure) worthless. Hence, only those procedures that are manageable for *most* (normal) people and *some* (realistic) issues will be accepted. If as a matter of fact *most issues* confronting most committees do not merit a more subtle decision procedure than, say, majority rule by a show of hands, then our proposal(s) might still be acceptable and valuable, i.e., we only require practicability (which I am assuming means *some kind* of superiority) for *some* fairly realistic issues.[4]

(3.4) The procedures must be *efficient* in the sense that they take account of all of the relevant information available to a committee for a given decision at a given time. What is required is not an everlasting search for relevant data, but the elimination of procedures that cannot process or make use of relevant data already possessed by committeemen.[5]

(3.5) The *influence* of each committeeman should be *proportionate to* his relative competence. This condition requires a more lengthy explanation and some defense, and I shall begin with the former.

We suppose a committee decision is to be reached by "combining" the decisions of all of its members. If the committee operates on democratic principles, each member's decision influences the final outcome (the committee decision) in exactly the same way. Each member receives one vote and if it is cast at all, it carries as much weight or has as much influence *formally* (or *legally*, or *arithmetically*) on the final outcome as every other vote. (Informally or in fact, of course, every group seems to have leaders and followers, and both types of people influence each other in more or less subtle ways.) The committee decision itself then is usually determined by the majority of the voters. (3.5) implies that this democratic procedure is acceptable if and only if every voter is exactly as competent as every other. According to (3.5), each member's vote should carry only as much weight or have as much influence on the committee decision as his competence merits. Moreover, since the composition of and the issues confronted by committees varies, (3.5) suggests that the status of a committeeman's competence should be regarded as *relative* to both of these variables.

---

[4]There is some evidence that "group decision-making" in political parties through *prima facie* democratic processes is merely a "ritual" or "ceremonial" performing a legitimizing rather than a decision-making service; e.g., in Robert A. Dahl, *Who Governs?* (New Haven, Conn., Yale University Press, 1966), pp. 112–114. My impression is that most of the university committees I have served on have been providing the same (perhaps important and necessary) service, a service that would not seem to require a very subtle procedure.

[5]I include this remark for those who might expect this condition to generate problems similar to those of Carnap's inductive "principle of total evidence"; e.g., A.J. Ayer, "The Conception of Probability as a Logical Relation," in S. Körner (ed.), *Observation and Interpretation in the Philosophy of Physics* (New York, Dover Publications, Inc., 1957), pp. 14–17.

In view of the vast amount of literature devoted to the problem of equality,[6] my defense of (3.5) will probably seem much too brief and primitive. It is as follows. As the influence of a committeeman increases, the chances of committee decisions being similar to his increase (provided, of course, that other things are equal and stable). As the competence (ability, rationality, etc.) of a committeeman increases, the chances of his decisions being "correct" increase. Hence, as the influence and competence of a committeeman increase, the chances of committee decisions being "correct" increase. Similarly, it is easy to see that as the influence and incompetence of a committeeman increase, the chances of committee decisions being "incorrect" increase. According to (3.5), acceptable procedures must contain some provision for the distribution of influence according to relative. competence. Therefore, insofar as this condition is met, the chances of committee decisions being "correct" will be increased and the chances of them being "incorrect" will be decreased. While this is not a guarantee that a committee will make "correct" decisions (or even *more* "correct" decisions *more* often), it does seem to be a necessary condition of adequacy for an acceptable group— decision procedure.[7]

Notice that the argument we have just presented does not commit us to the view that in all, most, or even some situations there is a "correct," more or less "correct," etc., decision which *is known* or even, practically speaking, *could be known* by certain committeemen. Of course in certain Adds (e.g., logic and mathematics) there are independent and explicit criteria of "correctness" for the solutions of most problems. So in these fields one frequently can and does *know* whether or not his decision is "correct." However, in many of the most interesting and important fields (e.g., human welfare, morality, law, religion, etc.) one seldom has such knowledge. But it does not follow that there are no "correct," "incorrect," etc., decisions to be made with respect to the various sorts of evaluative problems that arise in these fields. Indeed, following long line of different types of "objectivists" and a somewhat shorter line of naturalists,[8] I believe that in one way or another evaluative

---

[6]A review of this literature may be found in George L. Abernethy (ed.), The Idea of Equality (Richmond, Va., John Knox Press, 1959).

[7]Cf., "To have no voice in what are partly his own concerns is a thing which nobody willingly submits to; but when what is partly his concern is also partly another's, and he feels the other to understand the subject better than himself, that the other's opinion should be counted for more than his own accords with his expectations...." John Stuart Mill, *Considerations on Representative Government* (New York, Harper and Brothers, 1867), p. 181. More recently James W. Protho and Charles M. Grigg found that while roughly 96% of the people in their survey (of registered voters in Ann Arbor, Michigan and Tallahassee, Florida) agreed that "every citizen should have an equal chance to influence government policy," there was nearly a "total absence of consensus" on the view that "in a city referendum, only people who are well informed about the problem being voted on should be allowed to vote." "Fundamental Principles of Democracy," *The Journal of Politics*, vol. 22 (1960), pp. 282–285.

[8]This shorter line includes such illustrious names as M.R. Cohen, John Dewey, Herbert Feigl, R.W. Sellars, and most recently, Henry Margenau. The latter's *Ethics and Science* (Princeton, N.J., D. Van Nostrand Company, 1964) may be regarded as an outline of the sort of view I have adopted.

problems (including problems of conflict of interest, etc.) can be analyzed in ways which permit one *to make* decisions that are "correct," more or less "correct," etc., and occasionally *to know* which are which. If it should turn out that a naturalistic theory of value is untenable, then it might well be necessary to make a sharp division between procedures that are applicable to evaluative problems and those that are applicable to nonevaluative problems; In that case, the argument presented above would be applicable only to procedures designed for nonevaluative problems. Nevertheless, until "all the returns are in," I shall continue to line up with the naturalists.

Weighting Voters

Even if one is persuaded by this argument for, which I am, it does not take us very far. For it is one thing to say that we *ought* to distribute influence according to relative competence and it is quite another to *know how* to do it.[9] The remaining paragraphs of this section will be devoted to the latter problem, i.e., the problem of implementation.

Suppose we have a committee with n voting members:

$$M_1, M_2, \ldots, M_{\mathrm{n}}$$

Each member's vote will be assigned a *weight of influence* (or, for short, a *weight*) W which satisfies the following condition:

(4.1) The weight of every committeeman's vote will be a real number greater than or equal to zero, i.e.,

$$W_{\mathrm{t}} \geq 0 \, (i = 1, 2, \ldots n)$$

In view of (3.5) it is imperative that the weight of every member's vote is proportionate to his relative competence. The crucial question is: How are we going to measure relative competence? Clearly the usefulness of our amalgamation proposals will be severely curtailed unless a fairly plausible answer to this question is

[9]Mill's suggestion for "weighting" voters in a "universal but graduated suffrage" included the administration of "a trustworthy system of general examination," consideration of "the nature of a person's occupation," "successful performance" of a trade, "graduates of universities," and excluded "sex" or "any pecuniary qualification." *Op. cit.*, pp. 182–192. Some writers have admitted unequal "weightings" into their formal theories without tackling the problem of how such "weights" could be obtained; e.g., Germain Kreweras, "A Model to Weight Individual Authority in a Group," in S. Stemberg, V. Capecchi, T. Kloek, and C.T. Leenders (eds.), *Mathematics and Social Science I* (Paris Mounted and Co., 1965), pp. 111–118; and William H. Riker, *The Theory of Political Coalitions* (New Haven, Conn., Yale University Press, 1962), pp. 257–258.

produced. The solution offered here is not new[10] and it is *at best* fairly plausible. Its greatest virtue is its apparent ease of application, i.e., it is relatively convenient.[11] We shall explain it with the help of a concrete example.

Consider a committee with three members:

$$M_1, M_2, M_3$$

The committee is supposed to select an appropriate logic text for use in a freshman course. The usual (democratic) procedure is to give each committeeman one vote which he may cast as he sees fit. He may vote for this or that text, or abstain altogether. Following this democratic tradition, each of our committeemen will also be given exactly one vote. However, instead of asking each member to cast his vote on some question before the committee (e.g., the selection of a logic text), we shall ask each of them to *distribute* the weight of his vote (which is unity) among each of the committeemen. The distribution of a given member's vote should be such that it indicates the relative competence of every voter in the judgment of that committeeman.

More precisely, we are asking *first* that each member *weakly order* every voter in accordance with his relative competence. That is, every committeeman is supposed to try to decide for all of the members whether

(i) M_i is more competent than M_k or M_k is more competent than M_j or M_k and M_k are equally competent,

and

(ii) if M_i is at least as competent as M_k and M_k is at least as competent as M_j then M_i is at least as competent as M_j.

And *second* we are asking that every member try to assign a number to every voter in accordance with his rank order to serve as an *indicant*[12] of his relative competence. These numbers will be called "*initial* weights of influence" (or, "*initial* weights"). Moreover,

[10]Roughly the same procedure was used by J. Sayer Minas and Russell L. Ackoff in "Individual and Collective Value Judgments," in Maynard W. Shelly, II and Glenn and L. Bryan (eds.), Human Judgments and Optimality (New York, John Wiley and Sons, Inc., 1964), pp. 351–359. A considerably more complicated (though not necessarily more reliable) nine-step procedure may be found in my unpublished paper "Split Weight Option Voting".

[11]A number of doubts about its "greatest virtue" are raised in section "Objections and Replies: Weighted Voting".

[12]"The difference between an *indicant* and a *measure* is just this: the indicant is a presumed effect or correlate bearing an unknown … relation to some underlying phenomenon, whereas a measure is a scaled value of the phenomenon itself. Indicants have the advantage of convenience. Measures have the advantage of validity. We aspire to measures, but we are often forced to settle for less". (Italics added.) S.S. Stevens, "Mathematics Measurements and Psychophysics," *Handbook of Experimental Psychology*, ed. by S.S. Stevens (New York, John Wiley and Sons, Inc., 1951), p. 48.

(4.2) Every initial weight will be a real number w in the closed interval from 0 to 1, i.e.,

$$0 \leq w \leq 1$$

and the sum of the assignments that may be given *by* every committeeman will be 1.

The following matrix illustrates a possible result of (4.2).

FIGURE I

	M_1	M_2	M_3	w_i
M_1	1	0	0	1
M_2	$\frac{1}{3}$	$\frac{1}{3}$	$\frac{1}{3}$	1
M_3	$\frac{1}{2}$	$\frac{1}{2}$	0	1
W_i	$1\frac{5}{6}$	$\frac{5}{6}$	$\frac{1}{3}$	$3 = n$

Here M_1 has assigned himself an initial weight of 1 and left nothing for M_2 or M_3. We may assume then, that in the opinion of M_1 the other members of the committee do not know anything about logic texts. Or, to put the point another way, we may assume that M_1 believes the committee decision has a better chance of being "right" if it is similar to his own decision. M_2 believes his opinion is worth no more and no less than the others. So he distributes his initial weight equally among all the voters. M_3 figures that M_1 knows about as much as M_2 about logic texts and that he (M_3) just does not know anything. So he distributes his initial weight equally between M_1 and M_2.

If a committee has n members then it has n votes to be distributed or, possibly, withheld. Then, by definition:

(4.3) The weight of every committeeman's vote equals the sum of the initial weights assigned to him by all members of the committee, i.e.,

$$W_j = \sum w_{ji} \; (i \text{ and } j = 1, 2, \ldots, n)$$

for the jth committeeman according to each (ith) member.

In Figure I, the weight of M_1 equals the sum of the initial weights in the column below M_1, namely, $1\frac{5}{6}$. The weights of M_2 and M_3 are $\frac{5}{6}$ and $\frac{1}{3}$, respectively. The sum of these weights is $n = 3$, which happens to equal the maximum number possible for this group because no one withheld any of his initial weight.[13]

Notice the efficiency of the voting procedure prescribed for these committeemen in comparison to the usual (democratic) procedure. For example, consider M_3's position. Given the usual procedure, if M_1 and M_3 disagreed on a text then M_3 would have to *either* abstain altogether *or else* go along with M_1 or M_2 But in *both*

[13]To simplify the illustrations, no weight is withheld in any of them.

cases he would be merely making the best of a bad situation. His "real" judgment is that M_1's views are about as reliable as M_2's. However, the voting procedure forces him to act as if he had nothing at all to contribute (i.e., he abstains) or else to act as if he preferred the view of M_1 or M_2. In short, the usual procedure suppresses that modicum of competence that the committee recognizes in M_3. On the other hand, our procedure of weighting voters takes account of M_3's ability. It allows him to make a contribution that reflects his own best judgment. It is *not* a judgment about the question at issue (i.e., about the best logic text), but about the relative ability of the other members of the committee to judge that issue. It is what many writers regard as a typically administrative decision.[14] It is a decision about the ability of certain personnel to judge a certain issue, rather than a technical decision about the issue itself. The legitimacy and usefulness of administrative decisions can hardly be doubted, since it is difficult to imagine a highly complex organization such as an industrial corporation, university, or government agency without many people responsible for such decisions, viz., the administrators or managers. Therefore, if all other things are equal, then insofar as the procedure we are recommending provides a more efficient treatment of such decisions than the usual procedure, the former should be regarded as superior.

According to (4.1)–(4.3), the weight of each committeeman's vote must be a real number in the closed interval from 0 to *n,* i.e.:

$$0 \leq W_j \leq n \, (j = 1, 2, \ldots, n)$$

If every committeeman distributes his initial weight in equal amounts among all of the members of a committee then each one will receive an initial weight of *l/n* from every member. Since there are *n* members, the result of such a distribution will be a *democratic weighting* with every committeeman's weight:

$$W_j = 1 \, (j = 1, 2, \ldots, n)$$

Formally, this result is indistinguishable from an *anarchic weighting* in which everyone keeps all of his initial weight. The different attitudes of democrats and anarchists toward legitimate government is reflected by the different paths leading to the equalitarian weights. The democrat assigns each committeeman the same weight and, therefore, is obliged to use numbers of supporters as a legitimizing criterion. The anarchist assigns only himself a weight and, therefore, is obliged to use his own preferences as a legitimizing criterion.

---

[14]E.g., "In the field of organization, the knowledge on which what we call responsible control depends is not knowledge of situations and problems and of means foe effecting changes, but is knowledge of these things … the *crucial* decision is the selection of men to make decisions." Frank H. Knight, *Risk, Uncertainty and Profit* (New York, Harper and Row, Inc., 1965), pp. 292–299.

If every committeeman distributes his initial weight such that the weight of a single member, say, M_d is

$$W_d = n$$

the result will be a *delegatory weighting,* In effect the complete responsibility for the committee decision has been delegated to M_d. If the latter could be *born* into the position, there would be some justification for regarding this pattern as a *monarchic weighting.*

If the distribution of initial weights is such that the total weight of fewer than half of the voters is greater than half of the total weight of the whole committee, the result is an *oligarchic weighting.* More precisely, if there are m committeemen such that

$$\sum W_i > n/2\,(i = 1, 2, \ldots, m)$$

although

$$m < \text{n}/2$$

the weighting is oligarchic. If the composition or membership of the set of m committeemen varies as the issues before the committee vary, it might be more appropriate to refer to the weighting as *polyarchic.* In practice, many organizations that operate *formally* with democratic weightings, operate *informally* with polyarchic or delegatory weightings.[15]

Finally, if the distribution of initial weights is such that the weight of a single member, say, M_0 is

$$W_0 = 0$$

the result is a *disfranchising weighting.* Notice that no one can be disfranchised unless he chooses to be.

Obviously these weighting patterns are not mutually exclusive in pairs. While no pattern can be both oligarchic and democratic (or democratic and disfranchising), every delegated pattern must be oligarchic. Moreover, a priori there seems to be no good reason to suspect that the patterns defined here exhaust the interesting possibilities, i.e., these weighting patterns are probably not exhaustive.

More importantly, perhaps, it should be emphasized that it is *not* being claimed that the specification of the type of weighting pattern employed in a committee is *sufficient* to characterize the committee as, say, democratic. It is true, however, that the specification of the type of pattern is *necessary* for such a characterization.

---

[15]A classic description of a polyarchic system may be found in Dahl, *op. cit.*

Weighted Voting

Now that we have a procedure for weighting voters, the question is: How should the weights be used to reach committee decisions? This question can be neatly divided into the following two questions:

(A) How should weights be applied by voters?
(B) What proportion of the total weight (n) available should be required for a committee decision?

The latter question (B) has received considerable attention by legislators and philosophers, and we shall not attempt to improve upon traditional discussions here.[16] Instead, we shall focus on the former (A) and try to present some options that have received little or no attention. In particular, we shall consider six voting schemes. For each of the schemes it will be assumed that the decision (item, solution, policy, candidate, etc.) which receives the greatest support or has the largest weight will be accepted as the committee decision. Roughly speaking, this assumption is equivalent to answering (B) with: a plurality or simple majority is required for a committee decision. This is not an especially profound or unproblematic answer, but it will be adequate for our purposes. Above all it should be remembered that (A) and (B) are quite different questions, and that success or failure with either does not imply success or failure with the other.

Question (A) is vague. It might be answered by such disparate remarks as: In accordance with their consciences; with caution; happily; all together; in bits and pieces; etc. The last two replies suggest the sense in which we are interested. To begin with, we might apply weights as follows:

Total weight scheme: Each committeeman puts the total weight of his vote on a single decision (candidate, option, etc.), or he withholds all of it.

For example, suppose the weights assigned to a five-membered committee are:

FIGURE II

	M_1	M_2	M_3	M_4	M_5
W_i	1	0.5	1.3	0.7	1.5

and there are three alternative decisions to consider

D_1 D_2 D_3

Then on the total weight scheme, the result of a vote might be:

[16]An excellent review and criticism of some of the alternatives may be found in C.L. Dodgson (Lewis Carroll), "A Discussion of the Various Methods of Procedure in Conducting Elections" reprinted in Duncan Black, *The Theory of Committees and Elections* (Cambridge, Cambridge University Press, 1963), pp. 214–222.

FIGURE III

	D_1	D_2	D_3
M_1	0	1	0
M_2	0.5	0	0
M_3	1.3	0	0
M_4	0	0	0.7
M_5	0	1.5	0
Total	1.8	2.5	0.7

That is, M_1 puts all of his weight behind D_2, M_2 puts all of his weight behind D_1; and so on. The result is that D_2 becomes the committee decision because it has the most support.

The total weight scheme is perfectly straightforward. Each man either applies all of his influence (i.e., the total weight of his vote) to a single decision or he withholds all of it. However, sometimes a committeeman regards certain alternative decisions as equally acceptable. Or, faced with three or more options, he is frequently able to weakly order them. If *any* of the members of a committee are able to weakly order the various alternatives before them, then it would be useful (i.e., more efficient) to give them the option of dividing the weight of their votes according to their preferences. This involves two closely related assumptions. In the first place, it must be granted that weights of influence, which are already indicants of relative competence, may also be used as indicants of preferences. And secondly, it must be granted that people's preferences are comparable, e.g., if M_1 and M_2 rank D_1 above D_2 and the latter above D_3 we would *grant that* they both "feel about the same" about the three decisions *instead of* insisting that, say, M_1 prefers D_1 to D_2 much more than M_2 prefers D_1 to D_2, and so on.[17] While the dual role of weights of influence seems harmless enough, we shall have more to say about the weak ordering and interpersonal comparisons of "utility" in section "Objections and Replies: Weighted Voting".

Given the above assumptions, we might employ a:

Split weight option scheme: Each committeeman distributes the weight of his vote among the decisions in accordance with his preferences, or he withholds any part or all of it.

For example, consider the five-membered committee above, faced with the same three decisions. A possible result of the split weight option scheme for the voters in Figure II might be:

FIGURE IV

	D_1	D_2	D_3	W_i
M_1	0.5	0.5	0	1
M_2	0.5	0	0	0.5
M_3	0.8	0.5	0	1.3
M_4	0	0.2	0.5	0.7
M_5	0.5	1	0	1.5
Total	2.3	2.2	0.5	$5 = n$

[17] A suggestive graphic representation of this problem is given by Nicholas Rescher, "Notes on Preference, Utility and Cost," *Syntheses*, vol. 16 (1966), p. 333.

Here M_1 distributes the weight of his vote between two equally attractive (acceptable, plausible, preferred, etc.) decisions D_1 and D_2; M_2 keeps his vote intact; and so on. The result is that D_1 narrowly becomes the committee decision.

A major advantage of the split weight option scheme over the total weight scheme is that the former *takes account* of discernible preferential differences while the latter cannot take account of such differences. Or, to put this important point in a slightly different way, a committee decision based on the split weight option scheme is a function of more subtle or precise judgments than a committee decision based on the total weight scheme. Hence, the former scheme is more efficient than the latter.

Instead of allowing committeemen to divide their weights to indicate their preferences, we might provide each voter with an additional unit to distribute. More precisely, we might let each voter assign every decision (item, policy, etc.) a real number U in the closed interval from 0 to 1 called a "utility," with the sum of the utilities assigned by each member equal to or less than one. Here the term "utility" means nothing more than the value (desirability, satisfactoriness, etc.) of a decision according to a committeeman. An example of the result of such assignments might be

FIGURE V

	D_1	D_2	D_3	sum
M_1	0.5	0.5	0	1
M_2	1	0	0	1
M_3	0.7	0.3	0	1
M_4	0	0.3	0.7	1
M_5	0.4	0.5	0.1	1

If U_{ij} *is* the utility of the *i*th decision according to the *j*th member then the total *weighted-utility* of that decision for that member is:

$$U_{ij}W_j$$

Now we may define the:

Total weighted-utility scheme; Each committeeman assigns every decision a total weighted-utility (i.e., the product of the total weight of influence of his vote and the utility he assigns to each decision).[18]

For example, given the utility assignments in Figure V and the weights of influence in Figure II, we have

FIGURE VI

	D_1	D_2	D_3
M_1	(1) (0.5)	(1) (0.5)	(1) (0)
M_2	(0.5) (1)	(0.5) (0)	(0.5) (0)
M_3	(1.3) (0.7)	(1.3) (0.3)	(1.3) (0)
M_4	(0.7) (0)	(0.7) (0.3)	(0.7) (0.7)
M_5	(1.5) (0.4)	(1.5) (0.5)	(1.5) (0.1)
Total weighted-utility sum	2.51	1.85	0.64

[18]This is basically the scheme recommended by Minas and Ackoff, *op. cit.,* pp. 355–356.

The result of applying the total weighted-utility scheme with the given numerical assignments is a clear victory for D_1.

Although the split weight option scheme is less cumbersome than the total weighted-utility scheme, it is easy to show that the two schemes are equivalent. Using the former, a committeeman M_j would distribute the weight of his vote W_i such that every alternative D_i receives a certain proportion of it, say, x_{ij} where

$$\sum x_{ij} \leq W_j \; (i = 1, 2, \ldots, n)$$

for an n-membered committee. Using the latter, M_j would distribute his unit of utility U_j among the members in *the same proportions*. So, for any member Mj and any alternative D_i:

$$\frac{x_{ij}}{W_j} = \frac{U_{ij}}{1} = U_{ij}$$

Hence:

$$x_{ij} = U_{ij} W_j$$

But x_{ij} is the index of M_j's support for D_i according to the split weight option scheme and $U_{ii}\ W_j$ is the same index according to the total weighted-utility scheme. Therefore, the two schemes are equivalent.

To obtain greater uniformity in our utility assignments, we might employ the sort of marking system introduced by Jean-Charles Borda.[19] We would assign 0 utility to the least preferred alternative, 1 to the alternative immediately above that, 2 to the third highest, and so on until we reach the end of the, lot. Equally preferred alternatives are assigned the same number. For convenience, we shall call such indicants "Borda-utilities." The preferences ranked in Figure V would be indicated as follows in terms of Borda-utilities.

FIGURE VII

	D_1	D_2	D_3
M_1	1	1	0
M_2	1	0	0
M_3	2	1	0
M_4	0	1	2
M_5	1	2	0

Notice that while alternatives with Borda-utilities of n have exactly n *ranks* below them, they may have more or less than n *alternatives* below them. For example, M_2 distinguishes two preference levels. So the top level has a Borda-utility of $n = 1$, and there is one level but two alternatives below D_1.

[19] "Mémoire sur les elections au scrutin," *Histoire de l'Académie* (1781). For a thorough examination of Borda's views see Black, *op. cit.*, pp. 59–66, 156–159.

Now we may define a:

Weighted Borda-utility scheme: Each committeeman assigns every decision a weighted Borda-utility (i.e., the product of the total weight of influence of his vote and the Borda-utility he assigns to each decision).

For example, given the Borda-utility assignments of Figure VII and the weights of influence of Figure II, we have:

FIGURE VIII

	D_1	D_2	D_3
M_1	(1) (1)	(1) (1)	(1) (0)
M_2	(0.5) (1)	(0.5) (0)	(0.5) (0)
M_3	(1.3) (2)	(1.3) (1)	(1.3) (0)
M_4	(0.7) (0)	(0.7) (1)	(0.7) (2)
M_5	(1.5) (1)	(1.5) (2)	(1.5) (0)
Weighted Borda-utility sum	5.6	6	1.4

Hence, the result of applying the weighted Borda-utility scheme with the given numerical assignments is a victory for D_2.

If we provide additional units such as utilities and Borda-utilities to be distributed *and* allow committeemen to split the weight of their votes, then we may define a:

Split weight utility scheme: Each committeeman assigns every decision a split weight utility (i.e., the product of some or all of the weight of influence of his vote and the utility he assigns to each decision)

and a:

Split weight Borda-utility scheme: Each committeeman assigns every decision a split weight Borda-utility (i.e., the product of some or all of the weight of influence of his vote and the Borda-utility he assigns to each decision).

Using the Borda-utility assignments of Figure VII and the weights of influence of Figures II and IX illustrates a possible result of applying the latter scheme:

FIGURE IX

	D_1	D_2	D_3
M_1	(1) (1)	(0.5) (1)	(0.5) (0)
M_2	(0.5) (1)	(0.2) (0)	(0.5) (0)
M_3	(1.3) (2)	(0.3) (1)	(0.8) (0)
M_4	(0.7) (0)	(0.7) (1)	(0.7) (2)
M_5	(1.5) (1)	(1) (2)	(0.5) (0)
Split weight Borda-utility sum	5.6	3.5	1.4

Hence, the result of applying this scheme with the given numerical assignments is a victory for D_2. (Notice that every committeeman is permitted to multiply the Borda-utility he assigns *to each decision* by a number no greater than his total weight.)

By a line of argumentation analogous to that used to show that the split weight option and total weighted-utility schemes are equivalent, it may be shown that the split weight utility and split weight Borda-utility schemes are both equivalent to the former two schemes. Thus, in view of the unnecessary labor involved in the additional computations required for the application of the latter three in comparison with the split weight option scheme, there is no doubt that the other three schemes will never be practicable.

The following matrix summarizes the six schemes we have considered.

	No additional units provided	Additional units provided
Use all or No weight	Total weight	{ total weighted-utility weighted Borda-utility
Use some all, or No weight	Split weight option	{ split weight utility split weight Borda-utility

The total weight scheme comes about by answering question (A), (How should weights be applied by voters?) with "as a whole" and not providing any additional units to be distributed. If (A) is answered by "as a whole or in parts" and no additional units are provided, the result is the split weight option scheme. The remaining entries in the matrix arise analogously.

Objections and Replies: Weighting Voters

The constructive work of this essay has now been completed, and it is time to appraise our results in the light of the adequacy criteria introduced in section "Criteria of Adequacy". Six solutions to our basic problem (viz., How should the decisions [with respect to some issue] of the members of a committee be amalgamated for the committee decision to be determined in the most acceptable fashion?) were suggested in section "Weighted Voting". Each of these six employed the procedure for weighting voters that was described in section "Weighting Voters". So, if there are no acceptable procedures for weighting voters, then the practical value of the six schemes of weighted voting must be nil. It will be convenient then, to consider objections to the procedure for weighting voters prior to and in isolation from objections to particular schemes of weighted voting.

How does our procedure for weighting voters fare with respect to our five criteria, viz., (3.1) freedom from coercion, (3.2) internal consistency, (3.3) practicability, (3.4) efficiency, and (3.5) influence proportionate to relative competence? Taking the least problematic first, our procedure seems (to me) to satisfy the conditions of freedom from coercion, internal consistency, and efficiency. But the other two requirements require some discussion.

To begin with, it might be objected that our procedure violates (3.5) because it begins with an equalitarian distribution of influence in the form of a single vote worth exactly one unit. That is, *before* anyone's competence is estimated, every committeeman is given a vote whose initial weight is equal to that of every other. But according to (3.5), such a distribution is permissible only if the competence of every committeeman is equal to that of every other. However, at this (first) stage in our procedure we do not know how competent any committeeman is. Hence, we cannot justify an opening equalitarian distribution. Moreover, if we *could* justify such a distribution then the whole procedure of weighting voters would be a waste of time, because they would all receive the same weight always. But the first step in our procedure must be either unjustified or justified. Therefore, it must either violate (3.5) or trivialize the whole procedure.

This dilemma is more apparent than real. The first horn is problematic but the second horn is based on a misunderstanding. Let us take the second horn first. Recall that in our procedure each committeeman is called upon to make two different *types* of decisions, one on the abilities of the other members and the other on the issue(s) before the committee. Our opening equalitarian distribution only presupposes that every committeeman is equally qualified to make the first type of judgment. If *this* assumption is warranted then all that follows is that every member's *opinion about any committeeman's judgment* about the issue(s) before the committee is equal to every other member's opinion. It does *not* follow that every member's *opinion about the issue(s)* before the committee is equal to every other member's opinion. Hence, the whole weighting procedure cannot be trivialized by an opening equalitarian distribution. So much for the second horn.

The first horn of the dilemma cannot be dispatched so swiftly. Indeed, we must grant immediately that we have no reason to suppose that the ability to judge the ability of personnel to judge more or less technical issues is equally distributed among all or most people. What we would like to substitute for an opening equalitarian distribution is a distribution based on some reliable independent test. But this raises the question: How should we select such a test? And this question seems to lead us straight to section "The Problem" of this paper (which has finally led us to the present point) *or* to an infinite regress of reliable independent tests of reliable independent tests *or* to some more or less arbitrarily final reliable independent test. No doubt the last alternative will be preferred by most people, and the haggling will be over the cut-off point. The opening equalitarian distribution suggested in our procedure is merely a convenient (admittedly early) cut-off point which should be adequate for most purposes. After all, even the usual democratic procedure (which is less efficient than any of ours) has been regarded as adequate for most purposes. If the *cost* of an erroneous committee decision is very high, we would expect much more elaborate precautions to be taken to increase the chances of arriving at a more acceptable opening distribution.[20]

---

[20]The relation between costs and precision in measurement is outlined in C. West Churchman, *Prediction and Optimal Decision* (Englewood Gliffs, N.J., Prentice-Hall, Inc., 1964), pp. 116ff.

Briefly, then, my reply to the first horn of the dilemma is as follows. The objection is sound but not totally destructive. It reveals a defect in our procedure which becomes more or less serious as the cost of errors increases or decreases, respectively, and which further research should attempt to eliminate or reduce as much as possible.

Supposing we had solutions to these problems, would our procedure then be practicable [condition (3.3)]? It seems that out procedure may be impracticable for *at least* eight reasons.

(1) Committeemen may find the task of weakly ordering their colleagues in accordance with relative competence too *complicated.* Competence is very likely multi-dimensional and the dimensions may be extremely difficult if not impossible to compare. For example, a certain committeeman may be very good at identifying, say, the pedagogical strengths and weaknesses of a textbook (e.g., the organization and presentation of new material, definitions, illustrations, exercises, etc.) but very bad at recognizing factual or formal errors (e.g., that this was discovered by so-and-so then, that most people call this a such-and-such, that it is misleading to refer to this as that, etc.). Should such a committeeman be assigned a high or a low weight? Should a committeeman who is good at *both* tasks be assigned a weight that is *twice* as great as that of a committeeman who is only good at one? Are the two skills "really" equally important? Even if these problems could be solved, the cost of solving them may be too high *given* the benefits obtainable from our procedure *and* the availability of other procedures. That is, it is not merely this or that complication in the abstract that may be objectionable. Rather, it is the fact that in comparison with other procedures, the cost of untangling the complications in ours may be too high and the likely rewards too low to vindicate its application.

(2) The determination of relative competence may produce *disputes, factions*, and *enemies* that might otherwise be avoided. For example, a member may not appreciate receiving a low weight from a voter to whom the former has just assigned a low weight. Since committee meetings will probably take more time with our procedure, we may expect greater fatigue, irritability, impatience, and ennui. Hence, even trivial issues may become highly problematic.

(3) Our procedure may be regarded as too *"brutal"* because it does not provide any face-saving safeguards for perennial "light-weights." Even if the weights are never made public (which merely requires the help of a discreet and honest assistant, or a machine), it is bound to occur to some people that in their *own* opinion the judgment of certain committeemen is almost always nearly worthless. What is worse, if the split weight option scheme is used and everyone must be informed of their colleagues views about their relative competence, then perennial "light-weights" are going to be repeatedly embarrassed and probably embittered.

(4) Our procedure may breed *irresponsibility* in those who, for a certain issue, have been assigned a fairly low weight. The low weight assigned to a committeeman may have the effect of a self-fulfilling prediction, i.e., everyone expects him to

contribute very little; so he expends very little effort and, consequently, he has very little to contribute.

(5) Committeemen may nullify the opportunity to determine the relative competence of their colleagues by employing a *minimax loss* strategy. According to this strategy, a voter should distribute his initial weight to insure himself the smallest possible loss. His options are to give away none of it, give away part of it, or give away all of it. Clearly, he can protect himself against any loss at all by simply keeping his vote all to himself.[21] However, if everyone employs this strategy, then the result is an anarchic weighting. And if enough people employ this strategy often enough, our procedure would have to be regarded as redundant.[22]

(6) It is likely that committeemen will *misjudge* the relative competence of their colleagues. They will commit "errors of leniency" (i.e., assign more weight to those they like), "central tendency" (i.e., avoid assigning extreme weights of 0 or 1), "logic" (i.e., assign similar weights for skills that seem to be "logically related"), "contrast" (i.e., assign weights roughly inversely proportional to those they assign themselves), and "proximity" (i.e., assign similar weights for skills that are considered at roughly the same time or in the same context).[23] They will fall prey to the "halo effect" (i.e., assign weights in accordance with their "general impression" of the individual rated)[24] and the "Matthew effect" (i.e., assign higher weights to the "biggest names" regardless of their particular competence in a given situation).[25] They will be influenced by "prestige considerations,"[26] and, as the ambiguity of the situation increases, by social pressure to "conform."[27] Hence, instead of indicating relative competence, our weights will be meaningless numbers misleadingly suggesting precision and accuracy.

---

[21]Similarly, it has been argued that "A second vital reason for seeking the condition of political equality is a strategic calculation. Like so many important decisions, this one, too, is a calculated risk. Reduced to its boldest terms, our strategy comes to this: we cannot be confident of continued membership in an elite group whose preferences would be counted for more rather than less." Robert A. Dahl and Charles E. Lindblom, *Politics, Economics and Welfare* (New York, Harper and Row, Inc., 1963), p. 43.

[22]Other possible strategies may be found in my *Principles of Logic* (Englewood Cliffs, N.J., Prentice-Hall, Inc., 1969), ch. 8.

[23]Detailed discussions of these errors may be found in J.P. Guilford, *Psychometric Methods* (New York, McGraw-Hill Book Co., 1954), pp. 278–280.

[24]*Ibid.,* p. 279.

[25]Robert K. Merton, "The Matthew Effect in Science," *Science,* vol. 159 (1968), pp. 56–63.

[26]Robert E. Lane, "Political Personality and Electoral Choice," *American Political Science Review,* vol. 49 (1955), pp. 173–174.

[27]E.L Walker and R.W. Heyns, *An Anatomy for Conformity* (Englewood Cliffs, N.J., Prentice-Hall, Inc., 1962), pp. 92–95. Further problems may be found in Bernard R. Berelson, Paul F. Lazarsfrfd, and William N. McPhce, *Voting* (Chicago, University of Chicago Press, 1962), p. 232, and Paul F. Lazarsfield, Bernard Berelson, and Hazel Gaudct, *The People's Choice* (Ithaca, N.Y., Cornell University Press, 1960), pp. 80ff.

(7) There is some evidence that less competent people are less influential than more competent people anyhow.[28] So an attempt *formally* to weaken the former and strengthen the latter is unnecessary.

(8) If a committeeman believes that some other member of a committee is especially competent, then, rather than giving the latter some of his weight (losing formal influence and flexibility certainly and informal influence possibly), he would be wise to keep all of his weight and simply allow himself to be guided by the other member's decision. After all, from the former's point of view, the final result of giving the latter his weight to put behind a certain decision is no different from putting it in the same place under the other member's supervision. Hence, because committeemen have something to lose by distributing their weight and nothing to lose by keeping it, few or no distributions should ever occur.

Let us consider each of these objections in turn.

(1) It must be granted that *some* people may find the task of weakly ordering their colleagues in accordance with relative competence virtually impossible. That is why our procedure does not *require* such an ordering from anyone. The ordering is *requested*, and if most people cannot satisfy the request, most of the time, then our procedure cannot be expected to accomplish anything most of the rime. Nevertheless, our procedure provides an opportunity to use whatever resources happen to be available, which seems to make it superior to procedures without this provision. Moreover, and fortunately, there is no evidence of a widespread human inability to perform such tasks. On the contrary, while it is difficult to appraise the relative competence of this or that scholar in a certain area, such appraisals are very common. Thousands of employers are required to do just that, and they are frequently promoted for doing it well and discharged for doing it poorly. Hence, the real question seems to be: Are the rewards of untangling the complications in our procedure high enough to justify the costs? And in the absence of a definite issue, committee, and alternative procedure this question seems to be unanswerable.

(2) There seem to be good reasons for believing that our procedure will not create an inordinate number of disputes. In the first place, people frequently judge the merits of candidates for various positions of leadership, and our procedure is merely an extension of this common practice. In the second place, certain

[28]E.g. "The structure of interpersonal relations within legislative systems functions to place legislators with high degrees of skill and conscientiousness in the center of the legislative system and to increase their influence, and to isolate legislators with low degrees of skill and conscientiousness on the periphery of the legislative system and to decrease their influence." Stephen V. Monsma, "Interpersonal Relations in the Legislative System: A Study of the 1964 Michigan House of Representatives," *Midwest Journal cf Political Science*, vol. 10 (1966), p. 363. This article also contains a long bibliography. An instructive criticism of earlier attempts at formulating indices of "influence" may be found in Ralph K. Huitt, "The Outsider in the Senate," *American Political Science Review,* vol. 55 (1961), pp. 566–575.

precautions may be taken to reduce the chances of disputes. For instance, one should avoid using our procedure in situations in which the likelihood of misunderstanding is known to be high, e.g., in meetings involving people with quite specific and, perhaps, antagonistic *roles* such as labor and management representatives,[29] or officers and enlisted men.[30] Perhaps committeemen might be impressed with the idea that they are all part of a single "team" and that the less energy they expend attacking each other the more they will be able to expend on the issue before the committee. Again, the reward and punishment structure might be designed to militate against such phenomena, i.e., let the "payoffs" go to those who do not get involved in disputes and factions, and the penalties go to those who do.[31]

(3) The third objection seems to suggest a nice problem of balancing the demands of morality against those of rationality. Fortunately, that is not the case. The problem is one of balancing the demands of one moral prescription against those of another. On the one hand, committeemen are morally obliged to try to avoid embarrassing their colleagues. On the other, they are morally obliged to try to make as "correct" a decision as possible. Hence, the question they must ask themselves is this: Is the moral cost of embarrassing (and, perhaps, embittering) some members greater than, equal to, or less than the moral cost of making a less "correct" decision. If it costs more (i.e., seems to create more feelings of guilt) to identify and isolate the "light-weights" than it does to accept a slightly "incorrect" committee decision, then a committeeman ought to accept the latter; otherwise he ought to choose the former, unless the costs are equally balanced. In the latter case he might flip a coin.

It would be a mistake to assume that "lightweights" *must* be embarrassed or embittered. While there is a wealth of evidence to support the view that they will probably respond that way,[32] there is also evidence that the reaction of individuals to participation in or exclusion from decision-making that affects their lives is significantly influenced by their *expectations.*[33] Hence, someone who expects "the other fellow" to be responsible for this or that may be

---

[29]Mason Haire found that "management and labor each sees the other as less dependable than himself … and … deficient in thinking, emotional characteristics, and interpersonal relations …" in "Role-peroeption in Labor-management Relations: An Experimental Approach," *Industrial and Labor Relations Review,* vol. 8 (1955), p. 215.

[30]Paul F. Lazarsfeld, "The American Soldier," *Public Opinion Quarterly*, vol. 13 (1949), pp. 383–386.

[31]A number of other techniques are described in Richard E. Walton and Robert B. McKersie, "Behavioral Dilemmas in Mixed-motive Decision Making," *Behavioral Science,* vol. II (1966), pp. 381–384.

[32]Lester Coch and John R. P. French, Jr., "Overcoming Resistance to Change," Human Relations, vol. 1 (1948), p. 532.

[33]William R. Dill, "The Impact of Environment on Organization Development," in Sidney Mailick and Edward H. van Ness (eds.), Concepts and Issues in Administrative Behavior (Englewood Cliffs, N.J., Prentice-Hall, Inc., 1962), p. 105.

perfectly happy to be assigned a lighter weight. Moreover, it should be noted again that if the variety of issues considered by a committee is large, the probability that a certain committeeman will always be judged a "light-weight" is small. Most people tend to be specialists by inclination and aptitude. Hence, if the issues before a committee *vary*, it is likely that no one will be a perennial "light-weight" *or* "heavy-weight," i.e., the *typical* weighting will probably be polyarchic.[34]

(4) It seems that we might suggest with equal plausibility that those committeemen from whom everyone expects a great deal will be encouraged to work harder and, consequently, will be able to contribute more than anyone expects. But this reply merely reproduces the same unwarranted assumption on which the objection is based. That is, there is no reason to assume that committeemen must be weighted long before the final vote on the issue is taken. Indeed, there is no doubt at all that the weighting should immediately precede the voting and that *both* should take place after a discussion of the issues. Moreover, every committeeman should be given an agenda far enough in advance of the meeting to provide some opportunity for him to become familiar with the issues. Given these tactics and the fret that our procedure allows committeemen to gain complete control of a committee decision, it would seem to be difficult for a person with average ability to justify an attitude of impotence.[35]

(5) The application of a minimax loss strategy is not incompatible with the assignment of initial weights according to judgments of relative competence, i.e., it does not entail an anarchic weighting. If someone regards a less "correct" committee decision as a greater loss than a certain amount of personal influence on that decision, then the mini–max strategy would lead him to distribute his initial weight in support of competence, rather than merely in support of himself. In effect then, he would be applying the strategy to the following alternatives:

(a) Keep everything and obtain less "correct" committee decision.

(b) Distribute part and obtain more "correct" committee decision.

The second alternative might well represent the smallest possible loss. The important unanswered question is: Will enough people value "correctness" more than personal influence to make our procedure effective?

(6) The evidence for these suggestions is fairly strong. So all we can do is try to devise ways to minimize the effects of such propensities.[36] One way to tackle

---

[34]This is suggested, but by no means proved, by Dahl's research in New Haven, Conn., *op. cit.,* p. 228. A more extensive investigation by Robert E. Agger, Daniel Goldrich, and Bert. E. Swanson suggests a number of other alternatives, *The Rulers and the Ruled* (New York, John Wiley and Sons, Inc., 1964), pp. 478–537.

[35]Robert E. Lane's investigation of the political attitudes of 15 "average" men led him to the conclusion that "people tend to care less about *equality* of opportunity than about the availability of *some* opportunity," *Political Ideology* (New York, The Free Press, 1962), p. 79.

[36]Guilford introduces techniques to estimate some of the types of errors we listed. They obviously require the assistance of a trained statistician. *Op. cit.,* pp. 280ff.

the problem is to construct a set of minimum standards according to which initial weights must be distributed. For example, in the case of the selection of a textbook, we might give so many points for having taken so many courses, for having taught so many, for having published so many related papers, etc. Other more reliable tests would have to be developed for other types of issues. A second way to attack the problem would be to have the committeemen present their "credentials" with precise and standardized descriptions to reduce vagueness and ambiguity. This would reduce the temptation to interpret perceptions in a more or less arbitrary fashion.[37]

(7) Insofar as events are bound to take place exactly as we prefer with or without our (formal) efforts, such efforts must be regarded as unnecessary. But the ultimate triumph of wisdom over ignorance is hardly inevitable. Hence, we seem to be obliged to take *some* steps to "further the cause of rationality and good decision-making." What I would like to suggest here is that the formalization of influence in some situations might be *a* step in the right direction.

(8) It seems clear that in some situations it would be wiser to *copy* a more competent member's voting behavior than to give him all or part of one's weight. However, in other situations, the latter strategy seems preferable to the former. For example, suppose that one is not only interested in the "correctness" of a committee decision, but also in appropriately allocating the rewards or punishments resulting from that decision. The distribution of weights could be used as a basis for fixing responsibility and for fairly allocating rewards and punishments. Similarly, weight distribution provides an explicit record of committeemen's views of one another's competence which could be useful for the choice of operating procedures and personnel. Again, it is often important to know whether a committee decision has received a certain amount of support on its own as it were *or* simply on the strength of its supporters. After all, to return to a point raised in section "Weighting Voters", it is one thing to endorse a particular alternative and quite another to endorse a particular person who endorses that alternative. A ten-membered committee decision with one knowledgeable supporter and nine administratively competent but technically ignorant supporters seems to have less support in some sense[38] than the same decision with nine knowledgeable supporters and one supporting administrator. While weight distribution (according to the procedure suggested here) might not alter the final number of points received for such a decision in either case, it would provide some intuitively useful extra bits of information whose value would tend to vary directly with the error and implementation costs of any decision. Of course, one could probably gather the extra information by additional research of some sort, but weight distribution always provides such

[37]There is no doubt at all that the (international and unintentional) ambiguity of politicians' claims is highly correlated with the erroneous interpretations of voters, eg., see Berelson, Lazarsfeld, and McPhee, *loc. cit.*

[38]The precise nature and plausibility of this "sense" is still rather vague to me.

information and always makes the subtle difference in the *kind* of support received by any alternative completely explicit.

Objections and Replies: Weighted Voting

After reviewing the objections and replies to the procedure of weighting voters, it seems fair to say that as yet neither a case for nor against it has been decisively made. There are still a number of loose ends to be tied up, some of which require empirical investigation more than logical analysis. However, in this section we shall assume that our procedure for weighting voters is more or less acceptable and ask: How do the various schemes of weighted voting fare in the light of our five adequacy criteria?

Taking the least problematic point first, I think that we may grant the internal consistency [condition (3.2)] of all six schemes. It is certainly true that if one requires some sort of piecemeal comparison of alternatives (e.g., pairwise comparison, triplewise, etc.) *and* assumes that both individual and group systems of preferences must be transitive, then all of these schemes are liable to generate the so-called "paradox of voting" in certain situations.[39] But it seems to me that there is no good reason to expect group systems of preferences to be transitive or to require piecemeal comparisons of alternatives. So the "paradox" is something of a red herring.[40]

It may be recalled that in section "Weighted Voting" we showed that the total weight scheme is inefficient [violating (3.4)] in the sense that it is liable to be unable to take account of available information. Similarly, the weighted Borda-utility scheme must be inefficient because Borda-utilities vary at regular intervals whether or not the preferences of committeemen vary that way. For example, if someone ranks D_1 above D_2 and the latter above D_3, then the Borda-utility of D_1 is twice that of D_3 whether or not the committeemen believes is twice as "good" as D_3. While we are not *bound* to use the whole numbers 0, 1, 2, 3, … as Borda-utilities, we are bound to use *some* regularly increasing set (e.g., $0, \frac{1}{3}, \frac{2}{3}, \frac{3}{3}, \ldots; 0, \frac{1}{4}, \frac{1}{2}, \frac{3}{4}, \ldots$) because it is this very regularity that distinguishes this scheme from the total weighted-utility scheme. Hence, whenever committeemen have preferences that do not vary at regular intervals, they will be unable to "feed" this information into the weighted Borda-utility scheme. Hence, it too violates (3.4). Since the split weight Borda-utility scheme provides some means of breaking the rigid Borda-utility mold (namely, by appropriately splitting one's weight), it does not violate (3.4). Furthermore, for roughly the same reason, neither do the other three schemes.

---

[39]An excellent review of the formal issues surrounding this paradox may be found in Yasusuke Murakami, Logic and Social Choice (London, Routledge and Kegan Paul, Ltd., 1968), chs. 5 and 6.

[40]I am in Complete agreement with Dahl and Lindblom, *op. cit.*, pp. 422–424.

The total weight scheme seems to be free of any peculiar problems of practicability [condition (3.3)]. However, as we saw in section "Weighted Voting", the total weighted utility, split weight utility, and split weight Borda-utility schemes are all impracticable because the labor costs of applying them are greater than the costs of applying the equivalent split weight option scheme. Furthermore, with the exception of the total weight scheme, they all presuppose (i) the ability of some committeemen to weakly order their preferences for various alternatives and (ii) the interpersonal comparison of utility. Both of these assumptions have been debated so exhaustively in the literature that it seems very unlikely that anything novel can be said here.[41] So, I shall restrict my "defense" to the following brief remarks. In defense of (i) it should be noted that people are frequently (though by no means always) able to weakly order their preferences, and that this must be regarded as favorable evidence for the view that, as far as this problem is concerned, our voting schemes will frequently be practicable.[42] In defense of (ii) it must be admitted that the very fact that fairly stable wage and price systems exist may be taken as evidence that some services and commodities must have roughly the same value for many people. That is, if people of roughly equal means are willing to pay the same price for a certain commodity or do the same work for the same salary, then it seems more likely that they are receiving the same rather than different amounts of satisfaction from the exchange. Hence, this second problem seems to be primarily one of constructing appropriate technical "devices" to obtain reliable measures of comparability. Nevertheless, neither economists nor psychologists have been able to produce such "devices" after many years of trying. So it would be gratuitous to assume that these schemes did not face a serious problem of practicability.

The total weight scheme seems to violate condition (3.1), freedom from coercion, because it does not allow committeemen to distribute the weight of their votes in accordance with their preferences. They might then, be forced to give more support to certain issues than they prefer or simply withhold all of their influence. Similarly, the weighted Borda-utility scheme is liable to be coercive when it is suppressing information.[43]

---

[41] I have entered the periphery of the arena in "Postulates of Rational Preference," *Philosophy of Science*, vol. 34 (1967), pp. 18–22, and "Estimated Utility and Corroboration," *British Journal for the Philosophy of Science*, vol. 16 (1966), pp. 327–331.

[42] It is worthwhile to note, I think, that the chances of performing this task seem to be increased by considering Bentham's seven aspects of the "satisfaction" attached to a particular decision, viz., intensity, duration, certainty, propinquity, fecundity, purity, and extent. On this point Wayne A.R. Leys' discussion in *Ethics for Policy Decision* (Englewood Cliffs, N.J., Prentice-Hall, Inc., 1952) is very helpful, pp. 13–32.

[43] A similar objection was raised by Condorcet against Borda's numbers in 1785 according to Issac Todhunter, *A History of the Mathematical Theory of Probability* (New York, Chelsea Publishing Co., 1946), pp. 433–434.

The split weight option scheme and its equivalents may be shown to violate (3.1) as follows. We have a three-membered committee in which each member has a weight of unity and a vote is to be taken to select one of four alternatives. If each member voted his "true" preferences, the result would be a victory for D_1 as follows:

	D_1	D_2	D_3	D_4	W_t
M_1	$\frac{1}{2}$	$\frac{1}{2}$	$\frac{1}{4}$	0	1
M_2	$\frac{1}{2}$	$\frac{1}{2}$	$\frac{1}{2}$	0	1
M_3	$\frac{1}{2}$	$\frac{1}{2}$	$\frac{1}{2}$	$\frac{1}{2}$	1
Total	1	$\frac{2}{3}$	$\frac{5}{6}$	$\frac{1}{2}$	

However, M_3 figures that "half a loaf is better than none" and that while his first choice is a lost cause, his second choice would win if he put all his weight behind it. By misrepresenting his preferences thus,

	D_1	D_2	D_3	D_4
M_2	0	0	1	0

he insures a victory for D_2, because the new total is:

D_1	D_2	D_3	D_4
1	$\frac{1}{2}$	$1\frac{1}{2}$	0

Hence, for M_3 to insure a victory for his second choice given the split weight option scheme and the particular distribution of preferences of the other members of the committee, he must vote contrary to his preferences. So, the split weight option scheme and its equivalents violate (3.1); which means that all of our schemes are liable to be coercive.

Since the procedure for weighting voters is designed to guarantee the satisfaction of condition (3.5) and since it has rather precariously passed inspection, one might be inclined to say that the six schemes employing it are also provisionally acceptable on this score. Unfortunately, such an inference would not be warranted, because it is undoubtedly the case that all of these schemes are liable to violate (3.5). If, for example, every member of a three-membered committee has a weight of influence equal to unity going into an election and two of them abstain, the third member's weight of influence on the final outcome would jump from a third to one! But short of violating (3.1) there is no way to prevent such "anomalies" from arising. Hence, after all is said and done, we still do not have a scheme that will guarantee the satisfaction of (3.5). Indeed, we now know that it is impossible to construct such a scheme without violating (3.1). Thus, we have arrived at a conclusion that is analogous to Arrow's General Possibility Theorem.[44] That is, it is impossible to construct a voting scheme such that for *every* individual under *any* circumstances, both freedom from coercion and the distribution of influence according to relative competence are *guaranteed.* Of course, given certain individuals and circumstances, influence may well be distributed according to relative competence without coercion. So (3.1) and (3.5) are certainly consistent. But no procedure can *guarantee* their joint satisfaction.

If we let "*p*" be short for "passes" and "*f*" for "fails," then the views presented in this section may be summarized in the following matrix. The last line has been added to facilitate comparison with what we have been calling the "usual (democratic) voting procedure."

Voting scheme	Condition				
	3.1	3.2	3.3	3.4	3.5
Total weight	*f*	*p*	*p*	*f*	*f*
Split weight option[a]	*f*	*p*	*f*	*p*	*f*
Total weighted-utility[a]	*f*	*p*	*f*	*p*	*f*
Weighted Borda-utility	*f*	*p*	*f*	*f*	*f*
Split weight utility[a]	*f*	*p*	*f*	*p*	*f*
Split weight Borda-utility[a]	*f*	*p*	*f*	*p*	*f*
Usual procedure	*f*	*p*	*p*	*f*	*f*

[a]Indicates equivalent schemes

As the table discloses, the weighted Borda-utility scheme is the weakest of the lot, and all of the others are equally acceptable. At any rate, they are equally acceptable provided that one regards each of the five adequacy conditions as equally important. If the conditions were weighted unequally then one of the voting schemes might prove to be superior to the others.

Conclusion

Insofar as we have succeeded in providing a more or less systematic basis for logical and empirical investigations of group decision procedures which permit formal or explicit inequalities among voters and votes, our more general task has been completed. Insofar as we have been able to throw some light on the relationships, strengths, and weaknesses of various more or less plausible solutions to the problem of selecting an acceptable group-decision procedure, our more specific

[44]Arrow, *op. cit.,* pp. 46–60.

task has been accomplished. Perhaps the most appropriate summary of our results on the latter score would be a loose paraphrase of a remark made by Sir Winston Churchill: The usual (democratic) procedure is a very bad form of government, but it is every bit as good as all the others."[45]

[45]I would like to express my gratitude to Sidney J. Herzig, George Yoos, William Hughes, and especially Thomas A. Schwartz for their help and encouragement.

Chapter 9
Analytic and Other "DUMB" Guides of Life

Alex C. Michalos

In a somewhat famous paper Professor A.J. Ayer claimed that 'in the sense in which probability is the guide of life … [I do not] … think that statements of probability can be logically true'.[1] Even if such a statement were based on all available evidence, he claimed that 'there is no sense … in which the proposition … can be superior to any of the others as a measure of probability. And this being so, there can be no practical reason why we should take it as a guide' (p. 14). In the discussion following his paper Professor Ayer was supported by P.K. Feyerabend (*ibid.* p. 21). Since then others have joined the chorus. In particular, Wesley C. Salmon has written that he has been 'unable to see, in spite of Carnap's patient efforts to explain, how such [analytic] statements could constitute "a guide of life"'.[2] Similarly, W.C. Kneale wrote 'if confirmation theory is to be the guide of life, confirmation itself must be defined by reference to the rationality of action in the future. But I do not see how in that case statements of the form c(h, e) = p can ever be analytic'.[3]

Contrary to these authors, I shall argue that analytic statements *do* as a matter of fact function as guides and that a fortiori they certainly *can* have such a function. Moreover, I shall show that some analytic statements are better guides than others.

Michalos, A.C.: 1970. Analytic and other 'dumb' guides of life. Analysis, 30, pp. 121–123, doi:10.1093/analys/30.4.121.

[1]A.J. Ayer, 'The conception of probability as a logical relation', *Observation and Interpretation in the Philosophy of Physics*, ed. S. Körner (New York: Dover Publications, Inc., 1957), p. 17.
[2]W.C. Salmon, 'The justification of inductive rules of inference', *The Problem of Inductive Logic,* ed. I. Lakatos (Amsterdam: North Holland Pub. Co., 1968), p. 40.
[3]*Ibid.,* 'Confirmation and Rationality', p. 61.

A.C. Michalos (✉)
University of Northern British Columbia, Prince George, BC, Canada
e-mail: michalos@brandonu.ca

A.C. Michalos, *Philosophical Foundations of Quality of Life*,
DOI 10.1007/978-3-319-50727-9_9

It is easy to see why someone would want to claim that analytic statements cannot be *prescriptive.* After all, they are (I would grant) vacuous, uninformative or completely void of empirical content. So if they do not tell us anything, they cannot tell us to do anything either. They cannot provide us with information as to how we should act because they cannot provide us with any information at all.

I think that this argument is absolutely sound. However, it is beside the point because guides of life are not *identical* to prescriptions. Or, to put this fundamental point in other words, many things function as guides without prescribing anything. Consider the following examples.

Statements (1) and (2) are analytic in the most straightforward sense of this difficult term, i.e. they have self-contradictory denials.

(1) 'p and q' truth-functionally implies 'p'.
(2) 'p' truth-functionally implies 'p or q'.

Nevertheless each of these statements has been and will continue to be used by students of logic as a guide in the derivation of conclusions from premises. (1), for example, may be used to guide a student to 'A' from 'A and B'. The student examines the patterns of (1) and of his premiss 'A and B', and writes down 'A' as his conclusion. Because (1) is analytic, it cannot prescribe anything. But for the very same reason, it may be used as a completely reliable guide for the student's behaviour. Given 'A and B' and some instructions (including prescriptions probably) about how to use statements like (1) in demonstrations, the student knows what to do, i.e., how to act or behave with respect to 'A'. Similarly, the student would be justifiably confident that 'A or B' is one of the statements that may be validly derived from 'A' given (2). Sentence (2) is his guide to the conclusion 'A or B' from the premiss 'A' just as surely as if (2) were an honest man giving him directions verbally. But unlike the honest man, (2) is mute. It literally cannot speak; it cannot tell anyone anything.

There are many other kinds of "dumb" guides. The lines on the paper on which I am now writing have no cognitive content. Hence they are totally uninformative in any cognitive sense. But they are being relied upon as guides to keeping my written sentences more or less parallel to one another. The sights on rifles function as guides to accurate shooting. Road maps would be not only useless but self-defeating if regarded as some sort of prescriptive device. They would apparently be prescribing us to go every which way from this town to that. On the other hand, they are excellent guides. Mathematical tables of square roots, common logarithms, trigonometric ratios, etc. do not prescribe anything, but are useful guides for behaviour. We use them in order to find out what numerical expression should be plugged into this or that formula.

These examples should be sufficient to demonstrate the truth of my claim that many things function as guides without prescribing anything. Analytic statements are merely one of the kinds of things that can play the role of "dumb" guides.

Interesting as this conclusion is, it is not the only point worth making about such guides. As I mentioned in the second paragraph, some analytic statements are unquestionably better than or preferable to others. For example, suppose a student is given (1) and (2), the premiss 'A' and is asked to derive 'A or B'. (1) and (2) are both analytic, but (1) is worthless for the student's problem. (2) is better than or preferable to (1) because (2) may be used as a guide to the desired conclusion, while (1) cannot be used given the premiss 'A' and the instruction to derive 'A or B'. This is just a trivial case of a fairly common type of occurrence among students of logic. Given a whole battery of useful rules, axioms, theorems and definitions, usually only some of them are useful for a given job. Recall the frequency with which this or that complicated substitution is made in a given theorem only to find that not only has the desired theorem failed to appear but that what has appeared is farther from the desired result than some line before it. While we are carrying out the complicated substitution we are fully conscious that we must follow a certain path, we must repeat this symbol here and that one there. Exactly what this path is depends on what theorem, axiom, definition or rule we happen to be applying.

Similar remarks could be made with respect to maps, mathematical tables, various charts and graphs, etc. A completely accurate table of square roots is completely worthless as a guide to trigonometric ratios. The periodic table cannot guide our inferences in the calculus of sentences. All guides have limited applicability, and many of them have equally limited reliability. The so-called synthetic probabilistic inference rules are in the latter class. They are not only liable to yield a conclusion that is true but irrelevant, but they may well yield a false conclusion from true premises.

It might be objected that the distinction between guides and prescriptions that I have been insisting upon here is ad hoc and misleading. It is ad hoc because it is merely the result of trying to save logically true probability statements. It is misleading because the two words are usually regarded as interchangeable; so I am drawing a line where it has not existed previously. The first objection is simply false and would have been *ad hominem* at best anyhow. The second is, I think, very near the truth. The two words are usually used interchangeably. But, as I have tried to illustrate with numerous examples, they, do not have *identical* intensions or extensions. Furthermore, the differences seem to be so great that once they are brought to one's attention, it is difficult to imagine any advantage in allowing them to remain suppressed.

Chapter 10
The Morality of Cognitive Decision-Making [Ethics of Belief]

Alex C. Michalos

Introduction

In this paper an attempt is made to clarify the fairly old idea of an ethics of belief and to show that at least one plausible version of such an ethics is inescapable.

Briefly, the positive thesis defended here is that insofar as one engages in an activity designed to discover truth or to avoid falsehood one is engaged in an activity which is essentially moral in the narrow sense of the word, i.e. it is not morally neutral. After specifying the question in the next section, the cases for and against a negative ethics of belief are presented in sections "The Case for a Negative Ethics of Belief" and "The Case Against a Negative Ethics of Belief". In the "The Case for a Positive Ethics of Belief" and "The Case Against a Positive Ethics of Belief" sections the cases for and against a positive ethics of belief are developed. Following this, in section "The Case Against Any Ethics or Belief" I offer a critique of *prima facie* plausible but faulty objections to any version of an ethics of belief.

The Question

The shortest and, I suppose, the historically most familiar way to put the question I want to consider in this essay is this: Is there an ethics of belief? A longer and philosophically more lucid way to put it runs thus: Is cognitive decision-making

---

Michalos, A.C.: 1976. The morality of cognitive decision making [Ethics of Belief]. In M. Brand & D. Walton (Eds.) *The Winnipeg Conference on Action Theory* (pp. 325–340). Dordrecht: D. Reidel Copyright © 1976, D. Reidel Publishing Company, Dordrecht, Holland.

A.C. Michalos (✉)
University of Northern British Columbia, Prince George, BC, Canada
e-mail: michalos@brandonu.ca

A.C. Michalos, *Philosophical Foundations of Quality of Life*,
DOI 10.1007/978-3-319-50727-9_10

subject to moral appraisal? The extra length of the latter question will be granted immediately. Its additional lucidity will take some time to explain.

By 'cognitive decision' I mean a decision *that* something is or is not the case. For example, one might decide that two plus three is five, that the tracks in the snow were left by a beaver or that sugar is water-soluble. Such decisions are traditionally contrasted with so-called practical decisions which are decisions *to do* something or to bring something about, e.g. to swim, to write a poem or to twiddle one's thumbs.

From a psychological point of view, when one makes either kind of decision some kind of disposition or mental set is voluntarily acquired. If the decision is cognitive, one believes that something is the case. If the decision is practical, one is disposed to behave overtly in some particular way in some circumstances.

From a logical point of view, we may say that the object of a cognitive decision is a proposition and the object of a practical decision is an action.

As our basic question is put above, it might be understood as a question about the moral propriety of (a) a decision process (the input or means side of decision-making), (b) an act of deciding (the output, product or end which terminates the process), (c) holding the belief (decision that) resulting from the act, (d) the propositional content of the belief held, or (e) all of these. As we shall see shortly, our predecessors have often slipped unwittingly from (a) or (b) to (c) and back.

The question of the relation of belief to physically overt action is, I suppose, still largely open. I have argued at length elsewhere that there is a logical gap between the two which is impossible to bridge, but no one need believe that for what is to follow. Briefly there are four possibilities. One might hold that a belief can be

(1) logically independent and irrelevant to every overt action
(2) logically independent but not irrelevant to every overt action
(3) not logically independent and irrelevant to every overt action
(4) not logically independent and not irrelevant to every overt action.

The first position (1) is defended by Levi and called 'critical cognitivism'.[1] The second makes the relation of beliefs to action contingent, and this is my view (as well as Martin and Leach). The third is silly if not logically absurd, and no one I know of holds it. The fourth is a natural resting place for pragmatists and behaviouralists of one sort or another, e.g., Clifford, James, Dewey and Lewis.[2] Very often it is difficult to determine whether a given author holds a second or fourth class view and, since I think the former is more plausible than the latter, I tend to assume people want to be counted there unless they reveal some fairly explicit preference for the fourth class. At one time or another the people whose names follow 'Clifford' above all seem to have opted for the fourth view. I shall return to these options shortly.

---

[1]Levi, I., *Gambling with Truth*, Alfred A. Knopf, New York, 1967.

[2]Clifford, W. K., *Lectures and Essays*, Macmillan and Co., London, 1886. James, W., *Pragmatism*, Meridian Books, Inc., New York, 1955. Dewey, J., *Essays in Experimental Logic*, University of Chicago Press, Chicago, 1916. Lewis, C. I., *Values and Imperatives,* J. Lange (ed.), Stanford University Press, Stanford, California, 1969.

'Moral' and 'ethical', as most philosophers know, may be contrasted with their complements 'nonmoral' and 'nonethical' or with their contraries 'immoral' or 'unethical'. In the case of contraries, goodness and badness are attached to the connotations, but not in the case of complements. In the latter 'moral' is contrasted with things like political, psychological, technical and so on. C.I. Lewis divided the moral or ethical into a wider class of principles dealing with action generally and a narrower class dealing with what we usually regard as morality proper. The wider class of moral concerns seems to be coextensive with what some people call 'praxiology' nowadays.[3] At any rate, the only thing that hangs on this distinction is one's understanding of Lewis's ethics of belief. In his view "... cognitive correctness is itself a moral concern, *in the broad sense of 'moral'*."[4] (Emphasis added.). Hence, little more will be said about his view here.

It is the narrower sense of 'moral' that is of primary interest in this paper. I take it that something is morally good if and only if it is good from a (narrow) moral point of view, good on moral grounds or good for moral reasons. Such a view, such grounds or reasons would include maxims like "One ought to be fair minded and treat people fairly or justly" (Principle of Justice), "One ought to be honest and speak the truth as one sees it, deceive no one" (Principle of Honesty or Integrity), and "One ought to be or do good rather than evil" (Principle of Benevolence). We need not be concerned with the justification or the operationalization of these principles, so long as we all find them acceptable, i.e. we believe that violations are *prima facie*, at least, morally wrong. However, it should be noticed that each one is formulated as a prescription for being a certain sort of person as well as for acting in a certain way. This was done following Frankena's observation that morality concerns both character and action.[5]

One other distinction is necessary before we can lay out our central set of options. The following quotation from James will serve as an introduction.

> There are two ways of looking at our duty in the matter of opinion ... *We must know the truth*; and *we must avoid error*... they are two separable laws.... We may regard the chase

---

[3]See, for example, Kotarbinsk, T., *Praxiology: An Introduction to the Science of Efficient Action*, Pergamon Press, Oxford, 1965, and my critique 'Efficiency and Morality', *The Journal of Value Inquiry* (1972), 137–143.

[4]Lewis, op. cit., p. 163. My impression is that Price understands Locke's "ethics of belief' in this wider sense too, although I think part of the time at least Locke was concerned with the narrower sense. See, Price, H. H., *Belief*, George Allen and Unwin, Ltd., London, 1969, pp. 130–156, and Locke, J., *An Essay Concerning Human Understanding*, Vol. II, Dover Pub., Inc., New York, 1959, pp. 413–427. The following remarks by Locke p. 413 for instance, do not seem to be offered merely in the interests of efficiency or ethical action in a broad sense.

> He that believes without having any reason for believing, may be in love with his own fancies; but neither seeks truth as he ought, *nor pays the obedience due to his Maker*, who would have him use those discerning faculties he has given him, to keep him out of mistake and error. (Emphasis added.)

[5]Frankena, W. K., *Ethics*, Prentice Hall, Inc., Englewood Cliffs, 1963.

for truth as paramount … or we may, on the other hand, treat the avoidance of error as more imperative, and let truth take its chance.[6]

Roughly speaking, the distinction James is suggesting is the sort that obtains between so-called affirmative action and equal opportunity employers, or between a mother who urges her son to try to find honest work and one who tells him to at least stay out of trouble. In other words, one might subscribe to a *positive* ethical maxim of cognitive decision-making such as "One ought to pursue the truth and believe it" or a *negative* maxim such as "One ought to avoid falsehood and disbelieve (or at least withhold belief from) it." Accordingly, we have four new options. One *might* hold that there *can* be logically coherent and plausible

(1) positive and negative moral maxims of cognitive decision-making
(2) positive but not negative maxims
(3) not positive but negative maxims
(4) neither positive nor negative maxims.

Moreover, since the maxims would provide the backbone of a moral code, anyone accepting the fourth (4) position would be opposed to an ethics of belief on logical grounds and anyone favoring such an ethical system would accept one of the other three positions.

Given the five alternatives of process, terminating act, product (belief), content, all these; the three plausible views of the relation of belief to action; and the four views about maxims; we have at least 60 possible ways to answer our question. (Actually, there are more than 60, since the negative maxim cited above is divided into two distinct types later and the agnostic position mentioned parenthetically is not strictly equivalent to a negative one.) Obviously I am not going to consider all of them. Instead, I will present the cases for and against those positions which have been more or less strenuously argued by our predecessors. This way we will be able to avoid red herrings, to keep our analyses tidy and, hopefully, to satisfactorily answer the question with which we began, i.e. Is cognitive decision-making subject to moral appraisal? In short: Is there an ethics of belief?

The Case for a Negative Ethics of Belief

By the phrase 'negative ethics of belief' I mean an ethical code based on a negative maxim like "One ought to avoid falsehood and disbelieve (or at least without belief from) it" or "One ought to avoid believing anything on insufficient or inadequate evidence." Strictly speaking, these two maxims are not equivalent unless it is assumed that *the only* way to avoid falsehood is to withhold belief in propositions for which one has inadequate evidence. In fact, in W.K. Clifford's classic defense of

---

[6]James, W. *The Will to Believe and Other Essays in Popular Philosophy*, Dover Publications, New York, 1956, p. 17.

such an ethics, this assumption is frequently, if not always, made. I will say more about these maxims later.

Clifford offers several different but closely related arguments which are as intriguing as they are vague.[7] For those to be considered below, it may be assumed that the relation of belief to action is at most contingent. That is almost certainly a weaker assumption than Clifford would have preferred, but it is strong enough to do the job.[8] I also assume, though Clifford does not make the distinction, that it is *prima facie* duties or obligations that are our concern rather than duties or obligations *simpliciter*. Finally, since he pretty clearly shifts from talking about *holding* a belief to acquiring it in the first place (i.e. the act of deciding that), I will try to straighten out his views with paraphrasing. The first argument we will consider (3.1) is not sound, but it is used so often in one form or another by Clifford that it is worthwhile to get it out in the open and dispose of it. The other three arguments in this section (3.2–3.4) seem to provide good reasons for the maxim of avoiding falsehood.

Clifford's most frequently used argument runs as follows.[9]

> 3.1. Because we are social beings, beliefs tend to be held in common.
>
> For any task men pursue in common with others, each man has a moral obligation to hold up his own end.
>
> If one holds a belief on insufficient evidence, one neglects that duty.
>
> To neglect a duty is to violate the Principle of Justice. Hence, it is morally wrong to hold a belief on insufficient evidence.

Clifford spells out the first premise of 3.1 thus:

> And no one man's belief is in any case a private matter which concerns himself alone. Our lives are guided by that general conception of the course of things which has been created by society for social purposes. Our words, our phrases, our forms and processes and modes of thought, are common property, fashioned and perfected from age to age; an heirloom which every succeeding generation inherits as a precious deposit and a sacred trust to be handed on to the next one, not unchanged but enlarged and purified, with some clear marks of its proper handiwork.[10]

Ignoring the flowery parts of this passage, it seems unobjectionable as do the first, second and fourth premises. It is really only the third premise that might create problems. Why should holding a belief on insufficient evidence count as neglecting one's duty to contribute a fair share of the labour necessary to sustain a collective good? Presumably what is required here is the assumption that the structure of

---

[7]Clifford, W. K., 'The Ethics of Belief', *op. cit.*, pp. 339–363.

[8]"Nor is that truly a belief at all" he writes "which has not some influence upon the actions of him who holds it." *Ibid.*, p. 342.

[9]A form of it appears on pages 342 and 344 in 'The Ethics of Belief', and also in James, *op. cit.*, p. 140 and in V. Tomas (ed.), *Charles S. Peirce Essays in the Philosophy of Science,* The Liberal Arts Press, New York, 1957, p. 16.

[10]Clifford, *loc. cit.*, pp. 342–343.

beliefs held by a community is bonded together by sufficient evidence also held jointly. Then, anyone holding a belief without sufficient evidence would, as it were, be guilty of trying to hold only the structure without holding the foundation too. Altering our metaphor slightly, imagine a tent held up by several people with one hand on ropes holding the roof on and the other hand on ropes holding the floor taut. Then one who dropped his floor rope would be guilty of jeopardizing the shape of the tent. Similarly, one who holds beliefs on insufficient evidence only does part of what one is required to do to keep the total shape of our beliefs intact.

Plausible as this argument may sound, I think it is question-begging insofar as it requires the assumption that the structure of beliefs held by a community must be bonded together by sufficient evidence—held jointly or not. To see that this is so, one need only ask: Why is sufficient evidence required to bond the structure of beliefs together? Why not merely some significant evidence or, indeed, some nonevidential reason like faith or hope? That, of course, is roughly the sort of question James put to Clifford in 'The Will to Believe'. Clifford would be assuming here precisely what has to be demonstrated, namely, that if one has a good reason for believing any proposition to be true then one must have sufficient evidence for it, i.e. sufficient evidence is *the only* warrant for believing a proposition is true.

Another argument suggested by Clifford arises from the following.

> Habitual want of care about what I believe leads to habitual want of care in others about the truth of what is told me.[11]

That is,

> 3.2. When one is careless about the reasons one has for the beliefs one holds, others tend to become careless about the reasons for the views they express toward one.
>
> As others become careless, they tend to supply one with falsehoods so one becomes surrounded by "a thick atmosphere of falsehood and fraud".
>
> To surround a person with "falsehood and fraud" is to violate the Principle of Honesty. Hence, it is morally wrong to be careless about the reasons one has for the beliefs one holds.

Beginning with the first two premises of 3.2, Clifford also suggests the following finish.

> 3.3. To encourage others to surround a person with "falsehood and fraud" is to violate the Principle of Benevolence.
>
> Hence, it is morally wrong to be careless about the reasons one has for the beliefs one holds.

The difference between 3.2 and 3.3 is that the former focuses on the evil of drowning a person in "falsehood and fraud" while the latter focuses on the evil of encouraging people to perform such an act. It's wrong to do it and to help people to do it.

---

[11] *Ibid.*, p. 345.

Although I have not run any controlled experiments to determine whether the effects posited in the first premise of 3.2 and 3.3 occur always, usually or hardly ever, casual observation seems to suggest that the effects occur often enough not to be swiftly discounted. There is, of course, a lot of evidence on the pressures for and likelihood of individual conformity to group norms which is at least indirect support for this premise.[12] The second premise is also basically empirical, though it presupposes that in fact careless thinkers have more false beliefs than careful thinkers. If this is not true, then one of the main prudential reasons one might have for being a careful thinker is lost. I presume it is true. Similarly, I presume the final premises of 3.2 and 3.3 are unobjectionable.

Again, Clifford argues[13]

3.4. Insofar as one holds beliefs dogmatically one is less inclined to give issues a fair hearing.

Insofar as one is less inclined to give issues a fair hearing one is inclined to violate the Principle of Justice.

Hence, it is morally wrong to hold beliefs dogmatically.

As the first premise is formulated, it is virtually analytic. To hold beliefs dogmatically is just to automatically reject contrary views and arguments, and that is certainly not compatible with fairness. Unless one insists that 'fair-mindedness' can only apply to the adjudication of conflicting interests among people, the second premise is also unobjectionable. I should think, however, that the burden of proof would be on the insister in this case. Accordingly, the conclusion of 3.4 strikes me as true.

A couple of pages later Clifford asserts that "Every time we *let ourselves believe* for unworthy reasons, we weaken our powers of self-control, of doubting, of judicially and fairly weighing evidence."[14] (Emphasis added.). This suggests a variant of 3.4 in which the error is not in holding the belief but in deciding that it is true, i.e. in voluntarily acquiring it.

The Case Against a Negative Ethics of Belief

As indicated earlier, William James sought to discredit what he took to be Clifford's position. In fact, as I also insisted, Clifford unwittingly presented arguments in defense of at least two different basic maxims for a negative ethics of belief. Furthermore, as will be explained shortly, it is only the maxim linking belief to

---

[12]See, for example, Hare, A. P., Borgatta, E. F., and Bales, R. F. (eds.), *Small Groups,* Alfred A. Knopf, New York, 1966.

[13]Clifford, *loc. cit.,* p. 342.

[14]*Ibid.,* pp. 344–345.

sufficient evidence that James opposes, not the maxim against belief in falsehoods. In the following passage James suggests three reasons for finding

> ... it impossible to go with Clifford. We must remember that these feelings of our duty about either truth or error are in any case only expressions of our passional life ... he who says 'Better go without belief forever than believe a lie!' merely shows his own preponderant private horror of becoming a dupe ... but I can believe that worse things than being duped may happen to a man in this world: so Clifford's exhortation has to my ears a thoroughly fantastic sound. ... In a world where we are so certain to incur errors in spite of all our caution, a certain lightness of heart seems healthier than this excessive nervousness on their behalf.[15]

The first suggestion, that "these feelings of our duty" are "only expressions of our passional life" seems to be tantamount to the admission that we have reached a level of analysis at which the giving of reasons necessarily gives way to the expression of attitudes. That hardly seems plausible even to James, since he does try to present reasons for his view. His second suggestion is that considering the evils which may fall upon a person in this world, believing a falsehood is among the least of our worries. I suppose this should only be taken relativistically (even assuming a contingent relation between belief and action), since the consequences of some beliefs turning out false might be the overturning of one's whole orientation toward life, one's whole *Weltanschauung*, and that could be serious indeed. Finally, he suggests that we are so prone to error that one ought to maintain "a certain lightness of heart" toward it—rather than become what Lyndon Johnson used to call "a nervous Nellie". I imagine neither James nor anyone else knows how prone to error most people are, but again, I would think that the claim must be taken relativistically at best.

Taking these arguments together, I do not think we get to the heart of James's position. The latter comes out most clearly in the following passages.

> There are ... cases where a fact cannot come at all unless a preliminary faith exists in its coming. *And where faith in a fact can help create the fact*, that would be an insane logic which should say that faith running ahead of scientific evidence is the 'lowest kind of immorality' into which a thinking being can fall. ... *A rule of thinking which would absolutely prevent me from acknowledging certain kinds of truth if those kinds of truth were really there, would be an irrational rule.*[16]

Thus, for example, one cannot have trusted friends unless one believes that they are trustworthy without sufficient evidence, i.e. without evidence that would guarantee their fidelity. Since a maxim proscribing belief on insufficient evidence

---

[15] James, *The Will to Believe*, pp. 17–19.

[16] *Ibid.*, pp. 25–28. The single quoted phrase is a reference to a quotation from T. Huxley which James cites on page 7 without telling us where it comes from. "... Huxley exclaims:" according to James "My only consolation lies in the reflection that, however bad our posterity may become, so far as they hold by the plain rule of not pretending to believe what they have no reason to believe, because it may be to their advantage so to pretend [the word 'pretend' is surely here redundant], they will not have reached the lowest depth of immorality.".

would "absolutely prevent" one from deciding that a friend was trustworthy without serious testing, such a maxim should be rejected.

What James has hit upon in this passage is a species of prudential or pragmatic reasoning leading to *belief.* Schematically it might be represented thus:

Pragmatic Schema

1. $p \left\{ \begin{array}{l} \text{only if} \\ \text{usually only if} \\ \text{probably only if} \end{array} \right\}$ *X* believes that *p*.
2. *X* would like it to be the case that *p*.
3. So, *X* believes that *p*.

This pragmatic schema is roughly similar to traditional maxims of practical reasoning, e.g.

> If ϕing is (usually, probably) a necessary condition of it being the case that *p* and *X* wants the latter, then *X* ought (rationally, prudentially) to ϕ.

For example,

> If believing that I can outrun Newberry is (usually, probably) a necessary condition of my being able to outrun him, and I want to be able to outrun him, then I ought (rationally, prudentially) to believe that I can.

However, the conclusion of our schema is not that one *ought to do* something, but that one believes something. Although the premises do, I think, provide good grounds for the practical conclusion, it is the cognitive conclusion that is most interesting. For here we have not evidential (e.g. straight deductive or (narrowly) inductive) grounds for believing that something is the case, but purely pragmatic, prudential or teleological grounds. We have good reasons for belief, but not good evidence! And that I find at once exciting and frightening. It is exciting because such grounds have been almost entirely neglected by epistemologists so far as I know,[17] and it is frightening because God knows *what* one might have good pragmatic reasons for believing. I wish I could pursue all the niceties of pragmatic schemata with you now, but that is both beyond me and the plan of this paper. So I will return directly to James.

---

[17]The so-called pragmatic justification or vindication of induction supported by men like Feigl, Kneale and Reichenbach could be regarded as a special case of the general pragmatic line of argumentation schematized above or of ordinary practical reason. For an analysis of pragmatic justification see Salmon, W. C., 'Should We Attempt to Justify Induction?', *Philosophical Studies,* 1957, pp. 33–48, and for a review of ordinary practical reasoning schemata see Rescher, N., *Introduction to Value Theory,* Prentice-Hall, Inc., Englewood Cliffs, 1969.

What surprises me about James's approach here is that he does not try to rest his case on moral grounds, following Clifford, for instance. Instead, he complains that it would be "an insane logic" and an "irrational rule" which would proscribe belief without sufficient evidence. But why, after all, isn't it just plain morally wrong to prevent people from deciding that their friends or indeed, their fellow citizens are trustworthy prior to tests? "Don't trust anyone until he has proven worthy," is the sort of maxim which, if followed, would virtually destroy the social fabric of any community. One must trust the butcher not to color the meat, the doctor to conscientiously prescribe therapy, the mechanic to fix exactly what is broken, the teacher to try to put decent ideas into our kids heads, and so on. Without such trust there can be no community, no social or moral life, no friendship and no love. A maxim with these consequences must be pronounced morally offensive, and that seems to be as strong an objection as one could raise against it.

In James's final shot against the negative maxim, he says

> … if we believe that no bell in us tolls to let us know for certain when truth is in our grasp, then it seems a piece of idle fantasticality to preach so solemnly our duty of waiting for the bell.[18]

In other words, there is no *logical* point in proscribing the acceptance of beliefs on insufficient evidence because no one knows when evidence really is sufficient. One might as well tell people not to believe anything at all or, on the contrary, to believe whatever they damn well please.

Although I think it must be admitted that there is no single, all purpose, sure-fire criterion of sufficiency for evidence, it is hardly the case that we are entirely at sea in this area. For all sorts of everyday occurrences as well as scientific research and judicial proceedings we are able to reach widespread agreement about what counts as sufficient evidence. Case by case, the problems are by no means insurmountable, although in general and in the abstract they may be.

The Case for a Positive Ethics of Belief

Briefly and roughly the conclusion reached in the preceding two sections is that there is a negative ethics of belief, i.e. cognitive decision-making can be morally right or good, wrong or bad. Furthermore, it was shown that James clearly saw that there is a difference between such a view and what I have called a positive ethics of belief, and he evidently opted for the latter. From what was said in the preceding section and the following remarks we may formulate the sort of argument he would want to use.

> The importance to human life of having true beliefs about matters of fact is a thing too notorious. We live in a world of realities that can be infinitely useful or infinitely harmful.

[18] *Ibid.*, p. 30.

> Ideas that tell us which of them to expect count as the true ideas in all this primary sphere of verification, and *the pursuit of such ideas is a primary human duty*. The possession of truth, so far from being here an end in itself, is only a preliminary means towards other vital satisfactions. … *Our obligation to seek truth* is part of our general obligation to do what pays. (Emphasis added.)[19]

That is,

> We have a moral obligation to try to preserve human life.
>
> "The possession of truth … is only a preliminary means …" toward that end.
>
> The pursuit of truth is often if not always necessary for its possession.
>
> Hence, "the pursuit of such ideas is a primary human duty".

In short we are obliged to pursue that course of action which, often enough, is necessary to obtain a morally prescribed end.

The first premise of this argument follows immediately from the universally recognised Right to Life. The second premise strikes me just about as it struck James, namely as "a thing too notorious". The third premise is phrased as it is to avoid the objection that one might after all just stumble upon the truth. Of course one might, but I do not believe that is the usual or most promising way to find it. Given these premises then, there does not seem to be any escape from the conclusion. That is, James has given us one good reason to accept a positive ethics of belief.

As James laments elsewhere, he and other pragmatists paid dearly for all their references to payments, cash value, practical consequences, working and utility. The cost, he suggests, was in the form of the "solemn attribution of… rubbish to us .. .".[20] I will not review the literature on the nature of the pay-offs actually or usually envisioned by pragmatists generally or James in particular. However, I should point out that if the reference to payment in the last sentence of the quoted paragraph above is understood in terms of the preservation of human life, then that sentence is roughly only a truncated version of the argument set out for him.

Another argument in favor of a positive ethics of belief runs as follows.

> If there is a moral obligation to speak the truth as one sees it then there is a similar obligation to try to see it as it is.
>
> There is a moral obligation to speak the truth as one sees it (Principle of Honesty).
>
> Hence, there is a moral obligation to pursue the truth, i.e. to try to see the world as it is.

This argument clearly stands or falls with the first premise. Suppose it is false. If one has no obligation to try to find the truth, then the obligation to speak the truth is pointless. "Believe whatever you like for whatever reasons you like but always say what you believe" is a silly commandment because there is no virtue, intellectual or moral, in speaking falsehoods or in some kinds of reasons. That is, not all reasons

---

[19]James, *Pragmatism,* pp. 134 and 150.

[20]James, W. *The Meaning of Truth: A Sequel to 'Pragmatism'*, Longmans, Green and Co., New York, 1909, p. 212.

are good reasons and not everything one likes is worth sharing. Thus, an unconditioned command to say whatever you believe cannot be a moral maxim, though it may be great for psychotherapy. Consequently, the first premise of this argument must be accepted and with it, the argument itself.

The Case Against a Positive Ethics of Belief

It might be argued that because, for example, a little philosophy makes one an atheist or at least an agnostic, one has no obligation to pursue the truth. Better to be a dogmatic believer than a doubter or a disbeliever! I do not doubt at all that one could imagine cases in which blatant dogmatism has better short run results (maybe even long run results) that are preferable to the results of disbelief or agnosticism. But to admit that is to admit nothing more than that the obligations and duties we are discussing are necessarily *prima facie* in character. There is a big step from this to the conclusion that we have a *prima facie* obligation to be dogmatic *because* sometimes dogmatism has more benefits than costs. If that line of argumentation were accepted then we would have similar obligations to lie and steal as well. In fact, the moral realm would be turned virtually up-side down. Accordingly, I reject this line without reservation.

The Case Against Any Ethics of Belief

At this point everything that I have to say in favor of an ethics of belief based on a negative and a positive maxim has been said. In the remaining paragraphs of this section then, I will present *prima facie* plausible objections to the position defended above and try to show that they are unacceptable.

7.1. The idea of an ethics of belief or of cognitive decision-making being moral or immoral is just so much self-serving sop. Only an academic mind or worse, a philosophic mind, would seriously entertain the notion that deciding that something is the case or holding on to a belief once acquired could be a moral act. No one else would be inclined to try to get moral credit for thinking straight.

Reply. This objection is obviously just an *argumentum ad hominem*. Of course an ethics of belief would have special relevance for academics of all kinds, philosophers, scientists or whatever. But that does not make the idea true or false, sound or silly. Our critics will have to aim higher.

7.2. Suppose it is granted for the sake of argument that there is, as some ancient philosophers might say, moral virtue in intellectual virtue. It still would not follow that cognitive decisions are moral or immoral. Recall, for example,

Lewis's view that the sense of 'moral' involved is wide rather than narrow. Alternatively, consider the following remarks by Thomas Aquinas.

> Other intellectual virtues [wisdom, science and art] can, but prudence cannot, be without moral virtue. The reason for this is that prudence is right reason about things to be done, and this not merely in general, but also in the particular, where action takes place. ... Consequently ... in order that he be rightly disposed with regard to the particular principles of action, viz., the ends, he needs to be perfected by certain habits, whereby it becomes connatural to man, as it were, to judge rightly about the end. This is done by moral virtue, for the virtuous man judges rightly of the end of virtue, because *such as a man is, such does the end seem to him.* Consequently the right reason about things to be done, viz., *prudence,* requires man to have moral virtue.[21]

In other words, Aquinas holds that morality can play a role in decision-making only insofar as beliefs are related to overt actions, i.e. only in the realm of what he calls 'prudence'. In that realm there *is* moral virtue in intellectual virtue, but that is only possible because the decisions made are not merely cognitive.[22]

Reply. Aquinas's view may be true, but it is question-begging to merely assert it in this manner. After all, what has to be shown is *not* that one can classify so-called intellectual virtues so that cognitive decisions never have any moral import, but that such a classification does justice to all the relevant facts or arguments. This sort of a justification has not been provided.

7.3. If cognitive decision-making has moral import then all good scientists, philosophers and mathematicians must be morally good. Ho, Ho, Ho! If that doesn't destroy the thesis once and for all, what else can?

Reply. This argument is a *non-sequitur.* One might just as well argue that anyone who performs lots of morally good actions is morally good. What if he is also performing lots of morally bad actions on the side? For example, he might be murdering people for money and giving all the money to his favorite charity. Or, what if he performs lots of morally good but trivial actions and one or two morally horrendous and highly significant actions? For example, he might regularly pay his grocery bills until one day he murders his grocer and every one else in the store. Clearly, the first premise of 7.3 will have to be tightened up in order to have any plausibility. Thus,

7.4. If cognitive decision-making has moral import then a mathematician doing his sums correctly (with no inclination or opportunity to share his results with others) is doing something that is morally right or good. That is, granted that he is not neglecting some duty or doing anything else on the side which is morally reprehensible, we must say that there is moral virtue in what he is doing. That is just an outrageous departure from common sense and ordinary

---

[21] *Basic Writings of Saint Thomas Aquinas,* Vol. II, A. C. Pegis (ed.), Random House, New York, 1945, p. 447.

[22] This is how E. Gilson interprets Aquinas too in *The Christian Philosophy of St. Thomas Aquinas,* Victor Gollancz Ltd., London, 1957, pp. 260–261.

usage. Imagine trying to persuade a man on the street that an accountant correctly multiplying 3728 by 261 is doing something that is as morally significant as telling his neighbour the true product!

Reply. In fact, of course, the last sentence is misleading. Insofar as both acts have moral significance they are in the same class, but it does not follow that each act has the same amount of moral virtue. The fact that all moral acts are praiseworthy does not imply that they are all equally praiseworthy. Whether or not finding the correct product would be as morally praiseworthy as truthfully giving the information to one's neighbor is a debatable question. Would giving the information to a total stranger merit more praise than giving it to a friend? I don't think one can answer such questions without considerable development of the cases.

For its relevance, if not for the sheer beauty of the prose, the following passage for Ferdinand Lundberg's classic *The Rich and the Super-Rich* is worth repeating.

> ... in the process of being educated there is always the danger that the individual will acquire scruples, a fact dimly sensed by some of the neo-conservatives who rail against the school system as "Communistic". These scruples, unless they are casuistically beveled around the edges with great care, are a distinct handicap to the full-fledged money-maker, who must in every situation be plastically opportunistic. But a person who has had it deeply impressed upon him that he must make *exact* reports of *careful* laboratory experiments, must conduct *exact* computations in mathematics and logic, must produce *exact* translations and echoes of foreign languages, must write *faithful* reports or *correct* readings and must be at least imaginatively aware of the world in its diversity, and who has learned these lessons well, must invariably discover that some element of scrupulosity — even if he hasn't been subject to moral indoctrination — has been impressed on his psyche. If he enters upon money-making in a world bazaar where approximate truths, vague deceptions, sneak maneuvers, half promises and even bald falsehoods are the widely admired and heavily rewarded order of the day he must make casuistic adjustments of his standards. The very process of laboriously making the adjustment, even if he succeeds, puts him at a disadvantage *vis-á-vis* the unschooled, who need waste no energy on such adjustments, who pick up anything lying around loose as easily as they breath. Some educated people can't make even a partial adjustment to the market bazaar, and their disgraceful bank accounts show it. They are, as even their wives sometimes kindly inform them, failures, though they are doing something conceded to be useful such as instructing children or enforcing the law. They can inscribe after their names a big "F" and go stand in a corner under a dunce cap as the propaganda dervishes scream about success.[23]

The rest of 7.4 is straightforward, but answerable. If one believes, as I and many others do, that it is logically possible to, say, dedicate one's life to learning and leave the comfort of human communities (with all that such a severance implies) and be or become a good person by doing just that, then there is nothing outrageous or extraordinary about the thesis being defended here. In short, if hermits can be morally good and can continue to perform morally praiseworthy acts in their hermitage, then the thesis of the moral significance of cognitive decision-making must be not only logically coherent but true as well.

[23]Lundberg, Ferdinand, *The Rich and the Super-Rich*, Bantam Books, New York, 1968, pp. 107–108.

7.5. As Campbell pointed out a while ago, no amount of nonmoral value can be added to produce moral value.[24] That means one cannot be morally praiseworthy or blameworthy for cognitive decision-making.

Reply. On some views of the nature of moral and nonmoral value, the former is constructed out of the latter. "Teleological theories" Frankena tells us "... make the right, the obligatory, and the morally good dependent on the nonmorally good."[25] Thus, considerably more than is said in 7.5 would have to be said in order to sustain the objection.

Conclusion

If the preceding analysis has been accurate then the answer to the question "Is cognitive decision-making subject to moral appraisal?" or "Is there an ethics of belief?" in the sense specified above is: Yes.[26]

[24]Campbell, C. A., 'Moral and Non-Moral Values: A Study in the First Principles of Axiology', *Mind* (1935).

[25]Frankena, *op. cit.*, p. 13.

[26]Several people have given me advice about this paper and I would like to thank them: Myles Brand, Charles Goodbrand, David Hall, William Hughes, Margaret Kumagai, John Leslie, Michael Martin, Jay Newman and Douglas Odegard, Ray Panavas.

Chapter 11
Meeting Current Needs

Alex C. Michalos

The latest book by one of Canada's most distinguished philosophers has been in the works for some time. So it is fitting that the Canadian Philosophical Association should have devoted a special symposium to David Braybrooke's *Meeting Needs* in our 1987 annual meeting. An earlier version of the review that follows was presented at that symposium and has benefitted from some replies from Braybrooke. As one might have expected, as we parted company after that symposium, we still had some fundamental disagreements.

Social indicators are statistics that are supposed to have some significance for the quality of people's lives. Researchers working in this field distinguish so-called objective indicators like crime rates, educational achievement rates, mortality rates and so on from so-called subjective indicators or personal reports of things like satisfaction and happiness with life as a whole, marital satisfaction, job satisfaction and so on. Since the social indicators movement began in the mid sixties, there have always been people who regard needs as relatively objective, relatively objectively measurable and relatively attractive as a starting point to develop a list of relatively objective social indicators. Many people have appealed to Maslow's work on a hierarchy of needs and have found his framework helpful for organizing their thoughts on the development of indicators. Most of the people who have appealed to a concept of needs have not been very concerned about providing a logically tidy definition. Indeed, much of the attraction of the idea of needs has been the belief that the idea is uncontroversial, that people like Maslow have produced a generally acceptable definition and that a social indicators research programme would be launched on relatively solid ground by proceeding from needs.

David Braybrooke, Meeting Needs (Princeton, NJ: Princeton University Press, 1987), pp. 344, $35.00, $12.50 paper. Page references are to this work.

Michalos, A.C.: 1988. Meeting current needs. Dialogue, 27, pp. 507–515.

A.C. Michalos (✉)
University of Northern British Columbia, Prince George, BC, Canada
e-mail: michalos@brandonu.ca

A.C. Michalos, *Philosophical Foundations of Quality of Life*,
DOI 10.1007/978-3-319-50727-9_11

Needless to say, most of the people working in the field of social indicators are not philosophers and most of them have no idea of how much ink has been shed on concepts of need, on distinctions between needing, wanting, preferring, choosing, deciding, on logical and normative implications obtaining among these ideas and others related to ethics and social/political policy, and so on. I have looked at a lot of the philosophical literature and have added some pages to it myself in my *Foundations of Decision-Making*.[1] After explaining my proposed definition of course-of-life and adventitious needs following Braybrooke's lead a decade earlier, I said that

> One of the reasons that people engaged in arguments about wants have a tendency to try to pass off their wants as needs is that the latter are generally supposed to involve more serious and inescapable hardships when they are not met. Hence, their appeals are strengthened. But one of the reasons such manoeuvres can typically be successfully repelled is that needs cannot be defined without making assumptions about what are to count as equilibria states and excessive departures from them. *Thus, appeals to needs tend to generate the same sorts of haggles that are generated by appeals to wants* (*FDM*, 37, emphasis added).

After reading Braybrooke's book, I would add to that last remark: If you do not believe me, read Braybrooke's book on needs. And to David, I must say: I told you so.

In a few places Braybrooke tells us that he is trying to give us an account of "the concept of needs" which makes explicit its usage in English (77–78). He typically talks about "the" concept rather than "a" concept. He wants to give us an account which he regards as a set of hypotheses about the common usage of the concept (62–63). He also says he is primarily interested in the normative use of the concept to assess social policy (7–8). He does not want to define a concept but to give an account of its use (77–78). I think he has successfully captured most of the complications, nuances and implications of a concept of needs familiar to most people. I am sure he has given us a more thorough analysis than anyone else has of an idea of needs, and I am sure he has anticipated most of the general and particular criticisms that will be raised against the project. Indeed, after every chapter he gives us a brief dialogue between a critical reader and a not-yet-repentant author in which most of my own criticisms are found and answered, not persuasively of course, but answered.

I certainly would not "reject the concept of needs" now any more than I would have before I read this book. However, I am even more convinced now than I was before I read this book that no appeal to a concept of needs is going to solve any social or political problem. Where issues are controversial, appeals to needs will simply be mired in the controversy, and where issues are not controversial it does not matter if appeals to needs are made or not. Moreover, as an empirical hypothesis, I would suggest that David has the cart before the horse regarding needs talk. That is, I suspect that appeals to needs tend to look effective in just those cases

---

[1]Alex C. Michalos, *Foundations of Decision-Making* (Ottawa: Canadian Library of Philosophy, 1978). Hereafter cited as *FDM*.

where agreement can be reached about what is to be done, what should be possessed or what is to be provided. Put another way, I suspect that people negotiate what it is they think should be the case for whatever reason and then they describe that as what is needed. So, what David regards as successful appeals to needs or successful working of the concept I suspect is at least as often a kind of official sealing of a negotiated agreement. The sequence is not typically: x needs y, we discover that x needs y, therefore we say that x should have y. Rather, it is: we think that x should have y, therefore we say x needs y. Perhaps even more typically: x wants y, therefore x says y is needed. For examples, the Mulroney government has argued for the need to de-index pensions, to cut back unemployment benefits, to allow the pharmaceutical industry to have greater profits, and to privatize relatively profitable Crown Corporations. All of these alleged needs (and many more examples could be given), it seems to me, are simply ideological desiderata of Progressive Conservatives.

The only claims about needs that are epistemically warranted are those that are negotiated according to the practices, principles, methods, beliefs, etc., of some community of people. These epistemic practices, principles, etc., as social studies of science continue to show, are loaded with a variety of social, political, cultural and ideological features. The only claims about needs that can be assumed as non-controversial are those that have been properly warranted. Hence, the only claims about needs that might provide Braybrooke or similarly inclined social indicators researchers with a set of relatively non-controversial building blocks for social and political policy making are all and only those which have already survived suitable value-laden, theory-laden epistemic substantiation. In such cases, of course "the concept of needs works well" when it works at all to oil the wheels of negotiated settlements, but its work consists merely in giving a name to an accomplished fact, not to producing or even revealing the fact. It is useful and beneficial for people to be able to signify some kinds of negotiated agreements by calling some things needs or by saying that this or that is needed. However, if the argument I have just given is sound, it is a mistake to claim that the concept of needs has some important substantive role to play in the formation of a relatively non-controversial and relatively objective set of basic agreements regarding social and political policy making. The concept is useful at the output side rather than the input side of policy making.

So much for generalities. Now I would like to make some detailed remarks about various claims in the book in order to substantiate my charge that Braybrooke has taken a notoriously messy idea or group of ideas related to the word "need" and, metaphorically speaking, picked an unsightly pimple into a raging case of acne.

In various places he talks about needs, wants, preferences, wishes and interests as if these are different things, but he only defines needs. There is a list of needs, a criterion for generating some new needs and the repeated assumption that needs take precedence over preferences, but no definition of preferences. It appears as if "preferences" simply functions as a name for things that in principle can always be justifiably over-ridden by things called "needs". But he grants that some preferences can be more important to people than some needs. So, it would be helpful to have a definition of needs that might allow one to see exactly why preferences are subordinate to needs. More importantly, as I said in my *FDM,* one cannot tell how good one's explication of a concept is when it is defined in isolation. If we all knew what we all meant by the key words he uses, like needs, wants, preferences, etc., then there would be no need for or point to providing definitions. But we do not know any more about the others than we do about needs. So what we have is a package of ideas about needs which may not fit well with careful definitions of wants, preferences and so on when equally thorough definitions of the latter are given.

We are told his list of basic needs is necessarily incomplete. However, it includes #6, "the need (beyond what is covered under the preceding needs) for whatever is indispensable to preserving the body intact in important respects" (36). That does cover everything that will ever come up related to the body, and I wonder why he did not just generalize it to whatever is indispensable to preserving people intact in important respects. I also wonder why the need for sexual activity gets put into the pot of things governments are supposed to provide for citizens (36). Granted that some inmates of some prisons have sometimes been allowed to have sexual activities (as Braybrooke noted in the symposium), it is unlikely that anyone suddenly discovered that people have a need for sex. I appreciate sexual activity as much as anyone and would rank it very high on my list of things important to a good life, but it hardly measures up to food, water and oxygen as a need. Or does it? There is a problem here regarding a shift from talking about what is needed for a relatively typical life (species-wise, culture-wise, etc.) to talking about what is needed for a relatively good life (species-wise, culture-wise, etc.). What is needed *ought* to be possessed at least in order to have a good instance of a type and at most in order to have a good instance of an ideal type (which is, as an ideal, good). In either case, someone has to evaluate something and get others to agree in order to talk persuasively about what is needed. Well, as I said, one can always haggle about what is needed.

The criterion used to determine what is needed is roughly what is required to allow one to perform the basic social roles of parent, householder, worker and citizen such that one's performance or functioning is not "deranged" (48). Braybrooke is aware that roles vary for individuals and cultures, but he still stays with these sociologically constructed definitions of needs (58–59). At this point in his account he seems to let language and roles do the work of people making decisions under constraints and with certain aims in view. His general approach is to try to draw relatively objectively specifiable needs out of language and roles which he seems to regard as relatively objective too. Having a concept of needs implies who has what needs, and average people who speak English have a concept of needs (38–39). It is fairly naive ordinary language philosophy. Hard questions about who really speaks the language, what features have been built in, what concepts with what biases, serving what purposes are part of the language, etc., are just ignored. It would not be so troublesome if only philosophy were at stake, but Braybrooke wants to make public policy out of common usage, wants to get recommendations about who needs what on the basis of how some of us construe the language. That could be dangerous. Given the notoriously male-biased language that we use and the science springing up comfortably along side it through the years, that could be, as it has been, especially dangerous for women.

Besides having basic needs relativized to people's language, they are also relativized to "available resources" (59–60). We are not told what it means to be available or a resource in this context, but available seems to mean that the resource can (in every sense of this ambiguous term) be used right now by the people deciding who needs what. Relativizing needs to available resources is a radical departure from any reasonable usage of the term needs. It tends to make his further assumption more plausible, namely, that if someone says x needs y then the same someone has accepted responsibility for providing y for x. But I find the latter assumption completely implausible. Consider the latter assumption.

Braybrooke has a Principle of Precedence which says that needs take precedence over preferences. He holds that if someone accepts the principle then that person accepts some responsibility for meeting the needs referred to for some reference population (61). But no argument is given for this claim. When I test it against my Cleveland/Chicago/Guelph English usage (now there is a splendid basis for public policy), I find it false. There were other claims of this sort that I found questionable but Braybrooke claimed in the symposium that he never made. So I am happy to abandon those objections. However, I would like to hear how he reconciles his claim on 91 that x could need y without anyone conceptualizing it *with* his claim that x needs y means that someone has the concept and attributes the need to x, which seems to be his main position.

Braybrooke claims that one advantage needs have over preferences is that the former do not involve any aggregation problems. Once things are defined as needs, he says, "the tendency is to put them beyond politics" (67). The most cursory inspection of what issues are debated in the House of Commons, in our provincial legislatures and in the news media reveals that practically all the politicking is over who needs what compared to who needs what else. To let a single case do the job of many here, consider the Halifax group known as Mothers United for Metropolitan Shelter (MUMS). Everyone knows people need shelter and most Haligonians know Halifax has too few housing facilities for relatively poor single parent mothers and their families. The various levels of government in Nova Scotia have refused to provide the needed housing. Their arguments are typically that there are other needs more pressing. Governments typically argue that there are always more needs than can be provided for. They typically provide less than most people think is needed. I do not have the numbers in front of me, but if you look at the yearly Gallup polls asking Canadians what a family of four needs to live on and look at what the several governments together provide, you will find that poor Canadians do not get what most Canadians think the poor Canadians need. The NDP typically argues for greater subsidies for those in need, while the Tories typically claim either that the needy have their needs met or that other needs are at least as pressing. So, the NDP and the Tories spend a lot of time arguing about exactly what is needed and what must be provided by whom for what reason. It is only in some philosophical treatises where needs are regarded as beyond politics.

The conceptualization of needs is essentially related to social arrangements, politics and conventions (83–99). But Braybrooke still thinks such ideas have some special political bite. He claims that social arrangements can be ruled out by applying his list of basic needs (86–87). Even if this is true, it does not imply that the list is prior to politics or enjoys some sort of a priori, relatively objective status. Warranted lists, again, have to be negotiated by a community, with all that such negotiation implies. In particular, the acceptability of lists floats on a sea of negotiated epistemic agreements as indicated above. So social arrangements never confront naked, unsocialized lists any more than individual persons nakedly confront naked facts. That much Kant and the later pragmatists got right.

At one point Braybrooke asserts that the stronger the convention concerning a defined need, the better the case for the need (103). Again, this just commits him to a radical relativization of needs.

On page 111 we read that the concept of needs always wears normative vestments. My own understanding of the use of the word "need" indicates that there is a relatively non-normative and a normative use. Most of the people working in medical and bioethics seem to assume and argue for a notion of needs that is essentially normative, like Braybrooke has and I did in my *FDM*. But some people (including notably some working in bioethics) hold the view that, although x needs y implies that without y x will not have something that most other members in x's class or of x's type have, such absences do not entail any evaluative status. Instead of saying what most of us say, namely, that x will suffer some deterioration (an obvious evaluation), they simply say that x without y will, for example, vary from the statistical average of x's type by more than two standard deviations or something like that. Maybe from x's point of view such a deviation would be regarded as a deterioration, as bad, and calling for improvement, etc. Maybe from some interested biologist's or ecologist's point of view similar evaluations might be made. Still, it is not necessary for any particular person's or group's definition of a need to carry the same evaluative baggage that most of ours carries. Although it is no criticism of Braybrooke's account that it does involve evaluation essentially, it is worthwhile to point out that there is an alternative, allegedly non-evaluative notion of needs in circulation that merits some consideration and is not considered in this book.

Braybrooke grants that as a result of conventions, social arrangements, derivations and other things there may be interminable fruitless disputation about needs (118). But when he tells us how he intends to "deal" with such problems, he seems to deal with them by giving away the store. He says we must regard his list, minimum standards provision, criterion and principle of precedence (i.e., virtually his whole theory or set of hypotheses, as he called them) as a "schema capable of more expansive use". In more than one place he became so laid back about his account and so amenable to "expansion" that I wondered if there was any point to it. Even "strict final priority" (i.e., these needs must take precedence) in appeals to needs gives way to "role-relative precautionary priority" (i.e., these needs conditionally must take priority) as he tries to provide an account that is more realistic. But, like his imaginary reader who admits to becoming dizzy (127) with all the comings and goings of this and that feature of his account, I suspect Braybrooke's baby is deep in the drain even before all the bathwater is out of the tub.One would hope that after a thorough analysis of a concept is given, we would have a clearer idea about it, indeed, a better idea. In carnapian terms (although people seldom talk this way any more), one would hope that a careful analysis of an explicandum would allow us to propose a crisp, logically tidy and clear explicatum. That certainly does not happen here. On the contrary, the end result of this analysis reminds me of those relatively useless debates in the fifties between the formal language and the ordinary language philosophers. The latter seemed to think that things were going well insofar as they were talking like most other people. The former thought things were going well insofar as most people were talking like them. Neither group had much to offer to public policy making.

Braybrooke thinks that a major advantage of appealing to needs instead of utilities, happiness or satisfaction is that it is relatively easy to measure the former (164–165). His language in this part of the book is similar to that of many of us who have argued for social indicators and against relatively abstract and obscure notions of utilities. We say things like find out who lacks a roof over her head, etc. and see to it that such things are provided. Unfortunately, the dispute that arose in the fifth century B.C. regarding who was happy or well-off arose again in the sixties. While Democritus and his followers thought that a happy person was one who felt contented, satisfied or at peace, others thought a happy person was one who had all the things that contributed to such feelings, for example, good health, good family relations, friends, a job, and so on. In the social indicators literature, as suggested above, some people still lean toward one or the other point of view. Some opt for so-called objective indicators to the exclusion of all others, some opt for so-called subjective indicators and some, like me, opt for both. For our purposes it is enough to remark, I suppose, that if people have most of the good things in life and also feel good about their lives, they are well-off. Put differently, if as a good moral consequentialist you are committed to improving the human condition, you cannot go wrong if you aim to improve both the relatively objective conditions in which people live and their relatively personal subjective feelings about their lives.

In fact, social indicators researchers have demonstrated many times, with many national and smaller probability samples, in many countries that people's feelings of happiness and satisfaction with various aspects of their lives are not highly correlated with the relatively objective features of their lives. They certainly *are* correlated and because they are it would be wrong to simply forget about what is going on in the world and concentrate on what is going on in people's heads. But the correlations are typically low, so low that if one cares at all about what people feel and think about their lives, one really has to ask them to find out. If one is at all inclined to make public policy about one's society on the basis of a realistic assessment of what is going on in that society, it is difficult to avoid survey research involving questions about how people actually feel about various aspects of their lives. It is difficult to avoid all the haggles, ordering of interests, preferences, levels of satisfaction, and so on that are very similar to the haggles so familiar to older welfare economists and utilitarians. I am certainly sympathetic to those who, like

Braybrooke, want to get away from relatively abstract and obscure theoretical disputes to useful research for public policy. But such movements are essentially relative and frequently more apparent than real.

I read Braybrooke's text and shake my head. It seems so far from anything that might be used by any politician, so far from any of the concrete issues that people fight about in public life. I ask myself *what does this tell us to do* about day care, our unfair taxation system, the elimination of poverty, and so on. I ask myself *what can I do better* regarding these vital issues of public policy now that I have finished reading this book. The answers, I think, are not much, if anything at all. In the symposium Braybrooke said that I "could not have picked better examples" for him to prove that his book really did have an important message for contemporary policy makers. The message was then announced as a series of questions about who had what day care needs, who needed what tax relief and so on. The announcement completely confirmed my original judgment. There are now and have been for some time interest groups, political parties and plenty of individuals claiming that this or that system of day care is needed, that this or that group needs tax relief, and so on. If the main contribution of this book is to raise questions about who needs what, it is a contribution that benefits no one. The questions have already been put, and many answers have been proposed. It is time to choose an agenda and act. On this score this book does not meet current needs.

Chapter 12
A Reconsideration of the Idea of a Science Court

Alex C. Michalos

In August 1976 the U.S. Task Force of the Presidential Advisory Group on Anticipated Advances in Science and Technology published an interim report on something they called "The Science Court Experiment."[1] It struck me immediately as a potentially sound idea needlessly and perhaps hopelessly encumbered by some pretty poor philosophy. It seemed to be exactly the kind of idea that ought to receive but has not yet received serious attention in the philosophic literature on science and technology.

My plan is to present an outline of the proposed Science Court Experiment, and then to offer replies to several prima facie plausible objections to it. Although proponents of the Court may occasionally suspect that with friends like me they really don't need any enemies, I must admit (insist) that I'm engaged in a salvaging effort. I still think that we have witnessed the birth of a good idea. It just needs a little love and attention from the proper nursemaids.

The following outline has been written and circulated by the chief architect of the Science Court Experiment, Arthur Kantrowitz.

Michalos, A.C.: 1980. A reconsideration of the idea of a science court. In P.T. Durbin (Ed.) Philosophy and Technology: An Annual Compilation of Research, Vol. 3 (pp. 10–28). Greenwich, Connecticut: JAI Press.

[1]Task Force of the Presidential Advisory Group on Anticipated Advances in Science and Technology, "The Science Court Experiment; An Interim Report," *Science* (August 1976), pp. 653–656.

A.C. Michalos (✉)
University of Northern British Columbia, Prince George, BC, Canada
e-mail: michalos@brandonu.ca

A.C. Michalos, *Philosophical Foundations of Quality of Life*,
DOI 10.1007/978-3-319-50727-9_12

Outline of the Science Court Experiment

This is an abstract of the procedures with a fuller explanation to be found in the Interim Task Force Report (*Science*, August 20, 1976). One procedure, #15, has been added since the Interim Task Force Report.

Initiation

1. The experiment will begin with agreements between the Science Court Administration (SCA), the host institution and the funding institution concerning the plans for the experiment.
2. The first step will consist of contacts with regulatory agencies and others to search for a suitable issue. The first issue will be presumed to be bipolar and will be presumed to be a value-laden decision which must be made by the agency and in which the scientific facts are apparently in doubt.
3. An agreement with the regulatory agency to supply necessary legal powers for uncovering nonpublic information if necessary.

Organization

4. The SCA, equipped with an issue and funds, will seek Case Managers (CMs) for each side of the issue. The work of the CMs will be funded by the SCA.
5. The SCA will issue suggested procedures, suggested referees, and a panel of prospective judges.
6. The CMs will review these suggestions. The experiment will go forward only after both CMs agree on the referee, the judges and the procedures. A signed agreement to proceed will commit the SCA, the funding agency, the regulatory agency, the CMs, the judges, and the referee.

Suggested Procedures

7. The CMs formulate a series of factual statements which they regard as most important to their cases. Such statements must be results or anticipated results of experiments or observations of nature. The statements should be ranked in order of importance assigned by the CM.

8. The judges examine each statement to determine that it is a relevant scientific fact.
9. The CMs then exchange statements. Each side is invited to accept or challenge each of the opponents' statements.
10. The list of statements accepted by both sides will constitute the first output from the S.C.
11. Challenged statements are first dealt with by a mediation procedure in which attempts are made to narrow the area of disagreement or to negotiate a revised statement of fact that both CMs can accept.
12. The mediated statements are added to the S.C.'s output. Those statements which remain challenged are then subjected to an adversary procedure.
13. CMs prepare substantiation papers on statements remaining challenged and transmit these to the judges and the opposing CMs starting with the first (most important) challenged statement.
14. The substantiation is cross-examined by opposing CMs and judges and contrary evidence is presented and cross-examined.
15. A second attempt to negotiate a mediated statement is made and if successful this statement is added to the Science Court's output.
16. If this is not successful the judges write their opinions on the contested statement of fact.
17. This procedure is repeated for each of the challenged statements.
18. The accepted statements plus the judges' statements constitute the final output of the procedure. (See Fig. 12.1.)

In the remaining paragraphs I will largely ignore the sections of the outline headed "initiation" and "organization," and focus attention on the section headed "suggested procedures," For ease of reference I have numbered all the objections, but the order is not significant.

Obj. 1 The term "Science Court" is a misnomer because

(a) most of the examples used to illustrate the need for and operation of the court are drawn from technology and medicine (e.g., banning saccharin, Red Dye No. 2, legalizing marijuana).
(b) use of the term "court" implies a verdict or a value-laden decision.[2]

Reply: There's no need for argument here on either score. We can think of the term "science" as merely an abbreviation for "science, technology and medicine." This may trouble linguistic purists but it need not trouble us. The procedure described by the Court's proponents may be applicable to problems that straddle disciplines or fields of study. For example, the question of whether or not saccharin is carcinogenic may be regarded as belonging to science, medicine, medical science

[2]A. Kantrowitz, "The Science Court Experiment; Criticisms and Responses," *Bulletin of the Atomic Scientists* (April 1977), p. 44.

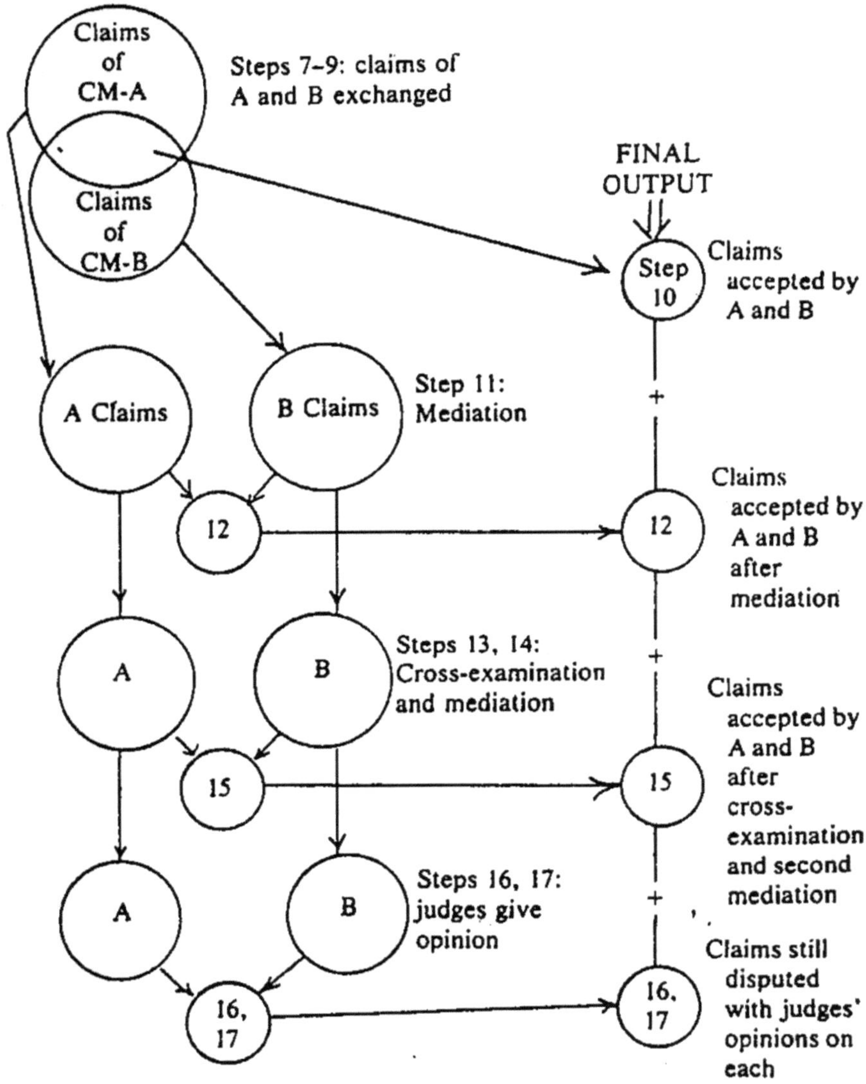

Fig. 12.1 Output decision-points of the science court

or even technology. As long as we have an abundance of prima facie suitable cases for such an institution, we need not worry much about borderline cases.

The question of the term "court" implying "a verdict or a value-laden decision" is only a symptom of a deeper problem that proponents of the Science Court have with values. So instead of attacking the symptom, I think we should go right after the disease.

Obj. 2. The Science Court cannot work because facts cannot be separated from values.[3]

Kantrowitz's writings are speckled with assertions that in one way or another require a separation between facts and values. For examples, he claims, "The Science Court will restrict itself to stating facts."[4] "Scientists take great pains to separate the factual statements they make from any of their personal values."[5] "We can do a better job of separating facts from values if we address ourselves to that goal."[6] "How will we actually go about eliminating values and irrelevancies from factual statements...?"[7] "I personally do not believe it is possible for scientists to have deeply held moral and political views about a question and simultaneously maintain complete objectivity concerning its scientific components."[8] "It is the old issue of the separation of facts from values, and I submit that this separation of facts from values can always be made."[9] "It bears repeating that the Science Court will stop at a statement of the facts and will not make value-laden recommendations."[10]

Reply: These are certainly ideas whose time has come, somewhere around 1935, I should imagine (for those of us with short memories). This is the stuff of which Vienna Circles are made. But a circle by any other name finally leads nowhere.

It's difficult to know where to begin arguing with someone who seems to be committed to the view that evaluations are worthless or, what is almost as bad, that allegedly value-free claims are somehow better than value-laden claims. On the face of it people with such views seem to have no appreciation for logical absurdity in the strict sense of self- contradictoriness. After all, it is patently self-contradictory to affirm, for example, that evaluations are worthless, but this evaluation of the worthlessness of ail evaluations is true. If this value judgment is true then the principle of the worthlessness of evaluations is false. Similarly, if it is true that allegedly value-free claims are somehow better than value-laden claims then one who says so would be better advised not to say so. He ought to know better on his own principles. In short, it is plainly logically impossible to say anything good or bad about anything without saying something that is value-laden. It is just literally absurd to pooh-pooh values in the interests of good science, good methodology, good sense, good manners or good God almighty.

---

[3]E. Callen, "The Science Court," *Science* (September 1976), pp. 948–951; L. Lipson, "Technical Issues and the Adversary Process," *Science* (November 1976), p. 890.

[4]Kantrowitz, *Bulletin* (see Footnote 2), p. 44.

[5]*Ibid.*, p. 46.

[6]*Ibid.*

[7]*Ibid.*, p. 47.

[8]A. Kantrowitz, "Controlling Technology Democratically," *American Scientist* (September–October 1975), pp. 506–507.

[9]*Ibid.*, p. 507.

[10]Task Force, *op. cit.*, p. 653.

Obviously, I have come not to praise this feature of the Science Court, but to bury it. However, I intend to breathe some new life into the Court out of the ashes of this fact-value problem. The reply I want to offer to the fact-value dichotomy objection is this: It's a red herring. The distinction between facts and values is not essential to the main purposes of the Court and it's a pity it has been given the center of the stage. The main purpose of the Court, as I see it, is to arrive at a *timely and authoritative agreement* about issues broadly classifiable as scientific. The idea is to design a procedure that will give elected representatives access to the most reliable and valid information relevant to such issues as soon as possible. Although it has been called a court, it is plainly in the family of special task forces, commissions and boards of inquiry. Just as we often describe such institutions as ad hoc fact-finding bodies, it is natural to think of the mandate of a Science Court in the same way. Nevertheless, just as task forces, commissions and boards of inquiry tend to focus on what is important, whether it's overtly value-free or value-laden, we ought to think of the Science Court in the same way.

Apart from the fact that the objection is misleadingly beside the point of the main purpose of the Court and the fact that it's logically impossible to say anything good about anything without an evaluation, it is also proper to maintain a certain amount of humility in the presence of notoriously thorny epistemological problems. From an epistemological point of view, there is no way of distinguishing what is *generally agreed to be* the case from what *is* the case. Logically or conceptually, of course, there is a difference. It's roughly the difference between epistemology and ontology, i.e., the difference between warranted assertion and the real furniture of the world. It is virtually a truism that the most soundly warranted of empirical claims may turn out to be false. But there is nothing analogous to this epistemological truism at the level of ontology. What is indeed the case cannot turn out to be not the case in the same way, at the same time and so on. This is not to deny the possibility of change, just the possibility of things existing with contradictory attributes. Whenever we arrive at what we are inclined to say *is* the case, I think it finally has to be admitted that we have merely arrived at an epistemological resting place. What we know is always subject to error, correction, criticism and so on. If what we think we know is never shown to be in error then it may be fairly said that *for all we know,* we know what is the case—not merely what is generally agreed to be the case. Still, there's no great triumph here since we began with "for all we know," a nice epistemological caveat.

If you agree that in the last analysis we can't distinguish facts from what are generally agreed to be the facts, then I think you have a good reason to regard the fact-value dichotomy as largely inconsequential. From an epistemological point of view one is in exactly the same boat in the case of values that one is in the case of facts—assuming one could distinguish them. The most one can hope to do is get general agreement about this or that evaluation. There is no way to cross the logical gap between this epistemological position and the ontological ground one hankers for. Just as there is no way to demonstrate that what we all agree is the case is the case, there is no way to demonstrate that what we all agree is good is good in and of itself. Maybe there are naked facts and naked "objective" values in the world to be discovered, but there does not seem to be any way to reach them. Logically, I just don't see any way to bridge the gap from epistemology to ontology, and I don't see that we are at all better or worse off with values than we are with facts—supposing they could be distinguished. Thus, it would seem to be a waste of time and effort to make a big deal out of determining facts only and scrupulously avoiding values. It would be wiser just to try to figure out what we all think is true, well supported or worthy of belief, whatever its ontological makeup happens to be. Instead of raising misleading criticisms like "That's a value judgment!" as many scientifically trained people are inclined to do, one ought to say "That's unwarranted!" Then the air is cleared immediately for rational debate over the reasons underlying one's claims, instead of being swiftly engulfed in the metaphysical fog of yet another unproductive fact-value debate.

Obj. 3. A Science Court would overemphasize facts and underemphasize important values, thus becoming a misleading and possibly harmful institution.[11]

Reply: In view of my remarks in response to objection 2, little more has to be said here. The fact-value dichotomy is inessential to the Court, and what is finally emphasized or ignored will be almost entirely a function of problem-specification, search procedures and personnel. These elements will require much more attention than the question of what is factual and what is not.

Obj. 4. The proposed Court procedure is unworkable because good people will not be willing to "risk interruptions in their careers and possible damage to their reputations to join in a procedure that is as yet untried and undeveloped."[12]

Reply: Kantrowitz's own reply to this objection is that "the motivation to participate must stem from an enthusiasm for bringing before the public and policy-making officials the best possible formulation of the state of scientific fact when such formulations are needed for urgent policy questions."[13] Presumably the "enthusiasm" is based on patriotism and pride.

I have never seen an investigation of the quality of commission and task force researchers compared to run-of-the mill researchers. The fact that there have been some splendid commission and task force reports shows that it is possible to get good people to shift their research interests in the public interest. Whenever a new bandwagon is formed, it's likely that a lot of people are inclined to join because they have nothing to lose, either because they are so close to the bottom or to the top in some self-selected hierarchy. But this is completely compatible with the possibility of getting first-rate people to venture into new areas.

Obj. 5. The procedure will be unworkable because it involves a winning and a losing side, and no one of any stature is going to risk public exposure as a loser.

[11] Kantrowitz, "The Science Court Experiment: Criticisms and Responses," p. 46.

[12] *Ibid.*, p. 47.

[13] *Ibid.*

Reply: Insofar as the scientific enterprise is regarded as an ongoing and self-regulating activity, no researcher has to be characterized as a loser. Instead, they may enjoy the luxury of thinking of themselves and even being thought of by others as participants in a more or less creative battle against ignorance. That's not only a wonderful image to face in the mirror every morning, it's also a terrific ego defense mechanism. It stands in sharp contrast to the image of an advocate throwing all his professional weight into a fight and being personally publicly pulverized. Nevertheless, two important points should be kept in mind.

First, it should be remembered that three out of the four decision or output points in the procedure do not identify a winner or loser. In step 10 a "list of statements accepted by both sides will constitute the first output." In step 12 "mediated statements are added to the output." In step 15 "a second attempt to negotiate a mediated statement is made and if successful is added to the output." Finally, "the judges write their opinions on the contested statement of fact." By the time this final output emerges everyone should have had enough clear or quasisuccesses to be able to stand a little reversal.

In the second place, it should be possible to orchestrate the proceedings of the Court so that it is clear that all participants are engaged in research in the public interest. Logically I'm sure that's possible, but of course the force of the objection was not logical but psychological. Unfortunately, the empirical evidence for the objection is not available yet.

Obj. 6. The Court procedure is unworkable because all the knowledgeable personnel will be committed to one side or the other of any live issue.[14]

Reply: This objection fails to distinguish the types of knowledgeable personnel required by the Court, namely, case managers (advocates), referees and judges. Case managers should be knowledgeable advocates for a particular position. They should combine a Popperian zeal for criticism with a Carnapian penchant for justification. In the best of all possible worlds they would be as critical of their own views as they are of those of the other side. In such a world much of the force of the fifth objection would be dissipated. The trouble is, of course, that the real world may be a long way from this ideal fantasy land. However, we shouldn't try to slay more than one dragon at a time. The main problem with respect to biased advocates was considered in the previous objection, and that's where the matter has to rest.

So far as referees and judges are concerned, bias is intolerable. The job of the referee is to see that the decision procedures agreed upon by both sides are scrupulously followed, and the Task Force has even suggested that referees should be "advised by legal counsel."[15] The job of the panel of judges is, again, to "write their opinions on the contested statement of fact."[16]

---

[14]Kantrowitz, "Controlling Technology Democratically," p. 506.

[15]Task Force, *op. cit.*, p. 653.

[16]Kantrowitz. "The Science Court Experiment: Criticisms and Responses." p. 45.

Judges and referees should be scientists in the broad sense of the term used here, but not specialists in the particular issues to be debated by the Court. Since contemporary science and practically every other field today tends to be dominated by specialists, it shouldn't be difficult to find people who are very good at something that is structurally, logically, methodologically and/or conceptually similar to issues going before the Court. For example, it should be easy to find chemists, epidemiologists or pharmacologists willing and able to serve as judges in cases involving the carcinogenic effects of saccharin, even though their own research has not dealt with that particular chemical.

Obj. 7. The Court is unnecessary because we already have too many commissions, task forces and special boards.

Reply: I really like the spirit of this objection, and I don't think it represents a serious problem. Although many advisory bodies come into being and seem to persist long after there is anything useful for them to do, some don't. In Canada, for example, royal commissions on the drug industry, taxation and farm machinery have come and gone. The U.S. Commission on Obscenity and Pornography had a short life. So we might think of the Science Court as analogous to such short-run commissions of inquiry rather than to standing committees or boards. Indeed, if we think of the Court primarily as a *procedure* rather than an *institution,* much less a structure literally set in concrete, we probably come closer to giving it an adequate characterization. It's entirely possible that the Science Court procedure could be used as the operating procedure of a commission, task force or board of inquiry. Since it's roughly a mixture of Delphi, adversary and mediation tactics, several of its features would be suitable for other boards of inquiry and possibly even familiar to board members.

For the record, I should mention that Kantrowitz has claimed that "it would be expected that periodically repealed procedures would be necessary with the advance of scientific knowledge, in contrast with 'single jeopardy' in some legal court proceedings."[17] Although this suggests a standing body or institution of some sort, I think the force of most of his writing is on the side of a decision-making procedure. He has also claimed that at the Leesburg Colloquium on the Court "the consensus was that we should really be planning a procedure rather than an institution."[18]

Obj. 8. The Court is unnecessary at best and harmful at worst because its output will only be used if it's compatible with policies preferred by those in power.

Reply: This is an objection that applies as well to virtually all research institutions. Even if one accepts its premise as generally true, it's difficult to accept its conclusion. Insofar as the objection applies to all research institutions, the result would be the dissolution of research in the interests of preventing its misuse. That may be wise in specific instances, but it can't be plausibly recommended as a

[17]*Ibid.*, p. 44.
[18]*Ibid.*

general policy. As a general policy it's roughly equivalent to insisting that wisdom is always on the side of flying by the seat of your pants, a pretty silly proposition, to be sure.

Obj. 9. The Court will be self-defeating because it is based on an adversary procedure, and such procedures have as their aim not the discovery of truth but the resolution of disputes without violence.[19]

Reply: This is a false dichotomy. The pursuit of truth and the resolution of disputes are neither exclusive nor exhaustive aims of courts of law or of the proposed Science Court. If we have learned anything since the Popper-Carnap controversy in the fifties it is that truth or proximity to the truth are not necessary or sufficient for the acceptability of all scientific hypotheses in all circumstances. Our scientific journals are stuffed with trivially true hypotheses tortuously defended with exotic experiments and magnificently sophisticated statistical machinery. It is clear, however, that very often a wide variety of considerations like relevance, explanatory power, internal and external coherence, and so on must be weighed in order to determine the most acceptable hypothesis at a given point in time. So the model of a court procedure for decision-making in the realm of science broadly conceived strikes me as eminently reasonable. Indeed, as I have argued at length elsewhere, I believe rational decision-making generally is more appropriately characterized by the model of a judge weighing considerations in a trial than of a druggist weighing chemicals in a laboratory. The richness of most decision-making situations just tends to be obliterated in the druggist model.

It is also important to remember that the idea of a Science Court has emerged as a response to contemporary conflicts in science broadly conceived. It is precisely because we have had and will continue to have so many serious disagreements over scientific-technological issues that the idea of the Court has had initial plausibility. Nuclear energy, solar energy, SST, space shuttles, Red Dye No. 2, monosodium glutamate, saccharin—the list is virtually endless. Clearly we cannot subject our people to a continuous barrage of quasi-popular, media-polished claims and counterclaims about all the benefits and costs of this or that scientific theory or technological device. The result would be confusion at best and decision-making controlled by the loudest voices, at worst. The best hustlers might lead us to the worst calamities. The idea of having an adversary procedure with rules of evidence and fairness instead of a steady diet of media events seems to be just what's required for the kinds of conflict resolution envisioned by the Court's proponents.

Obj. 10. The adversary procedure proposed for the Court will be self-defeating because it will tend to polarize issues and exclude intermediate positions.[20]

---

[19]N.E. Abrams and R. Stephen Berry. "Mediation: A Better Alternative to Science Courts," *Bulletin of the Atomic Scientists* (April 1977), p. 51.

[20]*Ibid.*, Kantrowitz, "Controlling Technology Democratically," p. 508; P.M. Boffey, "Experiment Planned to Test Feasibility of a 'Science Court,' "*Science* (July 1976), p. 129.

Reply: Such a procedure could have the effects mentioned in this objection, but there is no good reason to think that it must have those effects. It's true that in the design of the original procedure it is assumed that the issue investigated will be bipolar. I assumed that this was a matter of simplicity and convenience, rather than a limitation in principle. In principle and in fact ordinary courts are not limited to the adjudication of bipolar issues. So the Science Court doesn't have to be limited that way either. Furthermore, since each case manager will be producing and reviewing several relevant statements, I doubt that the exclusion of intermediate positions is likely. If I had to bet, I would bet that the procedure will be threatened more by an overabundance of more or less relevant views than by polarization around a couple. One of the most difficult problems of group decision-making is getting members to collectively pursue a manageable set of aims, rather than individually taking off in different directions. So 1 think the constraints built into the Science Court procedure will be remedial for the sort of behavior most likely to occur.

Obj. 11. The Court will turn out to be self-destructive because lawyers will eventually have more to say than scientists about its proceedings and then respectable scientists will abandon it.[21]

Reply: Since the vast majority of participants in the Court are going to be scientists, I doubt that lawyers will eventually have more to say. However, supposing that respectable scientists do abandon it, a couple different things can happen. On the one hand, the machinery could continue to crank out garbage, which in the worst of all possible worlds would be joyfully consumed by everybody with disastrous results. On the other hand, the machinery could crank out garbage which is immediately identified by its smell and thoughtfully committed to the nearest trash can. Hopefully, we would be nearer to the best than to the worst of possible worlds, but there's no guarantee of that. Still, these alternative scenarios are logically possible consequences of most decision procedures. So they don't represent special problems for the Science Court.

Obj. 12. The Court will operate as a loyal agent of whoever sponsors it; so its output is bound to be biased.[22]

Reply: I have no illusions about the ability of people to avoid bias in their everyday affairs or their scientific research. But a Science Court would not be any more exposed to this sort of aberration than any other research institution. On the contrary, the adversary procedure involved in the Court may contribute to the reduction of bias, as its proponents originally hoped.

Obj. 13. Judgments of the Court would be misleading guides to public policy because they would overemphasize technical and underemphasize all other dimensions of problems.[23]

---

[21] Abrams and Berry, *op. cit.*, p. 51.

[22] *Ibid.*

[23] *Ibid.*

Reply: This objection is a variant of the third, where the issue was put in terms of facts versus values. But this time it seems as if what's being resisted is the very idea of a division of labor in the review of scientific issues. Presumably such a division is precisely one of the central aims of Science Court proponents. In defense of the latter, it ought to be emphasized that Science Courts are not in any way exclusive of other decision-making institutions. There is no reason in principle why such Courts could not work in tandem or simultaneously with commissions, task forces, boards of inquiry, civil servants, elected representatives or anyone else. For this or that specific problem, the Court may provide an excellent auxiliary approach toward a solution.

The question is: Would such a suggestion fail by giving up more than proponents of the Court want and less than the opponents want? For all I know, the intellectual arteries of both sides may have hardened to the point where proponents and opponents see no need or possibility of accommodating the other side. Opponents may feel that the kind of technical decision-making apparently envisioned by Court proponents is really illusory. In economic jargon, they may believe that there are no real externalities; there are only costs and benefits which for one reason or another one refuses to face. Proponents may deny just that, or they may accept it and insist that there are good reasons for scientists or people with other special interests and expertise to treat some effects as external. In other words, they may just think, rightly I suspect, that not everyone can or should try to attend to every aspect of every problem. Some division of labor is necessary. In particular cases it may be difficult to decide how to cut the pie, but I don't think this operational problem is sufficient to reject the very idea of having a division. After all, lots of things are perfectly acceptable in principle although they are often tough to operationalize; a just society, for example.

Obj. 14. The Court would be self-defeating because its decisions would "seem to carry more authority than a conventional publication," and it would be extraordinarily difficult to alter them.[24]

Reply: This is another objection that seems to be based on a disagreement of principle rather than of any particular feature of the Court itself. One of the benefits of the Court, according to its proponents, is that it would produce authoritative decisions about scientific issues. The point is to create an institution that would bring diffuse sore spots to a head. The objection seems to be tantamount to the view that the proposed cure would be worse than the disease. If I can squeeze my metaphor a bit further, the objection seems to assume that scientific sore spots are self-limiting anomalies which ought to be allowed to run their course.

I don't think the objection comes to grips with the problem that Science Court proponents are trying to solve. The problem is that in the world of ordinary affairs decisions often have to be made sooner rather than later. Some of these decisions

[24] *Ibid.*, p. 52, Boffey, *op. cit.*, p. 129.

require scientific information that may be widely dispersed in the literature, very complicated and loaded with contradictions, If any old staff assistant is sent for the latest word in some area, he or she is likely to return with only half the story, and the result could be disastrous for public policy. The Science Court is intended to help reduce the risk of some such catastrophes. It represents a major screening device for scientific decision-making in the interests of preventing major and catastrophic consequences. The expected benefits of providing this type of public service seem to outweigh the expected costs of introducing some rigidity into the scientific enterprise.

Obj. 15. The Court would be unworkable because we have no criterion for deciding when a case has been conclusively established.[25]

Reply: Presumably this is a by-product of the view J have already granted that empirical claims are always in principle corrigible. However, the fact that it's always logically possible to falsify such claims is not a reason to doubt them or to say that they have not been established. For example, it would be silly for anyone to doubt that everyone dies, although it's logically possible that someone won't. Just as we have excellent reasons for believing that everyone dies, although it might be difficult to articulate the general criteria that have to be satisfied in order to reach that warranted certainty, we may have excellent reasons for believing more esoteric things. We manage to muddle through epistemological problems with the same facility that we muddle through political problems; Our paths are seldom logically tidy, but the human race would probably have gone the way of the dinosaur by now if our paths weren't more or less correct, more often than not.

Obj. 16. The establishment of a Court would undermine efforts to persuade working scientists to be more concerned with their broader social responsibilities.

There is a significant tendency for all human beings to try to put restrictions on the numbers and kinds of things for which they may be held responsible. In other words, almost everyone likes to pass the buck. So, whenever anyone suggests the need for a new institution, structure or organization designed to put an end to buck-passing, one may be justifiably skeptical. In the case of the Science Court, the fear is that while some of us will be occupied with the business of creating a purification system for scientific information, the vast majority of working scientists will still be busy creating an increasingly unmanageable cesspool. The problem is not structural or systemic, but personal. If individual scientists and their sponsors had the pursuit of truth and the avoidance of falsehood as their primary aim, there would be no need for a Science Court. Furthermore, the more we talk about the latter, the more the focus of attention is shifted from real to cosmetic solutions.

Reply: As you might imagine, the author of the previous paragraph is fairly sympathetic to this objection. But he doesn't, i.e., I don't, think it's decisive against the idea of a Science Court. It cuts too deep and it poses a false dichotomy. If it

[25]Abrams and Berry, *op. cit.*, p. 52.

were accepted as a decisive consideration in rejecting the idea of a Science Court, it would be difficult to consistently avoid appealing to it whenever any new structural changes are proposed. In some measure I think it ought to be used fairly generally, but as a rule of thumb rather than a knock-down argument. One ought to be skeptical about organizational or institutional solutions to problems, all right, but healthy skepticism shouldn't prevent the consideration of every case on its own merits. Apart from that, however, one really doesn't have to choose a priori between designing systems or structures that facilitate one's aims and recommending responsible individual behavior. There can certainly be a conflict of interests between such designs and recommendations, but even *within* science and *within* the realm of morality there can be such conflicts. Sometimes it's just impossible to satisfy two scientific aims or two moral aims at the same time, but the existence of such conflicts doesn't demonstrate that, a priori, one must choose between any two scientific aims or any two moral aims. Particular conflicts of interest have to be resolved on the basis of the particular benefits and costs involved case by case, the hard way.

Obj. 17. The Court will be undermined by those who will use it to stall for time and those who will use it to hurry decisions that require more time.[26]

It is likely that representatives of industries that have sunk a lot of research and development resources into some new product will be anxious to have market clearance for it. So they are likely to press for a hearing by a Science Court, Once a hearing is granted, they are bound to have much more information about their product than anyone else. They will have a definite edge over competitors at the start of the hearing. Hence, the sooner they can force a decision, the more probable it is that their initial advantage will be maintained and that they will have their way. On the other hand, competitors who find themselves on the short end of such a battle may subvert the proceedings by delaying them until relevant facts emerge that tip the scales in their own favor.

Reply: Although one can solve the problem of delays with time limits, one can't solve the problem of rushed decisions that way. It is also not plausible to expect that every side of every issue will be defended with exactly the same amount of resources. So I think one has to assume that some issues will come before the Court with a handicap and others will come with an edge. The question is then: Can one compensate for such anomalies? Clearly some useful steps can and are taken in the interests of giving people an equal opportunity to defend their positions in ordinary courts. However, virtually every public opinion poll, specialist and official commission that has addressed the problem of equality in North American courts has concluded that rich people are better served than poor people. So, while one may design compensating devices for the resource-poor participants in a Science Court, it's not likely that they will be able to make full compensation.

---

[26]J. Primack in the U.S. Department of Commerce, *Proceedings of the Colloquium on the Science Court* (Washington. D.C., 1977), p. 233.

Nevertheless, I believe the safeguards built into the Science Court procedure give us more protection than available alternatives. This is basically the result of the hybrid nature of the Court. Bits of Delphi, mediation and adversary procedures have been blended together for maximum strength. Besides, it should be noticed that the third item of the proposal calls for the "necessary legal powers for uncovering nonpublic information if necessary" and the fourth item stipulates that case managers are to be funded by the Science Court Administration. If reputable judges can be found who have no special ax to grind and no particular bias in favor of anything but scientific probity, 1 don't see how we can go wrong. If one side has an enormous advantage over another when the hearings begin, that would certainly be taken into account in the final report. There is no reason why we cannot require the reporting of such essential facts in every case. Indeed, there is no reason why judges could not dismiss a case on the grounds that the sides are so poorly balanced that a fair, unbiased hearing could not take place. This would make much more sense than going through the whole exercise and then announcing that there was, after all, no way to make it fair.

Obj. 18. The proceedings of the Court will be biased by the resources of the advocates, their style, cleverness, determination and information.[27]

Even if all advocates are committed to nothing but scientific probity, they may be more or less persuasive than they should be. If it is assumed that there are some more or less neutral facts to be discovered, then in principle at least it's possible for advocates to prove too little or too much. Apart from this unwanted result, a stronger advocate may overwhelm a weaker one. The stronger advocate's report may receive more attention and dominate the view of the final report.

Reply: Broadly speaking, I suspect that the human resources referred to in this objection are normally distributed. That is, I think the chances of picking individuals with more similar than dissimilar relevant characteristics are far greater than the chances of picking individuals with the opposite characteristics. Even assuming that the draws are not random but very selective, I would expect to see the same sorts of advocates chosen. Certainly in the long run, if there is a long run, there will tend to be some convergence on people with characteristics that seem to yield generally satisfactory results in the Science Court environment. While one should expect more disparity in the short than in the long run, I can't see any good reason to expect much disparity in either case.

I think it should be emphasized again that judges have the option of dismissing cases in which there is little or no hope of a fair hearing. That may be putting a heavier burden on the judges than they ought to have to bear, but I don't see any escape from it. In ordinary courts I doubt that cases are ever dismissed on the grounds that one of the parties involved has resources that are vastly superior to those of the other. I imagine that the party with fewer resources just loses in one way or another. By refusing to take on such cases, the Science Court would be a bit

---

[27] *Ibid.*

better off than ordinary courts. Moreover, the public interest would be better served by having a court that occasionally dismissed cases than by not having a court at all. In the former situation we are informed that there is apparently no fair way to judge the issue, while in the latter situation we don't have such information. Thus, in the latter situation, which is what we have now, decisions may be made anyhow on the basis of a hopelessly biased hearing. Whether or not they are made depends on how this or that particular commission or board operates. On the contrary, the Science Court is being designed with the option of dismissal-due-to-inherent- unfairness being built into it.

Obj. 19. The Court procedure tends to reinforce the misleading impression of science as a field in which complete certainty is possible.[28]

Reply: This is roughly the opposite of the problem mentioned in Objection 15. There the worry was that we could not establish claims. Here the worry is that we will create a demand or expectation for certainty that we cannot deliver. Since the very point of using the Science Court procedure is to try to reach some sort of a consensus of views about issues that patently defy complete certainty, that are too complicated, fuzzy, open-ended and so on to be nailed down once and for all, I doubt that the Court will create a misleading impression. I believe that such an impression has been created by schoolteachers and texts, news media and some practicing scientists, and that these same people and institutions will have to play a major role in setting the record straight. The only way the Court might inhibit this activity is by creating the impression that usually there is no need for a Science Court because scientific problems tend to be clear, simple and solvable with complete certainty. That is, by insisting that the Court is designed to handle extraordinary problems, we have left the door open for the inference that scientific problems typically have characteristics just opposite of those brought before the Court. So the existence of the Court might lead to the problem cited in Objection 19 but in a roundabout fashion. I suppose it might; but I doubt that it would create more than a ripple in a sea of misleading impressions. What's more, there will be strong forces operating in the opposite direction. Presumably participants in the Court procedure will be fully aware of the uncertainties with which all scientific investigation is entangled.

Obj. 20. A Science Court would be dangerously elitist, operated by and for recognized authorities in various fields.[29]

All the nice talk about reputable scientists pursuing the truth in an unbiased way is really sop. A lot of money is going to be involved in the operation of the Court, perhaps one to ten million dollars.[30] No one is going to give that kind of money to

[28]J. Holdren, "The Nuclear Power Controversy," *Proceedings of the Colloquium on the Science Court*, p. 177.

[29]E. Callen in the *Proceedings of the Colloquium on the Science Court*, p. 217.

[30]J. Primack, *op. cit.*, p. 237.

Joe Blow. Indeed, proponents of the Court have never suggested that the Court should be run by anyone but extraordinary scientists. In the words of one participant in the Colloquium on the Science Court, "What we have had here for two days is a gathering of important leaders agreeing that important decisions should be made by important leaders… These leaders have told us why the judges have to be important leaders. Dr. Kantrowitz… said that, in the great public debates, too many scientists are going around the nation spreading wrong information. The science court is supposed to stifle those voices with its authority… What is sought here is stipulation as the facts."[31]

Reply: This is roughly the opposite of Objection 4, that "the best and the brightest" will not come forward to serve the public interest. Here the fear is that "the best and the brightest" will come forward, all right, but not necessarily to serve the public interest. In fact, there is a strong suspicion that they will merely serve their own interests. Again, I don't think there will be a serious problem of finding good people. However, the interesting thing about this objection is its fairly overt suggestion that one should not try to find exceptional people. Put in its boldest form, the suggestion would appear to be that scientific issues ought to be settled in a strictly democratic fashion, i.e., in a public debate among all interested parties. Although I find populism generally very attractive, I'm pretty sure it would be self-defeating if applied to many scientific issues. For example, how much light could an ordinary citizen be expected to shed on the question of whether or not saccharin is carcinogenic?

Perhaps the objector would want to allow only specialists of one kind or another to be advocates or judges, but have all participants drawn at random. If we didn't have some minimum requirements for specialists to satisfy in order to qualify for the pool, we could get some real duds. So we would have to have minimum requirements. For all I know a set of advocates and judges picked at random from such a pool of well-qualified people might produce excellent results. For purposes of experimentation, it would be worth a try. The risks of picking people with disparate resources and abilities might be increased with this procedure, but I don't know how much difference that will make. My guess is that if the advocates are worth their salt, they are going to consult recognized authorities and draw upon all available resources anyhow. So backing off from the attempt to select "the best and the brightest" immediately in favor of this more randomized procedure may not have a significant effect on results.

Obj. 21. Participation on other committees would be neglected because it would not have the prestige or other payoffs promised by participation on the Science Court.[32]

To take a single example, the U.S. "National Academy of Sciences has about six hundred permanent committees, each with probably twenty members."[33] If people

[31]E. Callen, see Footnote 3, above.

[32]J.R. Killian. Jr., in the *Proceedings of the Colloquium on the Science Court,* p. 287.

[33]R.O. Simpson in the *Proceedings of the Colloquium on the Science Court,* p. 37.

become enamored with the Court, it may be impossible to find people to serve on all these committees. On top of that, there are thousands of other committees that require scientific consultants.

Reply: I doubt that any well-qualified scientist is going to sit around waiting for the phone to ring. Besides, there are many more thousands of scientists than committees looking for scientists.

Conclusion

Having presented the basic objections to the idea of a Science Court and plausible replies to them, I think the ball is now in someone else's court. The idea seems to have survived some serious criticisms and to merit further attention. I hope, therefore, that the U.S. Task Force will be able to get the "experiment" off the drawing boards in the near future. I would also like to see some efforts in this direction in Canada.[34]

[34] I would like to express my thanks to Dr. Kantrowitz for kindly providing me with or directing me to most of the material referred to in this paper.

Chapter 13
Technology Assessment, Facts and Values

Alex C. Michalos

Introduction

The central thesis of this paper may be put thus: There are good theoretical and practical reasons to avoid any appeals to a fact-value distinction in the assessment of technology. Alternatively, one could say that in the assessment of technology any appeals to a fact-value distinction will be at least useless and at most dangerous and self-defeating.

The structure of my defense of this thesis is as follows. In section "Fact and Value: Ontology" I draw an ontological distinction between facts and values, and in section "Fact and Falsehood: Epistemology" an epistemological distinction between facts (truths) and falsehoods is drawn. In section "From Ontology to Epistemology" I present five illustrations of types of arguments that are frequently used to draw erroneous conclusions as a result of confusing the two distinctions drawn in sections "Fact and Value: Ontology" and "Fact and Falsehood: Epistemology". In section "From Ontology to Methodology" I consider possible, but by no means

---

Earlier versions of this paper were presented to the Research Group on Expertise and Lay Participation in Health Policy Decisions at the Institute of Society, Ethics and the Life Sciences, Hastings-on-Hudson, New York; the Morris Colloquium on Morality, Rationality and Environmental Crises at the University of Colorado, Boulder; and the Policy Studies Organization Workshop on Social Values and Public Policy, Washington, D.C.; as well as this German-American conference on the philosophy of technology. Obviously I have had plenty of good suggestions in all these places, including the Bad Homburg conference—for which I am grateful.

Michalos, A.C.: 1981. Technology assessment, facts and values. In P.T. Durbin and F. Rapp (Eds.) Philosophy and Technology (pp. 59–81). Dordrecht: D. Reidel. Copyright © 1981, D. Reidel Publishing Company, Dordrecht, Holland.

A.C. Michalos (✉)
University of Northern British Columbia, Prince George, BC, Canada
e-mail: michalos@brandonu.ca

A.C. Michalos, *Philosophical Foundations of Quality of Life*,
DOI 10.1007/978-3-319-50727-9_13

necessary, methodological advantages of distinguishing facts and values (i.e., making the ontological distinction). Then I briefly outline six theories of value (in section "Theories of Value") in order to show that one cannot simply talk about values as if everyone meant the same thing. The idea of a value, like the idea of a fact, is a theoretical idea, and a very controversial theoretical idea at that. In the light of the discussion in sections "From Ontology to Methodology" and "Theories of Value", I believe it is fair to say (in section "Rational Decision-Making") that appeals to a fact-value distinction in the assessment of any technology will be useless because of the controversial status of all theories of facts and values. What's more, such appeals will be practically or strategically dangerous or self-defeating because (a) the confusion in section "From Ontology to Epistemology" will probably not be avoided; (b) the appeals usually involve unwarranted appeals to authority (credentialing); (c) the appeals encourage belief in an epistemological handicap for all evaluations which is only warranted with some theories of value; (d) the appeals encourage belief in an epistemological robustness for all alleged factual judgments which is only warranted for some; (e) the appeals encourage unwarranted self-certification of allegedly factual claims. For all these reasons, then, I recommend that in all decision-making, including all decision-making involving technology assessment or any policy-making, one should avoid any appeals to an (ontological) fact-value distinction.

Fact and Value: Ontology

Sometimes people talk about questions of fact, factual issues, or factual matters in order to classify the questions, issues, or matters prior to attempting any answers or other assessments. For example, among all the issues related to the development and use of energy from alternative sources (e.g., coal, oil, gas, uranium, water, biomass, wind, etc.) there are supposed to be some straightforward factual matters such as how much energy is obtainable from a given amount of one of these sources, using a certain technology in a certain period of time. Even those of us who don't know the answers to such questions are willing to grant that these sorts of questions are factual, if indeed *any* questions are factual.

To say that a question is factual, involves an issue or matter of fact, is obviously not to say that the question is true. It is logically impossible for questions to have truth values, to be true or false. Normally, but not always, the same is true of exclamations (e.g., "Whoopie!") and commands (e.g., "Close the door.") I say "normally, but not always" because exclamations like "Fire!" may be regarded as doing at least double and possibly triple duty. One who yells "Fire!" may be regarded as asserting that there is a fire, expressing fear and deep concern, and urging listeners to do something—run for their lives, call the fire department or whatever. Only a linguistic purist would insist that "Fire!" cannot do all these jobs at once, and I doubt that many people would believe the purist.

It is not some sort of defect in questions, exclamations, and commands that they don't or normally don't have truth values. They have their own unique linguistic jobs to do. Declarative sentences do have truth values, and this is their distinguishing feature. Nevertheless, to say that a declarative sentence involves a factual matter or an issue of fact is not to say that the sentence is true. While it is logically possible for such a sentence to be true, saying that the sentence involves an issue of fact is not the same as saying that it's true. It is merely to classify the ontological category (ball park, pigeon hole) of the sentence. For example, the sentence "Canada has seven operating nuclear reactors" involves a factual matter but the sentence may be false. Similarly it may be false that the United States has fifty-four nuclear reactors, although the issue of the existence or non-existence of the reactors is a factual issue.

At least since Hempel's classic paper "Problems and Changes in the Empiricist Criterion of Meaning" in 1950 it has been known that there is not and is not likely to be any generally acceptable criterion of empirical meaningfulness. In other words, there is not and is not likely to be any rigorous criterion to apply that will allow one to decisively categorize sentences as empirically factual, sentences about matters of empirical fact or, briefly, factual sentences. We need not review Hempel's review of the demise of the verifiability, falsifiability, confirmability, etc., criteria. Before most of us, Hempel too was a teenage logical positivist. It troubled him as much as anyone to discover that nothing worked, that finally we had intuitions and hunches separating factual matters from metaphysics, theology, ethics and other things that frightened logical positivists. Still, that's where that story ends. You will not see a criterion of empirical fact. You will only see examples of sentences about empirical (sometimes logical) facts or factual matters. Here, as elsewhere, we can often agree on what or what not to do without being able to agree on why or reasons for doing it.

One may also talk about questions of value, evaluative issues, or evaluative matters in order to classify the questions, issues, or matters prior to attempting any answers or other assessments. For example, one may raise the question, "Is thermal energy from nuclear fission or burning coal more desirable from the point of view of site attractiveness?" That is, are coal-burning facilities more or less esthetically attractive than nuclear reactors?

Again, to say that a question is evaluative, involves an issue or matter of value, is obviously not to say that the question is true. It is merely to classify the ontological category of the question. A declarative sentence like "Nuclear reactors are esthetically more attractive than coal furnaces" involves an evaluative matter, but again the truth or falsity of the sentence doesn't follow from the mere fact that it involves an evaluative issue. Some people believe that such sentences are pseudo claims, that although the sentence is formally declarative, it cannot function as a declarative sentence (cannot have a truth value at all). However, even on this extreme view, to say that a sentence is evaluative, involves a matter of value or an evaluative issue, is still not to say that the sentence is true or false. Indeed, on this extreme view, it is logically impossible for the sentence to be true or false.

In short, according to some common usage, issues of fact may be contrasted with issues of value in a purely ontological classificatory sense. In this sense, truth or falsity is not at issue. Classifying a matter in this sense is not asserting the truth or falsity of the matter. Classifying an issue in this sense is logically prior to the question of truth or falsity, and the latter question may not even arise. For example, the question will not arise if one is only interested in getting a question classified as factual or evaluative, and the question will not arise when an evaluative declarative sentence is asserted and its assessor holds the extreme view that such sorts of sentences cannot have truth values.

Fact and Falsehood: Epistemology

Sometimes people use the term "fact" and its cognates as a synonym for "true." For example, people say things like "As a matter of fact there are several operating nuclear reactors in Ontario"; "It is a fact that there are nuclear reactors in Ontario"; and "In fact there are nuclear reactors in Ontario." The last sentence, for example, just means "In truth there are nuclear reactors in Ontario." The two before that may be expressed as "It is true that there are nuclear reactors in Ontario." Such usage of the term "fact" is not ontological but epistemological. The term is used not to designate an ontological category, but to designate an epistemological assessment or appraisal.

In the epistemological usage of "fact" it would be self-contradictory to talk about factual matters that were false. Factual matters in this epistemological sense are true, i.e., the sentences about the matters are true. For example, it would be self-contradictory for someone to say "In fact there are nuclear reactors in Ontario and it's false that there are nuclear reactors in Ontario." If in fact there are nuclear reactors in Ontario then it is true that there are such reactors there and it cannot also be false. Similarly, if in fact John is five feet tall then it would be self-contradictory to say "In fact John is five feet tall but he's not five feet tall."

Thus, in the epistemological sense of "fact," facts are contrasted with falsehoods, or, more precisely, factual sentences are contrasted with false sentences because "factual" is regarded as synonymous with "true." In this sense of "fact" to say "In fact nuclear reactors are visually more attractive than coal furnaces" is to affirm the truth of the claim that nuclear reactors are visually more attractive than coal furnaces. Clearly, those who believe that evaluative sentences cannot have truth values would insist that a sentence like "In fact nuclear reactors are visually more attractive than coal furnaces" must be self-contradictory. That is, if "in fact" is regarded as synonymous with "in truth" and evaluative sentences cannot be true or false, then it is self-contradictory to claim that it's true that nuclear reactors are more attractive than coal furnaces *and* it's not true or false. If it's not true or false, then it's not true.

It is the epistemological sense of "fact" that is intended when people talk about gathering relevant facts or undertaking a fact-finding investigation. If, for example, a journalist is sent out to dig up all the facts he can find about Cleveland's mayor, no one will expect the journalist to return with old shoes, chairs, and hubcaps. Nor would anyone expect to see the journalist bring a pick and shovel to work. What would be expected is a search for true relevant propositions or sentences about the mayor. In an ontological sense of the term, the mayor's shoes, chairs, and auto hubcaps are facts in his life, literally the furniture of his world. But gathering the facts about his life does not imply gathering up such furniture. (Anyone who wants to make something out of the difference between "facts in" and "facts about" is free to do so.)

It would be nice if we had a generally acceptable criterion of truth. There seems to be general agreement that Tarski's formal definition is sound: i.e., a sentence represented by "p" is true if and only if p; e.g., "John is sick" is a true sentence if and only if John is sick. As a meaning analysis of a common notion of truth, this seems to be unexceptionable. But it's obviously worthless as a criterion for determining which sentences are true and which are false. From the meaning analysis we don't find out how to prove that John is or isn't sick. (The problem is roughly analogous to knowing what it means to bake a cake, but not knowing how to do it.) To solve the criteriological problem of truth, I think one must appeal to some notion of coherence. Nicholas Rescher's *The Coherence Theory of Truth* is the most recent attempt to carry out such a program. It's not the sort of program one can expect to just carry out as one carries out the garbage. However, Rescher has taken significant steps forward.

From Ontology to Epistemology

Given the two common ways of talking about factual matters, an ontological way in which facts are contrasted with values and an epistemological way in which facts are contrasted with falsehoods, the stage is set for unwarranted inferences. It is easy to move from the assumption that an issue is a factual matter in the ontological sense of the term "factual" to the quite different assumption that the issue is factual in the epistemological sense of the term. In such cases, one starts with an issue that is ontologically factual and converts it into an epistemological fact, i.e., a truth or true claim, or a falsehood. Whether the conversion is intentional or not, the fallacy of equivocation is committed. One logically cannot derive epistemological appraisals of truth or falsity from mere ontological categorization.

As Edgar Bergen might have asked Mortimer Snerd, "How could anyone be so stupid?" And as Mortimer might have replied, "Wal, it's a lot easier in a crowd!" The fact (truth) is that several common ways of talking and thinking (in English at least) conspire to drive people to equivocate on the ontological and epistemological uses of the term "fact." For example, it often happens that when a group meets to discuss a problem, say, the development of an energy source, one or more members think it will be helpful to share some factual matters. If there is a thin edge of the wedge leading to complete consensus in a group decision-making situation, so the assumption goes, it must be at or near the factual side of things. So, by all means, let us lay out some of the facts as soon as possible. The move from factual matters to facts here can be a move from ontology to epistemology. Because factual matters (ontology) tend to be relatively unproblematic (relative to evaluative matters), the assumption goes, and factual matters are going to be discussed first, facts (epistemology) are going to be introduced first. The mere description of a claim as factual in the ontological sense tends to soften the path toward its acceptance as factual in the epistemological sense.

As a second example of how the equivocation arises, consider the case of expert advice given by scientists. Suppose it is granted that there really are experts on matters of scientific fact, e.g., chemical facts, physical facts, economic facts, etc. At a minimum that means that there is a body of factual (ontology) claims about which so-called experts know more than non-experts. To be an expert in, say, chemistry is just to know more about the factual claims of chemistry than most people know. Apart from the question of the truth or falsity of any factual claim of chemistry (or any chemical issue or problem for chemistry or matter of chemistry), most people I guess would be willing to grant that it is usually possible to distinguish such claims from many others. If I say, for example, that sugar is water-soluble, no one is going to quarrel about describing that as a fact of chemistry rather than a fact of sociology, economics, or arithmetic. Granted that these disciplines have fuzzy edges and no knock-down criteria of identification, it's not likely that the water-solubility matter is going to be resisted as a matter of chemistry. However, because there are some factual matters that clearly are in the province of chemistry (an ontological point) and there are experts on such matters, it is possible for the expert chemist to claim to assert chemical facts in the epistemological sense of "fact" and get away with it. The *non sequitur* runs: Smith is a chemical expert, x is a matter of chemical fact (ontologically speaking). So, if Smith claims that x is a chemical fact (ontologically yet) then x is a fact (epistemologically speaking, true). In short, Smith's credentials are doing the job (invalidly) that Smith's evidence should be doing (validly). We often tell students of introductory logic courses to beware of people with credentials in one field making claims in another field. We should also tell them to beware of people with credentials using those credentials instead of evidence to warrant claims in the field where the credentials are held.

There is another way in which an equivocation on the term "fact" occurs related to judgments that something is a matter of scientific fact. When one judges that some issue is scientific or is a matter of science, one might base the judgment on one's knowledge that there is a body of scientific literature about it. For example, one might think that the question of the thermal energy of coal is a scientific question because there is a recognized body of physical science literature dealing with precisely this question and related questions. The same person might think that the question of the visual attractiveness of a coal furnace is not scientific because there is (as far as he knows) no recognized body of science dealing with precisely this and related questions. Now he can reason invalidly: Science deals with facts (ontology). There is no science of visual attractiveness. So, there are no scientific facts (epistemology) of visual attractiveness. Thus, whatever one says about visual attractiveness cannot have the status of a scientific fact (truth). Whatever claims about visual attractiveness are, they cannot be true.

Besides noticing that the argument just presented involves an equivocation, it ought to be noticed that the criterion of scientific significance used in the preceding paragraph is far from rigorous or decisive. There could be no new sciences if the criterion of scientific significance required every allegedly scientific claim to have a recognized body of scientific literature devoted to it already. The scientific enterprise could never have begun if that had been the criterion of selecting scientific claims. Nevertheless, I don't doubt at all that many people do use such a criterion as a rough and ready guide to judgments about what is scientific. Since I have already said that there are no generally accepted, decisive criteria of scientific significance, I have no objections to people using rough and ready criteria. I only object if people use such criteria to pronounce all evaluative claims as in principle unscientific and hence untrue. After all, in such cases the principle is known to be defective and the inference is invalid.

A fourth way in which an equivocation on the term "fact" occurs is related to a defective argument for distinguishing empirical facts from values. It is sometimes argued that facts must be different from values because it is possible to get complete agreement on the facts of a situation (event, person, thing) but still have disagreement about its value. For example, we would be able to get complete agreement from virtually everyone watching me present this paper that I have a nose. The fact that I have a nose is literally as plain as the nose on my face. We could get agreement on its size, color, shape, physiological structure and so on. Nevertheless, the argument runs, it would still be possible to have disagreement about the physical attractiveness of my nose. Some people would say it's a nice nose, others that it's ugly, or plain, superb, classical Greco-Roman, and so on. In short, unlike the fact of my nose, the esthetic value of my nose is open to a variety of opinions. The fact (truth now) that I have a nose can be established beyond reasonable doubt, but the esthetic value of my nose remains doubtful forever. The preceding sentence is crucial. What is being contrasted in that sentence is not two ontologically distinct types of things. Rather, it is the epistemological status of factual claims that is being contrasted with evaluative claims. The issue is now one of truth versus something less than the truth.

To appreciate the weakness of the argument in the preceding paragraph, consider the following analogue. Values must be different from facts because it is possible to get complete agreement on the value of something but still have disagreement about factual aspects of it. For example, long before there was agreement on the facts about things like rainbows, sunsets, mountains, waterfalls and clouds, most people found such things not only attractive but often awe-inspiring. It would have been possible for two ancient Greeks (or two contemporary folks) to agree that a particular rainbow was beautiful while disagreeing on its origin, color, size, and shape. Anyone familiar with the history of science can probably multiply such cases easily. Anyone at all can probably think of many more cases in which complete agreement in evaluative issues comes at least as easily as agreement on facts. For example, we would be able to get complete agreement from virtually everyone watching me present this paper that I don't have a moral obligation to cut off my nose during the presentation. Similarly, nobody in his right mind would think that I would be physically more attractive at this minute with a bloody hole in the middle of my face instead of a nose. Nobody thinks I would look pretty with three noses, or four, and so on. Clearly there are as many evaluations or judgments of value as there are judgments of fact about which one can get virtually complete agreement. In principle there must be an infinite number; e.g., everyone will agree that I don't have two noses, three, etc., and everyone will agree that I would not be prettier with two noses, three, etc. There does not seem to be any ontological lesson to be learned about facts and values from counting heads regarding things people agree or disagree on readily. With a little thought one can cook examples to suit oneself.

While I am on this subject of agreement, I should take a few lines to address the frequently made assumption that if people cannot readily identify a good reason for some judgment, agreement or disagreement, then there must be an evaluation involved. In brief, people often argue: There is apparently no good reason to assert that p is the case. Therefore, the assertion that p is the case must involve an evaluation, a value, a value judgment or some such thing.

Instead of leaping to such a conclusion, one should at least consider the following seven other possibilities. The judgment that p is the case may involve (a) a perception that is not clearly identifiable; (b) an idea that is vague or open-textured; (c) principles or rules of inference that are obscure; (d) so many complicating factors to aggregate that, although one can intuit an appropriate judgment, one cannot clearly support it; (e) some premises that one cannot identify; (f) a mistake about some rule or premise; (g) a disagreement about facts difficult to discern.

A fifth and final way in which an equivocation on the term "fact" occurs is related to standard textbook treatments of rational decision-making or action on the Bayesian or estimated utility model. Briefly, according to this view decision-makers are confronted with a set of mutually exclusive and exhaustive possible future states of affairs and courses of action. Each combination of state of affairs and action yields an event with a particular value or utility. By quantifying these values, multiplying these quantities by the probabilities of the events that may occur and summing the products of every event attached to every action, one can obtain the estimated value of performing that action. A rational actor then is supposed to perform the available action that has the highest estimated value.

What seems to be built into the Bayesian procedure as just described is the assumption of a fact-value dichotomy in the form of a probability-value dichotomy. Rational decision-making and action on this model requires an amalgamation of two apparently ontologically distinct kinds of entities, namely, values and probabilistic facts or factual probabilities of some sort. But if probabilities have some sort of factual status and values do not, then there is a tendency to regard values as epistemological nonstarters. Probability assessments, the assumption goes, may be more or less accurate or true, but evaluations are simply given or not. The latter is especially the case when the values used in the model are based on revealed preferences which are uncritically given and accepted. Again, then, we have the unwarranted move from an ontological to an epistemological use of "fact."

On top of the objectionable equivocation just described, it should be noticed that it is a mistake to assume that probability assessments do not require evaluations and that evaluations do not involve probability (factual) assessments. I have discussed these connections in other places and will therefore be very brief. In order to measure any probabilities one must make decisions concerning one's universe of discourse, its appropriate description, the appropriate subset of the total universe to be used for any given problem situation, and the appropriate methods to be used to make all these decisions. These and other decisions involve assessments of the benefits and costs attached to alternative decisions; i.e., the decisions involve evaluations. Similarly, the evaluations required on the other side of the Bayesian model require epistemological assessments. For example, in order to form a preference for apples over oranges one must know something about both. Without building some sort of information or knowledge component into evaluation, it becomes impossible to distinguish the proverbial Fool's Paradise from Real Paradise. Conceptually, the difference between the two is either that the fool does not have any good reasons for valuing or preferring his Paradise while someone in a Real Paradise would, or that there are good reasons for believing the Fool's Paradise is not what he thinks it is; it is not, that is, the Real Paradise he thinks it is. For example, heavy smokers who believe they can go on smoking without damaging their lungs can only have the pleasure of a Fool's Paradise. In short, uninformed evaluations are worthless.

From Ontology to Methodology

I think that one of the reasons people believe that the so-called fact-value distinction is very important is that they have not distinguished the fact-value distinction from the fact-falsehood distinction. They believe that by determining the correct ontological status of an issue, as factual or evaluative, the truth status of the issue has also been settled. Given the particular views that some people have about evaluative issues (e.g., the people I characterized as having extreme views), evaluative sentences don't have any truth values. Hence, for people with such views, the ontological categorization of an issue as evaluative has the epistemological consequence that the concepts of truth and falsity will not be applicable at all. Against such extremists, it is pointless to try to establish the truth or falsity of an evaluative sentence. It would make as much sense as trying to establish the truth or falsity of a sneeze or a glass of beer. For these folks evaluative sentences, by definition, logically cannot have truth values. The sentences are epistemological non-starters and that's that.

If one is not an extremist on evaluative issues, then—unless one is a metaphysician interested in determining the ontological structure of the world—there is probably little of interest in the fact-value distinction. On the other hand, the fact-falsity, or better, the truth-falsity distinction is fundamental. If one can't distinguish truth from falsity, true sentences from false ones, then one runs the risk of eating stones, swimming in molten lead and making love to ostriches. Being able to distinguish truth from falsity really does have survival value in ways that being able to distinguish facts from values doesn't. So why fool around with the metaphysical question?

One answer is that it might be the case that if we got an issue correctly categorized ontologically, then we could address it with the right method. At any rate, we might be able to eliminate some methods as useless. For example, if one holds an extreme view of evaluative sentences, then once one knows that a sentence is evaluative, one knows that there is no method that can establish the truth or falsity of the sentence. This is indeed an extreme case, but it illustrates how one can use ontological knowledge to make methodological decisions. In this extreme case, the decision is simply to admit the inapplicability of every method. Given one's definition of evaluative sentences, no method is relevant to establishing their truth or falsity.

Suppose that you do not hold an extreme view. That is, suppose you believe that categorizing a sentence as factual or evaluative leaves the truth status of the sentence undecided but not undecidable. The question is: Can it help your epistemological task to know that the sentence involves an ontologically factual or evaluative claim? It might. It depends on the particular claim, your methodological resources (time, energy, strategy, money, logico-mathematical sophistication, etc.), your epistemological beliefs, and your value theory, to mention only a few salient variables. I wish there were a short answer. The only relevant short answer I can think of now is that correct ontological classification into the categories of matter of fact or value is no panacea. No one should imagine that a solution to the ontological-metaphysical problem would constitute a major epistemological breakthrough.

Consider some examples in support of the previous sentence. (1) The ultimate matter of the world is wave-like rather than particle-like. (2) Every innocent human infant should be tortured to death before the age of four months. (3) A human being wrote these sentences. (4) A morally good human being wrote these sentences. It seems to me, though this is not a knock-down demonstration, that sentence (1) is a factual claim whose truth is extremely difficult if not impossible to decide; (2) is an evaluative claim whose falsity will be granted by all but extremists and crazies; (3) is a factual claim as uncontroversial as (2); and (4) is more controversial than (3), less controversial than (2) and probably not as controversial as (1).

All I want to do with these four sentences (1)–(4) is illustrate and lend some support to my claim that solving the ontological status problem may leave one with enormous epistemological problems, depending on the particular claim to be assessed. I also said it depends on your methodological resources. For example, consider (5) It is wrong to torture all living babies to death and (6) The negation of a conjunction is logically equivalent to the disjunction of two negations. (5) is an evaluative sentence whose truth will be granted by virtually everyone who reads it, while (6) is a logical factual sentence (a sentence stating a logical fact or logical truth) whose truth will not be recognizable by everyone or even most people. Depending on one's training and methodological resources, the evaluative (5) and the factual (6) will be more or less easy to assess epistemologically.

Epistemological beliefs have a crucial role to play in determining how useful correct ontological categorization can be. I can't review the history of epistemological skepticism here. Suffice it to say that some folks believe there can be no certainty concerning the truth or falsity of empirical sentences. They may rest their case on so-called arguments from dreams, from illusions, from limited sense perception, from peculiar definitions of complete verification, and so on. If they are thoroughgoing skeptics, then there's no hope. They will regard empirical claims as inherently unjustifiable and hence doubtful. Alternatively, they may be less-than-thoroughgoing skeptics, holding that one might have complete certainty concerning empirical claims although such claims are inherently fallible. For example, they may say that sentences like "There's only one doctor in this town" can be known to be true with complete certainty, but they are still liable to be falsified. They are still fallible or corrigible but not doubtful. Although I find this view satisfactory, some folks don't. It depends on how one defines key epistemological terms like "knowledge," "certainty," "complete verification," and so on.

The last important variable I mentioned that determines how useful correct ontological categorization would be in determining the truth status of any sentence is one's theory of value. With some theories of value, the truth or falsity of evaluative sentences is a routine matter, provided that one is not a thoroughgoing epistemological skeptic. With other theories, as I have already suggested, "truth" and "falsity" just don't apply. In the next section I will review some basic alternative views of the nature of value.

Theories of Value

Before I begin my review of value theories, a couple of preliminary remarks will be helpful. In the first place, one must distinguish *things that have value* from *the value that things have*. Although virtually anything may be regarded as a thing that has value (or, briefly, a thing of value or a valuable thing), many people (especially social scientists) seem to focus on things like personal freedom, political efficacy, honesty, and self-esteem as examples. That's okay, as long as one remembers that strictly speaking sticks and stones and telephones, and anything else, may be regarded as valuable things in some sense of "value."

Just as theories of molecules, electricity, and democracy have as their subject matter molecules, electricity, and democracy, respectively, so a theory of value has value as its subject matter. Just as in molecular theory one gets meaning analyses of basic terms, measurement procedures, working principles and lawlike statements, a theory of value may be expected to have a similar battery of features. I have reviewed alternative views of the structure of scientific theories elsewhere. So here it is enough to say that there are over half a dozen views about what scientific theories ought to look like, ranging from mere unrestricted universal generalizations to axiomatic systems with logical and empirical vocabularies, rules of formation and transformation, and so on. Depending on what one means by the terms "theory" and "science," there have been more or less fully developed scientific theories of value. Perhaps the most fully developed theory we have had is that of Ralph Barton Perry in his classic, *General Theory of Value* (1926).

The alternative views of the nature of value that will be outlined below should be regarded as central features of possible (and more or less plausible) theories of value. Generally speaking, I describe the sort of meaning analysis that might be adopted for each view, and briefly suggest some of its salient strengths and weaknesses. I can't, of course, provide a thorough analysis and appraisal of any theory. Moreover, I do not try to press my own preference for any of the views. For the points to be made in the following section, it does not matter what theory of value one adopts. It only matters that one appreciates the variety of theories available.

When people say that something is valuable or good, just how should their remarks be understood? For example, how should one interpret remarks like "Jesus was a good man," "Clean air is valuable," and "There is some value in friendship"? We could, of course, retreat to a handy dictionary and get a standard lexicographer's definition of the key terms "good," "value," "valuable," and so on. But that would be an inappropriate response to the question. What we want to have is not merely correct English usage, but a more or less systematic or theoretical account of the meanings of these key words, and an account of the things referred to by these words—if there are such things.

Generally speaking, seven distinct kinds of answers have been offered to our question, each one suggesting a different view of the nature, essential being, or *ontological status* of value. The names used by different authors to refer to these seven different views vary a great deal, to put it mildly. Hence, it is vitally important that as you read this section, you must try to get each view fixed in your mind without becoming dogmatic about the labels used for the view. You should also not be surprised to find some people combining some of these views or elements of some of them to obtain hybrid forms.

The relations between the seven views are illustrated in the following diagram, which will be discussed in the remaining paragraphs of this section.

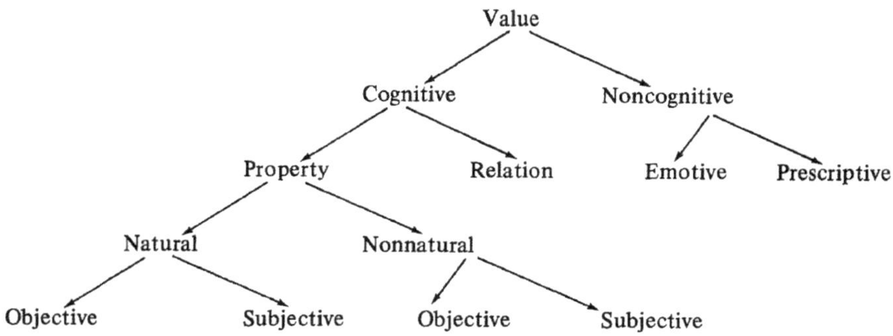

The first distinction to be drawn is that between cognitivism and non- cognitivism. In the *cognitivist* view the terms "value" and "good" designate something which is identifiable and namable, but not necessarily describable. Things that have value or goodness are thus similar to things that are yellow or sweet insofar as one can identify and name the qualities they possess, but cannot necessarily describe them in other words. In the *noncognitivist* view the terms "value" and "good" do not *designate* anything at all. Things do not have value or goodness on this view any more than "Such" is the name of something, or "Help me, please" describes any state of affairs.

As you can see from the diagram above, there are two species each of cognitivist and noncognitivist views of the nature of value. Since the division of noncognitivist views takes us to the *infimae species* or rockbottom of the righthand branch of our family tree, while the division of cognitivist views does not, I will consider the latter next.

Supposing that it is granted that "value" and "good" do designate something which is identifiable and namable, one might ask: Is value or goodness a property or a relation? From an ontological point of view, the difference between properties and relations is important. Consider, for example, the sentence "John is standing to the left of Frank." John and Frank do not seem to exist the way the relation designated by "is standing to the left of" exists. The *particular* relation seems to obtain (exist) when and only when John is standing to the left of Frank. Some people think that the *universal,* abstract entity, type or sort of relation designated by "is standing to the left of" has its own mode of existence, which Bertrand Russell called "subsistence" to distinguish it from ordinary existence.

I can't settle the old philosophical problem of the existence of abstract entities (Platonic forms, if you like—almost). But on a *relational* view, value may be thought of as a relation obtaining between at least two things (usually a person and a valued thing) *and* the relation may be regarded as a concrete particular or an abstract type of entity. I have not put two branches below "relation" on the diagram above in order to simplify the diagram. Strictly speaking, however, two branches could be drawn, one for the view that "value" designates particular relations and one for the view that "value" designates an abstract entity or universal relation. Similar divisions could be made for the view that "value" designates a property.

Whether value is regarded as particular or universal, insofar as it's regarded as a relation one will not be able to pick it out the way one picks out the terms of the relation. For example, suppose "Clean water is valuable" is taken to mean something like "There is a relation between clean water and people in virtue of which it is correct to say that clean water is valuable." We may be able to observe the clean water and the people (the two terms of the relation), but we can't observe the relation. Moreover, on this view, it is precisely that relation that provides the warrant for the attribution of value to clean water. Obviously, then, people who hold that value is a relation have special problems of characterizing the relation and giving criteria for identifying it. Here the ghost of David Hume looms large, because causal relations are prime candidates to figure in relational theories of value and Hume argued forcefully that such relations are nothing more than human artifacts, products of human imagination. Thus, relational theorists will have special problems establishing the truth or falsity of evaluative sentences. If they happen to be committed to abstract entities, they are even worse off. Or, turning things upside down, if one were an epistemological nominalist (believing there are no abstract entities) and if one became convinced that "value" designated an abstract entity, a relation-type, then one would be stuck with the view that value doesn't exist. For such people sentences like "Clean water is valuable" might be false or maybe meaningless, but certainly not true.

In contrast to a relational view, one might hold a quality or *property* view according to which "value" and "good" designate some sort of a property. On this view, value belongs to things roughly the way other properties belong to things, e.g., the way height, weight, triangularity, etc., belong to things.

Supposing it is granted that "value" and "good" designate a property of things that is identifiable and namable, one might then ask: Is value or goodness a natural property of the world or not? On the *naturalistic* view of value or goodness, this property or quality is as natural as water, mountains, headaches, and itches. Just as one does not have to design or make trees and toothaches, one does not have to design or make value or goodness. It just grows naturally, the way some tadpoles naturally become frogs and people naturally grow old, if all goes well.

On the *nonnatural* view ("supernatural" would do as well) of value or goodness, these qualities do not just emerge or evolve like flowers and snowflakes. They are somehow outside, above, or beyond the natural stream of things. They have roughly the same status relative to the world of nature that God and other supernatural spirits are supposed to have. One need not believe that there are any nonnatural or supernatural things in order to understand the point of view, I think. Nonnaturalists just happen to believe that value or goodness is not finally rooted in or grounded on anything in the physical, natural, or material universe.

There are two species of naturalism and nonnaturalism (supernaturalism) that merit attention. I will consider each in turn.

Naturalistic Objectivism

On what may be called a *naturalistic objectivist* view of the nature of value, to say that something is good or valuable is to say that something has some natural property in virtue of which the predicates "is good" or "is valuable" may be appropriately applied to it. For example, suppose one says that it is good to be kind to people, that kindness is worth a lot, or that kindness is a valuable characteristic for a person to possess. On the naturalistic objectivist view, such remarks have the status of genuine truth claims, i.e., they must be true or false. Moreover, they are true if and only if whatever is referred to by the subject of each remark has some property or attribute named by the predicate of the remark. Thus, for example, it *is* good to be kind to people if and only if kindness has some special property called "goodness." Similarly, Jesus was a good man, on this view, if and only if he possessed the particular property of being a good man. Accordingly, being good, having value or worth, on this view, is precisely analogous to being triangular or having the property of triangularity. Just as polygons can be triangular whether or not anyone knows or cares about it, someone or something can be good or valuable whether or not anyone knows or cares about it. Again, just as mountains can have snow and teeth can have cavities whether or not anyone knows or cares about it, someone or something can be good or valuable whether or not anyone knows or cares about it. Furthermore, it is true to say that something is triangular or good just in case that thing has the special properties named by "is triangular" and "is good," namely, the properties of being triangular and being good.

Naturalistic Subjectivism

On what may be called a *naturalistic subjectivist* view of the nature of value, to say that something is good or valuable is to say that somebody has some natural attribute, characteristic, or feeling in virtue of which it is appropriate to apply the predicates "is good" or "is valuable" to something. The term "somebody" might designate a single person, a small group, a culture, a nation, everyone in Western Civilization, or just human beings in general. As one moves from a single individual (i.e., naive egoism) to human beings in general, one's naturalistic subjectivism tends to become more plausible, but that is a long story that need not detain us now. The attributes, characteristics, or feelings possessed by the subject of one's naturalistic subjectivism might be, say, feelings of approval, satisfaction, pleasure, or favorable interest of some sort. Hence, for example, to say that kindness is worth a lot is to affirm something like the fact that Canadians approve of kindness, most people in the world approve of being kind, or that everyone you know approves of kindness. Supposing that one can recognize acts of kindness when one sees them, it would be true to say that they are good or valuable just in case Canadians do approve of them, most people approve of them, or everyone you know approves of them. It depends on how you specify the subject for your naturalistic subjectivism. If goodness or value is determined by, for example, ninety percent of Canadians having an empirically discoverable feeling of approval toward something, then that thing is good or valuable when and only when ninety percent of Canadians have such a feeling about it.

In short, then, naturalistic subjectivism and objectivism are alike insofar as both views hold that judgments of goodness, value, or worth are *genuine truth claims*, i.e., they are in principle determinably true or false. They are different views insofar as subjectivists locate the properties that justify evaluations in people while objectivists locate the justifying properties in whatever is claimed to be good or valuable. One way to keep the two views separate is to think of them as roughly analogous to two properties of sugar, namely, mass and sweetness. When one says that sugar has mass (ignoring relativity theory), one is talking directly about a property located in sugar. On the other hand, when one says that sugar is sweet, one is talking directly about the sensation of sweetness that is in people having the sensation, rather than in the sugar. "Sugar is sweet" is an indirect or roundabout way of referring to how sugar is perceived by people, while "Sugar has mass" is a direct way of referring to how sugar is. Just so with values. For naturalistic objectivists, "Sugar is valuable" is a direct way of referring to how sugar is, while for naturalistic subjectivists it's an indirect way of referring to how sugar is perceived or apprehended.

Nonnaturalistic Objectivism

On what may be called a *nonnaturalistic objectivist* view ("supernaturalistic objectivist" would do as well) of the nature of value, to say that something is good or valuable is to say that something has some nonnatural property in virtue of which the predicates "is good" or "is valuable" may be appropriately applied to it. The nonnaturalistic objectivist accepts everything that the naturalistic objectivist accepts about value judgments *except* their justification in natural phenomena. Things really do have goodness or value in them, but these are nonnatural or supernatural qualities inexplicably existing or, perhaps, existing by the will of God. The qualities do not just emerge like snowflakes and they are not natural the way my appetite for apple pie is natural. They are *something else*, and that's all there is to it!

Nonnaturalistic Subjectivism

On what may be called a *nonnaturalistic subjectivist view* of the nature of value, to say that something is good or valuable is to say that somebody has some nonnatural attribute in virtue of which it is appropriate to apply the predicates "is good" or "is valuable" to something. The nonnaturalistic subjectivist accepts everything that the naturalistic subjectivist accepts about value judgments *except* their justification in natural phenomena. It is the spiritual aspect of human beings that is the locus, ground, or origin of value in the world. Value exists insofar as people have feelings, attitudes, likes and dislikes, but human feelings, attitudes, likes and dislikes are not just natural phenomena like the pains or itches of cats and dogs. Human beings, on this view, have something in them that is not quite natural. Although the view does not logically entail theism, those who have spoken of the image of God in man have shared this view of the extraordinary status of human beings.

Again, nonnaturalistic objectivism and subjectivism are alike insofar as both views hold (1) that value judgments are genuine truth claims, and (2) that values are not grounded in natural phenomena. They are unlike with respect to where they locate the nonnatural properties that justify evaluations.

Before moving on to a discussion of the two kinds of non-cognitive views of value, some comments are in order about the strengths and weaknesses of the four views just considered. First, if objectivist views could be sustained then there would be a universal, objective, or absolute basis for evaluations. That would be marvelous indeed. It would mean, for example, that when people say things like "Abortion is wrong" or "Jesus was a good man" that anyone who doesn't agree with these judgments is seriously out of step with the structure of the world, either the natural or the supernatural world. Such a person would be mistaken in roughly the same way that someone who ate stones for nourishment would be mistaken. If one were a nonnaturalistic objectivist, then one would have special problems of characterizing the property designated by "value" and explaining how natural beings can have access to it. If one were a naturalistic objectivist, then one would have special problems explaining the fact that different people at different places or the same people at different times have quite different views about what is or is not valuable. (Recall the discussion in section "From Ontology to Epistemology".)

If subjectivist views could be sustained, life could be better or worse, depending on the views. Naive egoism makes every person his or her own court of last appeal, which would probably make life lonely, nasty, brutish, and short. It is also a consequence of this view that two people would not be affirming the same proposition if each judges that something is good or valuable, and they would not be affirming contradictory propositions if one judged that something was valuable while the other judged that it was not valuable.

G.E. Moore's famous "open question argument" was intended to undermine all naturalistic theories of value, but it could also be used against all forms of subjectivism. In either case, as Frankena showed some years ago, the argument is question-begging.

Emotivism

On what may be called an *emotivist* view of the nature of value, to say that something is good or valuable is not to affirm anything at all, but merely to express a feeling or attitude. Emotivists depart radically from all cognitivists because on the emotivist view assertions of goodness, value, or worth are not genuine truth claims, i.e., they cannot (logically) be true or false. Moreover, they cannot be true or false because they have the logical status of exclamations, not of declarative sentences.

Let us consider the view more carefully with the help of an analogy. Suppose I step on your toe. You might say "You're hurting me," or "Ouch," or you might just pull your foot out from under mine. If you just pull your foot back then you have made no claim that might be true or false. Similarly, if you just scream "Ouch!" or "Eeaah!" you have made no claim. On the other hand, the declarative sentence "You're hurting me" must be true or false, though for our purposes it does not matter which. What the emotivist view amounts to then, is just this: Sentences that appear *formally* as declaratives in which some property, namely, goodness or value, is being affirmed of something are *functionally* exclamations in which nothing at all is being *affirmed*, though something is being *expressed*. Thus, for example, when one says "Clean air is valuable," one should be understood exactly as if one were exclaiming "Hooray for clean air!" or "Whoopie! Clean air!"—neither of which is true or false. Therefore, and most importantly, it would be foolish to try to find any property in virtue of which the predicate "is valuable" may be appropriately applied because there is no such property. Since the sentence "Clean air is valuable" is not functioning as a declarative sentence, the predicate "is valuable" is not functioning as the name of some attribute in people or air or anything else. The fundamental assumption of all cognitivists is, according to the emotivists, just plain wrong-headed. Value judgments are not genuine truth claims at all; so it is pointless to ask why some are true and some are not.

Prescriptivism

On what may be called a *prescriptivist* view of the nature of value, to say that something is good or valuable is not to affirm anything at all, but merely to recommend or prescribe something. Like the emotivists, prescriptivists also depart radically from cognitivists because on the prescriptivist view assertions of value are not genuine truth claims. On this view such assertions have the logical status of commands, not of declarative sentences. Just as the prescription "Take two aspirins and go to bed" does not have a truth value, the sentences "It is good to be healthy" and "Better to be healthy than sick" are supposed to be without truth values. Apparent declaratives like "It is good to be healthy" should be interpreted functionally as prescriptions like "Promote healthiness," "Take care of your health," "Prefer health to illness." Again then, as is the case for emotivists, according to prescriptivists the fundamental assumption for all cognitivists is just wrongheaded. Value judgments are. not genuine truth claims at all; so it is pointless to ask why some are true and some are false.

The nice thing about noncognitivist views is that they provide an explanation for the apparent fact that people have not been able to discover and display the properties in virtue of which things are said to have or lack value. If "value" and "good" are not the names of any properties, there were none to be found. Noncognitivist theories also have the virtue of reminding us that evaluations often if not always are used as expressions of emotion and as prescriptions. Even if one rejects pure noncognitivism, it's difficult to reject these insights of the noncognitivist position. Evaluative sentences frequently seem to do double or even triple duty.

Rational Decision-Making

Two sections ago I raised the question: Can it help your epistemological task (the task of deciding which sentences are true and which are false) to know that a sentence in question involves an ontologically factual or evaluative claim? I answered that it might, and spent some time unpacking that answer. It might have been comforting to be able to say straightaway that yes, by God, once we know if we're confronted by facts or values we know where we are. At the very least some methodological roads are closed. Some kinds of answers will never be forthcoming, and so on. It might have been comforting, but it would not have been true.

The truth is that for some epistemological and evaluative views, the fact-value distinction is problematic and the gap between facts and values is logically unbridgeable. For thoroughgoing epistemological skeptics, the gap, insofar as it is recognized at all, is as serious as a pimple on a malignant tumor. For people holding a naturalistic theory of value, whether it is of an objectivist or subjectivist variety, there is no ontological distinction between facts and values. There are merely formally and functionally different ways to talk about and deal with facts, empirical or logical facts.

What I want to do in this final section is to suggest a useful procedural rule of rational decision-making. The rule is not, as far as I can tell, derivable in a strict sense from the preceding discussion. But it has emerged fairly directly in my own mind as a consequence of that discussion. The rule is just this: Forget about the fact-value distinction. It's almost always a red herring.

Whether the question at issue is epistemological, ontological, or axiological (i.e., a question of truth, being, or value) one is almost always wiser to tackle the question directly rather than to try to cut one's ontological pie into facts and values. Martin Luther King said that the trouble with resorting to violence is that then the issue becomes violence. I think that the trouble with resorting to metaphysics is that then the issue becomes metaphysical. Instead of fighting battles about whether something is true, good, or worth doing, one finds oneself fighting battles about credentials, either the ontological credentials of the issue before one (Is it a matter of truth or goodness or action?) or the credentials of the disputants. Instead of pressing the question "Are there good reasons for believing, preferring, or doing this or that?" the red herring question is raised "Is this a matter of values or facts?" The red herring question can have the effect of silencing voices and eliminating points of view that might happen to be right, or giving too much ground to those who are wrong. Neither error has to be risked if one insists that debate must focus on the issue of truth or falsity, or on what is to be done. Either one can substantiate one's case to satisfy most people or not. How one classifies the type of argumentation used is, I think, quite beside the point.

In the area of energy development decision-making in particular, I think that what we have been witnessing for the past few years is an attempt by some folks to have a greater voice in such decision-making. If one describes this effort as an attempt to get some values into energy policy development, then one may be drawing an imaginary line that some people will never be able to cross. On one side will be hardheads with the facts and on the other side will be softheads with values. It would be strategically wiser to describe the effort as an attempt to get a wider spectrum of issues considered or voices heard. Given our fuzzy understanding of facts and values as ontological categories, we have a stronger epistemological and moral warrant to describe the effort in this way. There will be facts and values (whatever both of these are) that everyone regards as relevant, some that everyone regards as irrelevant, and some about which people will disagree. If we can get agreement on what is true, good, or ought to be done, who but a metaphysician cares if we're agreeing on something factual or valuable or both? On the other hand, if we can agree that something is factual or valuable or both but can't agree on whether it's true, good, or ought to be done, then who but a metaphysician cares about that? In short, it seems to be a good idea for everyone but metaphysicians to forget about the fact-value distinction and get on with the pursuit of truth and the performance of good deeds.

Conclusion

In a roundabout way I think that all I have been arguing for here is humility in the interests of rational decision-making. I don't expect anyone to stop talking about facts and values as if I had laid these beasts of burden to rest. Indeed, I don't expect to stop talking about facts and values either. If I have managed to make it more difficult for some people—whether technology assessors, science policy analysts, or others—to use the terms glibly, and more difficult for them to be certain of the strengths of their own positions and the weaknesses of other people's positions, that will be enough.

Chapter 14
A Pragmatic Theory of Value

Alex C. Michalos

Introduction

In this paper I present a socio-psychological theory of satisfaction, called multiple discrepancies theory (MDT), and an empirical, Pragmatic theory of value based on it. MDT has emerged out of the social indicators movement since roughly the mid 60s. The Pragmatic theory of value has evolved out of the work of utilitarian philosophers and political economists beginning in the first half of the 18th century. Before explaining the two theories, it will be worthwhile to provide some background material.

Broadly speaking, social indicators researchers have used two explanatory models to account for satisfaction and happiness with life as a whole or with various domains of life (e.g., housing, friendships, transportation, health, etc.). In one model satisfaction and happiness with life as a whole are assumed to be determined by (to be linear functions of) satisfaction with domains of life. That is, it is assumed that one's general satisfaction with life is determined by one's satisfaction with such specific aspects as one's friendship networks, one's job, housing, and so on. When satisfaction with life as a whole is taken as a dependent variable and regressed on, say, half a dozen domain-type variables, a researcher is usually able to account for from at least half to two-thirds or more of the variance in that dependent variable. When happiness with life as a whole is taken as the dependent variable, the results are not quite as good.

This model has been used in several Western nations on a variety of samples (including national probability samples) with strikingly similar results. (See, for

---

Paper written in 1984, unpublished.

A.C. Michalos (✉)
University of Northern British Columbia, Prince George, BC, Canada
e-mail: michalos@brandonu.ca

A.C. Michalos, *Philosophical Foundations of Quality of Life*,
DOI 10.1007/978-3-319-50727-9_14

example, Andrews and Withey (1976), Andrews and Inglehart (1979).) Primary determinants of satisfaction with life as a whole include the obvious things such as health, housing, etc. There are of course differences too. In my research on rural senior citizens, for example, I found that domains involving interpersonal relations (e.g., spouse, friendship, family) were the primary determinants of happiness with life as a whole, while satisfaction with housing and health were the primary determinants of satisfaction with life as a whole (Michalos 1982). As one restricts one's sample to a single sex or age group, the primary determinants of life satisfaction tend to alter, as one would expect.

In another model, satisfaction and happiness are assumed to be determined by perceived gaps or differences between what one has and wants, has and thinks relevant others have, and has and has had in the past. Gap theoretic models have had less direct testing than the other analytic models, but the testing that has occurred has been fairly successful. I guess on average, about half the variance in our dependent variables (whether they are whole life or domain variables) can be explained using a gap theoretic model. In some work I did with rural people, using 22 variables to account for satisfaction with housing I could only explain about 30% of the variance in my dependent variable. With only 3 gap theoretic variables, I was able to account for over 40%. These 3 variables explained nearly 70% of the variance in satisfaction with transportation for my rural senior citizen sample. For reviews of this literature, see Michalos (1979, 1980a, 1982, 1983a, b).

Now, if you are familiar with the literature in the utilitarian tradition, especially Sidgwick's brilliant book on *The Methods of Ethics* (1874), you may already have a hint of the importance of this social indicators work for that older tradition. Using empirical research and multivariate statistical analysis we have been able to do things that Sidgwick did not know how to do, and even suspected could not be done. For example, we can measure reported satisfaction and happiness, the impact of satisfaction with various domains on life as a whole, the relations between satisfaction in diverse domains and trade-offs across domains, and the impact of conation, cognition and affect on satisfaction. Similar remarks may be made about the work of R.B. Perry and C.I. Lewis, the great naturalistic value theorists of this century. Perry's *General Theory of Value* (1926) is loaded with the empirical psychology of his day, but there was just not much available. Lewis's *An Analysis of Knowledge and Valuation* (1946) is practically void of social scientific research of his day.

The task I have set for myself for the next few years is to take the naturalistic program, especially Lewis's version of it, a step further. In the notes to follow I have tried to develop the bare bones of a pragmatic theory of value which is informed by the most current social science and responsive to the major objections to Lewis, Perry and Sidgwick. At this point I'm by no means sure about exactly what has to be stipulated as analytic, and what can be asserted and strongly confirmed or rejected on empirical grounds. It will take time to find all the pieces and put them in place. Obviously I welcome all the help I can get.

Satisfaction

According to multiple discrepancies theory (MDT),

H1: Reported net satisfaction is a linear function of perceived discrepancies between what one has and (a) wants, (b) thinks relevant others have, (c) the best one has had in the past, (d) expects to have after 5 years, (e) thinks one deserves and (f) needs.
H2: There is a rank ordering of impact of perceived discrepancies on net satisfaction, with that between what one has and wants taking precedence over all others.
H3: The perceived discrepancy between what one has and wants also serves as a mediating variable between all other perceived discrepancies and reported net satisfaction.

MDT incorporates the insights of aspiration theorists in H1 (a), social comparison theorists in H1 (b), expectancy theorists in H1 (d), equity theorists in H1 (e) and person-environment fit theorists in H1 (f). In the form presented here, especially H1, the theory has only been partly confirmed, as explained in the previous section and reviewed in the several studies cited there. Still, the confirmation that does exist is substantial.

H1 refers to reported satisfaction because the survey research procedures used to test MDT rely on personal reports. Although I usually omit the word 'reported', strictly speaking it is essential. Usually, I think, things are regarded and reported as satisfying if and only if on balance they are satisfying. So, typically 'satisfaction' has the force of 'net satisfaction', and 'dissatisfaction' has the force of 'net dissatisfaction'. Scales running from 'very satisfied' to 'very dissatisfied' presuppose that respondents are reporting net assessments. H1 and H2 refer to net satisfaction, but in practice the 'net' will be omitted.

According to MDT in H1, satisfaction is a natural property that emerges from or is caused by elements of conation, cognition and evaluation. These three elements may be present in different amounts in different occurrences of satisfaction.

There are two conative elements related to satisfaction, namely, wanting and needing. H2 asserts that the former has a more predominant role to play than the latter, since the perceived gap between what one has and wants always has a greater impact on satisfaction than any other perceived gap.

Following the analysis given in Michalos (1978), it is assumed that wanting and needing may be adequately explicated without appealing to any evaluative notions beyond those required for warranted assertability. Without rehashing my views, I should say that insofar as knowledge claims are claims which one is warranted in asserting according to some rules of epistemic evaluation, all such claims involve some evaluation essentially. In other words, strictly speaking it is logically impossible for there to be a body of knowledge (or any knowledge at all for that matter) independent of all evaluation. Since nothing counts as knowledge unless it has appropriate epistemic credentials, an appropriate epistemic warrant or briefly a good reason behind it, the idea of unwarranted knowledge is logically incoherent. From this point of view, in order for one to know that one wants or needs something, one must assume that some sort of an epistemic evaluation has been made or at least implicitly granted.

Some satisfactions require having a want or a need as a necessary condition. Satisfaction in such cases practically amounts to satisfying the want or need. Since wanting and needing may be given relatively affect-free dispositional analyses, no feeling or sensation has to accompany wanting or needing, or the satisfaction of a want or a need. Of course, some feelings or sensations may frequently or even usually accompany some wants, needs and their satisfaction. That is not precluded by anything asserted here.

There are two cognitive elements related to satisfaction, namely, what one thinks relevant others have and what one expects to have after 5 years. The first involves knowledge of the lives of others and the second involves estimates of future prospects. Each may be more or less reliable and valid. Usually what one thinks relevant others have has a greater impact on one's satisfaction than estimates of one's future prospects.

The two overtly evaluative elements related to satisfaction involve considerations of the best experience one has had in the past and what one deserves. Insofar as satisfaction is a function of perceived discrepancies based on such evaluations, any empirical theory of value that is based on satisfaction will involve some circularity. This is certainly an undesirable consequence. However, how undesirable it is depends on exactly how much satisfaction is a function of such evaluations. If, for example, it turns out that considerations of the best previous experience and desert have relatively little impact on net satisfaction, then satisfaction might provide a relatively sound basis for an empirical theory of value free of vicious circularity. If these overtly evaluative elements weigh in heavily, then some other empirical basis would have to be found.

Since I doubt that it is possible to have a value-free social scientific theory, I doubt that it is possible to have a value-free theory of satisfaction and, beyond that, a value-free empirical theory of value. In the latter case, one is clearly engaged in pulling oneself up by one's own bootstraps to some extent. Since the greater the extent, the sillier the enterprise, one must be conscious of the danger of vicious circularity at every step of the way.

One notable advantage of explaining satisfaction along the lines of H1 is that it allows one to distinguish a fool's paradise from a real paradise on the basis of the accuracy of one's perceptions and alleged knowledge. If, for example, one were poorly informed about the lives of relevant others, then one's perceptions of the gap between one's own circumstances and theirs might be severely inaccurate. If one's memory failed, then one's perceptions of the gap between one's present circumstances and the best one had ever experienced might also be inaccurate. The facts that people don't always know what they want or need also imply the possibility of inaccuracy and confusion. Moreover, even if one's knowledge base were relatively sound, one's capacity for assessing discrepancies might be more or less reliable and valid. Thus, a hypothetical fool would be fooled not by having the satisfaction resulting from misperceptions or erroneous beliefs. The satisfaction may be as real as anything else, but it has liabilities of which the fool is unaware. It is logically possible for a fool (and the rest of us I guess) to go through life without ever suffering as a result of having misperceptions or false beliefs, i.e., to live in error for a lifetime without suffering serious consequences. Still, insofar as one values truth at all, one would have to admit that real paradise would be preferable to a fool's paradise, i.e., that epistemologically well-warranted satisfaction would be preferable to unwarranted satisfaction.

The last sentence is so reminiscent of Mill's famous remark that it would be better to be Socrates dissatisfied than a pig satisfied that, a brief comment may be worthwhile. There are four relevant cases to consider, namely, those in which one's warrant or reasons are

(1) good and one is satisfied (Paradise)
(2) good and one is dissatisfied (Hell)
(3) bad and one is satisfied (Fool's Paradise)
(4) bad and one is dissatisfied (Fool's Hell)

I suppose there will be no disagreement about the judgment that paradise is the best of the four states. It seems that Mill would have preferred what I call hell to what I call a fool's paradise. Whether or not he did, someone might and if so, there might be no way for us to reach agreement. My view of knowledge or the possession of truth is thoroughly pragmatic. If the possession of truth yields no satisfaction or, as Perry might have said, satisfies no interest at all, then It is worthless. Such truth is literally without value as it is defined below. Inspecting the four cases above, it is clear that whether one has good or bad reasons for being satisfied, it is better to be satisfied than dissatisfied. That is, paradise is better than hell and a fool's paradise is better than a fool's hell.

The final feature of H1 that should be noticed is that although it makes no reference to positive affect or pleasure, the latter frequently accompanies satisfaction. It is possible to use the term 'satisfaction' so that it is practically synonymous with positive affect or pleasure. This is *not* the way I use the term. Positive affect or pleasure may be entirely absent from satisfaction, and in its place one might find a certain disposition, propensity or tendency to act in favour of, to support or to defend something. The case here is similar to that of liking, as the latter notion was analyzed in Michalos (1978).

Criteria of Adequacy

The question before us is: What criteria or conditions of adequacy should be stipulated for a pragmatic theory of value? In other words, according to what assumptions, rules or principles should this theory be appraised? As explained in Michalos (1978), some criteria are generally applicable to all theories and some are applicable only to specific theories. Moreover, some may be articulated quite formally, while others can be only informally indicated. I believe the following conditions must be satisfied by my theory.

(1) The theory should be internally self-consistent, i.e., free of logical self-contradiction.
(2) It should be externally consistent with well-warranted claims of common sense and science. Of course the term "well-warranted" is bearing a heavy burden in this requirement. Without attempting a lengthy analysis of this notion, let us agree that the claims of common sense and science range from the relatively indisputable to the highly disputable, and that external consistency merely requires my theory to be consistent with the relatively indisputable claims insofar as the latter are identifiable. The acceptance of this condition may be regarded as a rejection of the Cartesian idea that one ought to try to initiate research without any preconceptions. On the contrary, I accept the pragmatic view of a community of researchers as described by Peirce and Dewey, a community which provides a stock and flow of more or less well-warranted and fallible beliefs and practices. (I will have much more to say about this in my discussion of epistemic value.)
(3) It should provide a credible replacement or meaning analysis of fundamental evaluative terms, e.g., objective value, moral value, epistemic value (Lewis 1946, p. 466). If theoretical terms are introduced as explications (explicata) of terms in ordinary language (explicanda) then the former should bear some credible resemblance to the latter without being merely acceptable dictionary definitions.
(4) It should provide theoretical terms (explicata) and propositions that are generally more precise and more easily appraised than those it is supposed to be replacing, explicating or explaining. Perry (1926, p. 126) claimed that the "proof" of a definition of value is its success in facilitating the solution of all special questions of value. The data and difficulties of evaluations in ethics, esthetics and so on should fall into place in a coherent system.
(5) It should make all types of evaluations comparable and in principle commensurable. In other words, the theory should be such that all types of value are shown to be species of a single genus (Perry 1926, pp. 9–10).

It may be helpful here to distinguish *things that have value* from the *value that things have*. Anything may be regarded by someone as valuable or as something that has value, e.g., telephones, sex, justice and the English language. Usually, when people use the plural term 'values', they are referring to things they or someone regards as valuable. They may say something like 'Catholics regard marriage as a value' or 'Feminists regard free choice on abortion as a value'.

Such remarks may lead one to say that there are a wide variety or a plurality of values. Alternatively, one might say that there are a variety of valuable things and that all these things have some property in virtue of which they are regarded as valuable. This property (whatever it is) is what I refer to as the value that things have, and it is precisely this property that is the subject matter of my theory of value.

People who think that there are a variety of incommensurable values may regard this fifth adequacy condition as reductive and question-begging. However, it could only be so if their theory were well-warranted and mine were not, and if I were simply assuming that my theory is well-warranted. Obviously neither of these conditions is satisfied. My fifth requirement merely makes an aim of my theory explicit. It indicates one of the things such a theory should do. It does not prove that it is possible or even reasonable to try to construct such a theory.

(6) The theory should be such that value admits of measurement or quantification on at least an ordinal scale.

(7) It should be empirically testable. Given the comparability (5) and quantification (6) requirements, rigorous testability is virtually assured. This condition makes the need for such testing explicit. Although the definitions or meaning analyses of basic theoretical terms will be stipulated a priori, the theory must also generate particular and general (lawlike) propositions subject to empirical testing (Lewis 1946, p. 469). Insofar as the empirical testability of a theory may be regarded as a necessary condition of the latter's scientific status, the satisfaction of this seventh requirement may be regarded as contributing to the scientific status of the theory.

Generic Value

So far the basic elements of a socio-psychological theory of satisfaction have been presented, namely, the theory of multiple discrepancies or MDT. This is the empirical basis of the theory of value about to be presented. I begin with a definition of generic value.

D1: *Generic value* is identical to satisfaction.

The empirical theory of value that will be sketched here may be regarded as acceptable precisely insofar as every known species of value can be plausibly defined by appropriately qualifying this generic notion of value. Obviously I can not consider all or even most species of value in this brief paper. In fact, I will only present definitions of three important species, namely, objective value, moral value and epistemic value. A preliminary, but probably accurate, judgment about the likely output of the fully developed theory may be made on the basis of the acceptability of these three crucial definitions.

D1 is an analytic a priori stipulation. It is not proposed as an analysis of the meanings of words as commonly used. It is asserted as a basic definition of a key word in my theory. If it happens to be the case that most people use the words 'generic value' and 'satisfaction' as synonyms, that would make it easy for most people to accept D1. One might even want to regard D1 as an empirically accurate account of how those words are used by most people, if most people do indeed use the words that way. In that case D1 would be regarded as a lexical rather than a stipulative definition (Michalos 1969). Still, I regard D1 as stipulative, and that's the main point.

Insofar as satisfaction is a function of perceived discrepancies, so is generic value. That is, given H1, D1 implies that whatever value there is in the world is a natural effect of natural causes. Moreover, given H1, D1 implies that generic value is not simple nor unanalyzable.

Apprehensions of generic value are not incorrigible or indubitable. They typically involve judgments that are corrigible, and even pure affect may be corrigible. For example, it sometimes happens that tastes that seem immediately pleasant turn out to be unpleasant on closer inspection. Similarly, other experiences are not always immediately identifiable as of one sort or another. One's sensory receptors are just not infallible.

Generic value is ultimately or finally desirable for its own sake. In this respect, it is like intrinsic value as found in Lewis (1946, p. 382) and what is prized according to Dewey (1939, p. 5). Because it is a human quality rather than a quality of nonhuman things, it may be regarded as intrinsic to humans.

No assumption is made about the value of human beings or human nature itself. I think that the question of the moral value of human nature cannot be answered in a non-question-begging or non-self-contradictory way. Whether one says that human nature is morally good or evil, one must assume some criterion of moral evaluation. Suppose, for example, it is said that human nature is good insofar as it satisfied my Definition 8 (below). Then it is logically impossible for the definition to be satisfied by beings whose human nature is morally bad. Alternatively, suppose it is said that human nature is good regardless of any consequences emerging from that nature. Then clearly some other criterion than the satisfaction of D8 is being assumed. To simply affirm that the other criterion is acceptable while mine is not is to beg the question against mine.

Generic value may be used as a synonym for generic good. Then it would be reasonable to think of dissatisfaction as generic badness or evil. I guess one could talk about disvalue or negative value as identical to dissatisfaction. The word "disvalue" is pretty uncommon; so I try to avoid it. I will have almost nothing else to say about badness, evil or negative value, but it's easy to take what I say about value or goodness and construct parallel remarks about negative value or evil.

The satisfaction of any interest or want constitutes value, but not necessarily the same amount of value for every want satisfied. Wants that are more difficult to satisfy probably have greater positive affect when they are satisfied.

The satisfaction of morally evil wants also creates value, but obviously not moral value or goodness. In terms of satisfaction, one may say that the satisfaction of a morally evil want trivially constitutes satisfaction of a want and hence generic value. Still, it is trivially true that it is morally wrong to satisfy morally evil wants.

Since one may want knowledge, the satisfaction of this cognitive interest also constitutes generic value.

Objective Value

Since the flowering of logical positivism in the first half of this century, perhaps no idea has been more maligned than that of objective value. The attacks have been so severe that most people seem to reject the notion without the slightest bit of attention to it. Lacking even youthful defenders, its existential status is probably even lower than Santa Claus's. Hopefully, the next definition can begin to change things. D2 introduces the theoretic term 'objective value' in terms of a set of observable operations and an observable property, satisfaction.

D2: *If*

(a) any standard observer *i*
(b) in standard conditions
(c) performs a standard test on any object *o, then o* has *objective value* if and only if *o* produces satisfaction (generic value) for *i*.

D2 gives the general form of an operational definition of objective value. One might say that it gives a formal meaning analysis of the term 'objective value' in terms of generally specified operations or procedures, and a specific sort of result. To determine the objective value of any particular object one must particularize the operations, i.e., explain 'standard observer', 'conditions' and 'tests' for various types of objects.

Such definitions may specify meaning in a limited fashion, the limits being given by the sorts of tests available. Still, there are no better ways to define theoretic terms naming directly unobservable empirical properties. For example, the dispositional term 'weight' names a property which is empirical but not directly observable. One can specify tests and results that yield acceptable evidence that something has weight (or even some quantity of weight), but one cannot observe the presence of the disposition itself. Objective value has the same sort of dispositional existence. It is an empirical tendency, disposition or propensity to produce satisfaction (i.e. generic value) in certain specifiable conditions, just as weight is a disposition to move scale pans or springs under specifiable conditions.

So much has been written about observation and the difficulties of making sharp distinctions between observation and theoretical terms in natural languages, that a few remarks should be made about my assumptions. (A brief review of the literature may be found in Michalos 1980b.) The main point I wish to insist upon is that the observation term-theoretical term distinction involved in D2 is no worse than it is in any other operational definition. Put positively, it is at least as reasonable to operationally define objective value as in D2 as it is to define the standard textbook dispositional terms 'water soluble' and 'brittle'. The operationally defined term 'objective value' must have the same empirical status as 'water soluble' or 'brittle', for whatever that is worth. In short, I claim all and only as much empirical status and theoretical tidiness for objective value as I would for water solubility and brittleness.

No specific number of standard observers is required by D2. The idea is that *any* standard observer, past, present or future would be able to administer the test. More must be said about standard observers, specialists and experts. (See D3.) However, if observers are specialists or experts, the same universality would be assumed for them.

It's not likely that any number of standard observers can be traded off against specialists or experts. The latter have training and abilities that the former don't have, probably not even collectively. Among people equally likely to be able to perceive value in some field, majority rule may have to be used.

For some fields, then, it is assumed that 'standard observer' would have to be replaced by 'specialist'. The use of an expert would never be required in an operational definition. Expert testimony is a luxury rather than a necessity.

One might think of subjective value as being defined by an expression like D2 with some peculiarly specified (a) observer, (b) conditions or (c) tests. The rest of the definition would stand as is.

With D2 and standard tests of love, friendship, clean air, justice, beauty, liberty, etc. we can prove these things have objective value. For example, we can set up experimental situations in which individuals are asked to play the roles alternatively of friendly and unfriendly, constructive and destructive, clean and dirty, responsible and irresponsible, honest and dishonest, and so on. Then we can systematically measure the generic value that tends to be produced for the individuals of a variety of groups in which such role-playing occurs. In principle certainly and in fact almost as certainly we could build up a body of scientific hypotheses, facts, laws and theories of value. That is precisely the sort of long-range research program I have in mind.

D3: One is a *standard observer* if and only if

(a) one is not biased with respect to any relevant observations, and
(b) one's performance on standardized tests of basic cognitive and sensory capacities is at least within one standard deviation of the mean for all test-takers.

According to D3 (a), it is required that there should be no intentional misperceptions and that any unintentional errors should be random. It is assumed that standard statistical procedures may be used to measure nonrandom and random errors in measured perceptions. Thus, 'bias' is understood here as a matter of probabilities, not as a matter of morality, fairness or justice.

The assumption behind D3 (b) is that there are sufficiently reliable and valid standardized tests of intelligence, sight and hearing, for examples, to identify ordinary (normal) and extraordinary capacities. Infallibility and value-neutrality for such tests is never assumed here.

Standard observers are not ideal observers, experts or connoisseurs. On the contrary, they provide a basis for being able to identify experts.

The possession of some commonly held capacities is a necessary condition of having some kinds of experiences. Blind people cannot be expected to get any satisfaction from "looking at" paintings. Mentally retarded people cannot be expected to get any satisfaction from working problems in advanced calculus.

What's required is something analogous to the role played by the corner butcher in weighing meat. Nothing extraordinary is required of such a person to put a chunk of meat on a scale and read the results. Similarly, I would assume that such a person could serve as a standard observer for a wide range of tests for objective value.

Of course the corner butcher would be a poor standard observer to weigh subatomic particles, measure the speed of light or the value of a painting by Rubens. Any particular butcher may or may not be able to learn to manage the required tests, understand the theories, etc. Still, the point to be emphasized is that different species of standard observers will have to be identified for different fields or ranges of possible observations.

To insist upon different species of standard observers is not to insist upon experts yet, although ordinary language is troublesome here. I want to allow, for example, that physics students are not yet classifiable as experts, but may have enough training to know how to weigh subatomic particles. In other words, I want to allow for run-of-the-mill physicists or standard observers in the field of physics. Such people may be expected to perform within a standard deviation of the mean for all physicists. Then beyond these normal folks there will be a certain percentage of stars and duds, and I would like to reserve the name 'expert' for the stars.

So, I'm proposing various sorts of standard observers, beginning with ordinary folks, proceeding to ordinary specialists in certain fields and then experts or connoisseurs. I think that common usage would fudge my specialists and connoisseurs into one group called 'experts', and contrast these folks with ordinary people.

A butcher would be adequate to the task of weighing meat and to evaluating his scales to some extent. One could be expected to correctly perceive that one's scale is poor if, say, it always registered 3 lb. A butcher would know in broad terms what to expect from a good scale and some sure signs of a scale that was not good, worthless or without objective value as a scale. Again, however, such a person need not be accorded extraordinary capacities, certainly nothing to qualify as a specialist, expert or connoisseur.

Similarly, specialists in physics or painting may be expected to know in broad terms how to go about weighing subatomic particles and measuring the esthetic value of a Rubens. The physicist and art critic will know their subjects or specialties, know what to look for. Neither will set up shop in the dark, etc.

The appropriate definition and selection of standard observers is crucial from the point of view of the satisfaction to be obtained from any observation and from the point of view of the accuracy of estimations of that satisfaction. The problem here is, I think, endemic to epistemology. Standard definitions of weight, for example, could not be obtained if there were no more or less typical experiences of weight and more or less accurate estimations of those experiences. If people's experiences with and estimations of weight were entirely random, there would be no way to zero in on a standard definition of weight. Moreover, just as weight will be regarded as whatever our standard observers of weight say it is (for better or worse), satisfaction will be too. It happens, of course, that some standard observers and their stories come to be replaced by others, but I can't go into those problems here.

D4: One is a *specialist* in some field if and only if one has greater training, experience or capacity in that field than average standard observers.

According to D4, it is assumed that one becomes a specialist as a result of having above average education, training or studying, above average breadth of personal experience or above average natural powers or capacities for discernment. Different specialists might have different mixtures of such ingredients.

Specialists may be thought of as standard observers in special fields, specialized standard observers, standard observers of a special sort, or particular species of standard observers.

D5: One is an *expert* or *connoisseur* in some field if and only if

(a) one is a specialist in that field, and
(b) the reliability and validity of one's appraisals in that field are above average for such specialists.

According to D5, experts are essentially "a cut above" specialists. They represent a class of relatively extraordinary specialists, as measured by the reliability and validity of their usual output. Of course one would expect more disputes about the identification of specialists. One would expect to find borderline cases, conflicting judgments about who is better than whom, for what reasons, and so on. Insofar as such problems are unsolvable in any given field (art, science, law or whatever), the idea of an expert will be useless. A priori there is no way to decide exactly which fields will be more or less troublesome.

D6: *Standard conditions* obtain if and only if the conditions do not introduce any bias into the testing procedures.

One is inclined to opt for some stronger terms like 'optimum' or 'ideal' conditions, but the only necessary condition seems to be the elimination of bias. In practice that will mean that conditions are standard if there are at least no good reasons to think that the conditions bias test results in a certain way, or at most good reasons to think that the conditions do not lead to such bias.

Here again we face traditional epistemological problems that are not unique to evaluations, and again there will be clear-cut and borderline cases. For example, clear-cut standard conditions for the inspection of visual properties would include adequate lighting. It would be silly to try to get an objective assessment of what something looks like if the thing is hidden in a totally dark room, under a basket, behind a brick wall and under water. We have good reasons to think such conditions would bias what we see—to put it mildly. On the other hand, it might be difficult to decide on standard conditions for the inspection of adolescent behaviour under stress. What looks like a stressful situation to one person may not look like one to some other person. Still, all one can validly conclude from such difficulties is that there are going to be difficulties in getting agreement on some standard conditions for measuring the value of some things.

For the sorts of tests that will be relevant to measuring satisfaction, standard conditions would typically include random selection of standard observers (respondents). If special fields are involved (e.g., painting, motor vehicles) or special groups (e.g., elderly, poor) random selection would occur within specially defined observation areas.

Standard conditions will typically be reproducible, but the only virtue of reproducibility is to control against bias in experimental set-ups. So reproducibility does not have to be included in the definition of standard conditions.

D7: A *standard test* is

(a) unbiased,
(b) with a measurable degree of reliability and validity, for measuring the presence of some property.

There are hundreds of standardized tests in print for things like verbal and mathematical ability, perceptual acuity, and so on. D7 simply suggests a couple of key features such tests must have.

H4 lists some probable consequences of something or someone having objective value.

H4: If x has more objective value than y then, if all other things are equal, probably

(a) x produces satisfaction

(i) for more people
(ii) for a longer duration
(iii) with greater intensity
(iv) with higher probability (reliability)
(v) requiring greater cognitive demands
(vi) requiring greater conative demands
(vii) requiring greater affective demands

(b) x has

(i) greater inclusiveness
(ii) greater harmony (coherence, integration)

This multi-faceted empirical hypothesis replaces the traditional hedonic or felicific calculus. The features listed in H4 characterize things with objective value or the satisfaction obtained from such things. The operational definition of objective value, D2, is adequate as a definition for greater or less value. By D2 something has more or less objective value exactly in proportion as it produces (under standard conditions, etc.) generic value or satisfaction. H4 merely lists features that as a matter of fact probably characterize things with relatively greater objective value or the satisfaction obtained from such things. Although many of these features have been talked about since Bentham's early work, I know of no rigorous empirical tests of their connection to objective value. There certainly have been no tests of their connections to objective value as operationalized in D2.

I assume that current measures of satisfaction (e.g., the delighted-terrible scale) plus the Standard Gamble technique will be sufficient to measure satisfaction or generic value. The former gives us ordinal values which the latter can turn into interval values in principle.

Moral Value

Like objective value, the idea of moral value is of fundamental importance to a general theory of value. Any theory of value that could not provide an acceptable definition of moral value would be so impoverished as to be worthless. I propose the following:

D8: Something has *moral value* exactly insofar as it impartially maximizes each affected person's objective probability of obtaining the maximum average amount of objective value that is factually possible to obtain under the circumstances, and subsequently allows Pareto optimal increments.

A shorter and perhaps misleading formulation of D8 might run thus: Something has moral value insofar as it impartially maximizes the average amount of objective value going to each person, allowing subsequent Pareto optimal increments.

Several features of D8 require explanation. First, the roots of this definition are utilitarian, as the imprecise and somewhat misleading shorter formulation may reveal more clearly. According to D8, moral value or moral goodness is measured by the quantity and distribution of objective value or, goodness. Traditionally, utilitarians have recommended maximizing either *total utility* (in some sense) for a group or *average utility* for each member of a group. The latter includes a distribution requirement that the former omits, and has been vigorously defended by John Harsanyi in a number of publications, e.g., most recently in Harsanyi (1982). Without going into details now, it is fair to say that the main difference between Harsanyi's proposal and mine lies in my use of the idea of objective value. I will have much more to say about this later.

D8 includes two theoretical terms that were explicated at length in Michalos (1978), namely, 'objective probability' and 'factual possibility'. Without going into details, the former term is used to designate either relative frequencies or propensities, while the latter term is used to designate any occurrences whose descriptions do not contradict any true sentences. The ideas of interpreting probabilities as relative frequencies or propensities will probably be familiar to most readers. In the absence of objective probabilities, one would have to resort to some sort of personal or logical probabilities. The reference to impartial maximization in D8 is an abbreviated way of indicating two things, namely, equalizing and maximizing probabilities. What is required is not merely giving each affected person the same chance but the same and as good a chance as possible. In the best case, of course, each affected person would be certain to have an equal share of the total objective value available.

I invented the idea of factual possibilities in response to the problem of the multiplicity of kinds of possibilities that were identified by various writers, e.g., physical, logical, political and technological possibilities. One fundamental distinction that obtains no matter how many kinds of possibilities are identified is the distinction between occurrences that are impossible because they admit of no self-consistent description (e.g., Drawing circular squares.) and occurrences that are impossible because their descriptions are inconsistent with some true sentence(s). (e.g., 'I can fly by waving my arms' states a physical impossibility insofar as it cannot be true given the truth of certain physical laws and sentences about the structure of my arms.)

The phrase "under the circumstances" in D8 is included to allow for such things as the determination of appropriate regions of analysis in which to make relevant measurements and estimates. The trouble with definitions like D8 is that they usually give no hint as to when to start or stop counting effects; who is to be included, for how long, in what areas, etc. They also are usually silent on required levels of reliability and validity (consistency and accuracy) of measurements. I have explored these problems in a bit more detail in Michalos (1978), and will therefore not rehash my "solutions" here. I have not written my last word on these important matters, but I don't have anything new to add to that earlier discussion.

It is primarily actions that are said to have moral value, but D8 allows other things as well. I have argued in Michalos (1976, 1978) that beliefs and sets of beliefs as embodied in scientific and other sorts of theories are subject to moral appraisal. D8 makes such appraisal possible.

Maxims that have traditionally been accepted as moral or having moral significance (e.g., prescriptions for truth telling, proscriptions of lying) are moral according to D8 just so far as action in accordance with them tends to produce moral value. Again, giving people what is due to them (i.e., treating people justly or with equity) also has moral value.

The moral value of anything according to D8 lies in its probability of generating a maximum average amount of objective value for all those affected by it. In this sense, moral value is supreme among all species of value. It is supremely comprehensive by definition. The highest good is the greatest average good. This consequence of D8 is also of fundamental importance for the general theory of value sketched here. It is frequently held that moral value is supreme among all species of value, but arguments and theories of value that support this view are seldom produced.

Pareto optimal increments of objective value are such that their addition creates no disadvantage for anyone and some advantage for at least one person. I'm not sure if this has to be built into D8 as a moral requirement or if it's simply a matter of common sense. Why, after all, should anyone reject an opportunity to increase objective value for someone when (by hypothesis) it creates no loss of objective value for anyone else?

As defined in D8, moral value is in principle measurable. In fact, of course, rigorous measurement will frequently give way to estimates and "guesstimates".

To appraise something from a moral point of view is to appraise it from the point of view of its moral value. Any issue becomes a moral issue just so far as it is appraised from a moral point of view. This is another advantageous consequence of the present approach to morality, namely, that it provides a sufficient criterion for identifying moral issues which is broader than the application of moral maxims. It is often said that one knows one is faced with a moral issue when one has a generally accepted moral maxim that is directly applicable. For example, one knows that lying is a moral issue because one has the well-known maxim that says lying is morally wrong. On this view, moral issues exist insofar as relevant moral maxims exist. On the view recommended here, morality is not defined by the sum total of codified maxims but by the attempt to impartially maximize average amounts of objective value for all people affected by one's actions. From this point of view, one knows that lying, swimming, selling papers or singing are moral issues insofar as they are appraised from the moral point of view, i.e., from, the point of view of their capacity to impartially maximize average amounts of objective value. Thus, from this point of view, morality has profound heuristic value. It provides a priori guidance concerning the moral conduct of human affairs. Instead of providing merely prohibitions, it provides the basis for prescriptions about right action. In particular, D8 leads to the following two definitions.

D9: An act is *morally right* exactly insofar as it produces moral value.
D10: An act *morally ought to be performed* insofar as it is morally right.

According to these two definitions, insofar as one has good reasons to believe that one's act is morally right, one ought to perform it. By D8 one may in principle determine the moral value of actions. By D10 one has a prescription of what to do next.

Definitions 9 and 10 are, of course, analytic and a priori. If a morally right act produces moral value, which is the impartial maximization of objective value to all affected by it, then what is morally right will also be what ought to be done. There will be no morally better option.

Objections to Consequentialism

I use the term "consequentialism" to designate moral theories in which morally right conduct is a function of its contribution to morally good consequences. Classical utilitarian theories are consequentialist since they all involve the designation of something (e.g., an experience of pleasure, happiness or satisfaction) as good in itself and actions designed to maximize such things as morally right. The pragmatic moral theory that I am proposing is obviously consequentialistic, since it defines morally right action in terms of the probable maximization of average amounts of objective value. In the paragraphs that follow, it will be assumed that this theory has been articulated in enough detail to confront it with standard objections to consequentialism generally and to a variety of utilitarian theories. Generally acceptable replies to these objections are required in order to satisfy our criteria of adequacy.

1. *Integrity*. It has been argued that insofar as a moral theory focuses on the maximization of a certain kind of experience (e.g., happiness) regardless of any other aims or interests one may have, particular persons are robbed of their integrity, individuality or autonomy. All three of these terms are used, sometimes by the same author apparently as synonyms and by different authors apparently not as synonyms. For our purposes there is no need to try to give distinct explications for each term. Instead, we will proceed to an examination of some specific texts and work with the implicit definitions provided by each author.

Scheffler (1982, p. 9) puts the problem as follows.

> Utilitarianism … requires the agent to allocate energy and attention to the projects and people he cares most about *in strict proportion* to the value from an impersonal standpoint of his doing so, even though people typically acquire and care about their commitments quite independently of, and out of proportion to, the value that their having and caring about them is assigned in an impersonal ranking of overall states of affairs. It is *this* feature of utilitarianism which may be thought to alienate the agent 'from his actions and the source of his actions in his own convictions', and thereby to undermine his integrity.

Following up some suspicions of Kenneth Arrow about utilitarian theories "denying … individuality in a deep sense", Rawls (1982, pp. 180–181) wrote that

> … it is natural for Arrow to say that the *individuality* of persons is denied. All their conceptions of the good are publicly commensurable via a shared highest-order preference as the notion of a shared highest-order preference defines persons as what we may call 'bare persons'. Such persons are ready to consider any new convictions and aims, and even to abandon attachments and loyalties, when doing this promises a life with greater overall satisfaction, or well-being, as specified by a public ranking. The notion of a bare person implicit in the notion of shared highest-order preference represents the dissolution of the person as leading a life expressive of character and of devotion to specific final ends and adopted (or affirmed) values which define the distinctive points of view associated with different (and incommensurable) conceptions of the good.

Sen and Williams (1982, p. 4) claim that

> Essentially, utilitarianism sees persons as locations of their respective utilities–as the sites at which such activities as desiring and having pleasure and pain take place…. Persons do not count as individuals in this any more than individual petrol tanks do in the analysis of the national consumption of petroleum.

Insofar as these criticisms of utilitarianism have any validity at all, they must be applicable to my pragmatic moral theory too. According to the latter, every person is morally obliged to try to impartially maximize the probability of each affected individual receiving a maximum average amount of objective value. The requirement of impartiality is included precisely to insure that every person has the same status from a moral point of view. Indeed, it is assumed that equal respect for all persons, regardless of any of their particular attributes, is a necessary condition of giving them moral consideration.

Granted, then, that the criticisms regarding integrity or individuality apply to my theory as well as to the utilitarian theories attacked by the authors cited above, I would offer the following replies. First, insofar as any moral theory fails to respect all persons equally, it will fail to be an effective instrument for the resolution of conflicts of interest. Whether one regards conflict resolution as good in itself or as a good means of evenly maximizing average amounts of objective value for all disputants, it cannot be denied that morality frequently plays a significant role in such resolution. Thus, unless one is prepared to abandon this powerful instrument, one's moral theory must include some impartiality requirement.

Second, since the sameness or difference among things can only be determined with respect to specific properties and relations, and a person's individuality or integrity is a function of a wide variety of such attributes, the idea that personal individuality or integrity is undermined, denied, lost, dissolved or discounted by a single similarity is a fantastic oversimplification. One might as well argue that insofar as 25 million people are, most of them want to be and many of them chose to be Canadian citizens, their individuality or integrity has been denied, lost and so on. Any Rawlsian reasonable moral agents who regard justice and personal liberty as the highest goods would thereby undermine or deny their individuality or integrity. Clearly, such people have "a shared highest-order preference", whether it is justice or personal liberty or both, and therefore would become "bare persons" according to Rawls's definition. Thus, if this oversimplified view of personal integrity or individuality proved anything, it would prove far too much to be taken seriously.

Third, each of the three quoted paragraphs above appears to make utilitarian theories more demanding than other theories so far as personal interests are concerned. But this is simply special pleading. Scheffler makes it appear as if utilitarians have less freedom than adherents of other acceptable moral theories to look after their own "projects and people" they care about. Of course the operative word here is "acceptable", but it is not likely that Scheffler is right. It is easy to imagine cases in which, say, a Rawlsian contractarian has to choose between the rights of strangers versus her interests in her own "projects and people". For example, justice as fairness might demand that one walk a picket line along with one's striking colleagues, although one's family is put under some stress worrying about the consequences of such behaviour.

Rawls makes it appear as if utilitarians have to be willing and able to drop everything, abandon "convictions and aims, and even … attachments and loyalties" whenever an opportunity arises to obtain higher levels of satisfaction from such change. But the same may be said of someone who regards justice as fairness as the supreme good. Suppose, for example, that one planned to devote some resources to painting one's house Saturday. Then a friend comes by and explains that the main reason one can engage in that activity is because some Third World worker was coerced into producing the paint at exploitive wages. Justice would be served, he argues, by devoting one's resources to Oxfam instead of to painting one's house. Since the poor, exploited and underprivileged are virtually always going to be with us, one can always find a just cause which, morally speaking, ought to take precedence over the multitude of "convictions and aims, and even attachments and loyalties" that most people have.

It might be thought that a Rawlsian would have an advantage over a utilitarian in such cases because the former does not but the latter does have to seek out the best thing to do every moment of her waking life. But this is wrong on two counts. Obviously one cannot make the search for the supreme good the sole aim of one's life, neglecting food, shelter and everything else. To say that moral interests ought to take precedence over all others cannot reasonably be regarded as saying that moral interests ought to exclude all others. (As I explained in my account of moral value, the latter is supreme among all species of value in the sense of being supremely comprehensive.) Thus, no moral theory, including utilitarianism, should be given such an interpretation. So a Rawlsian would have no advantage on this score. In the second place, however, the case before us is one in which the agent was confronted with virtually endless "opportunities" to act on her conviction that justice is the supreme good or on some less important conviction. No search was or would ever be necessary. Such "opportunities" or, more properly, moral dilemmas are always before us. The fact that most people fail to recognize such dilemmas and do not drop everything to seriously practice what they preach should not delude one into thinking that the dilemmas are not there. One does not have to be a utility maximizer to fail to live up to one's moral Principles. (I will have more to say about a pragmatist's interpretation of moral principles and character later.)

Sen and Williams make it appear as if utilitarians are guilty of separating people from their feelings, and then entirely neglecting the former in their calculations of moral goodness. In their striking metaphor, they make the absurd suggestion that people are as irrelevant to the determination of levels of happiness as "petrol tanks" are to "the national consumption of petroleum". Since there are no disembodied feelings and happiness exists exactly insofar as happy people exist, Sen and Williams have seriously misrepresented the utilitarians' position. The classical utilitarian formula recommends the greatest happiness for the greatest number, which makes the concern for the spread of happiness among the greatest number of people as explicit as it could be. The alternative formula, recommending the greatest average happiness for the greatest number, maintains the original concern to distribute happiness as broadly as possible and, to avoid unwarranted and inefficient distributions, as evenly as possible. Again, the concern with the equal treatment and well-being of all people could hardly be more explicit.

I think the preceding paragraphs have demonstrated that the specific criticisms against utilitarian theories on the grounds that they subvert personal integrity or individuality are unsubstantiated. The criticisms are without foundation so far as utilitarian theories themselves are concerned, and they fail to establish any sort of special liability for such theories compared to nonutilitarian alternatives. Before we move on to other criticisms, it will be worthwhile to briefly review an apparently plausible but really dangerous way to try to accommodate the "problem" of individuality or integrity.

Following Sidgwick, Scheffler (1982, pp. 15–16) noted that utilitarians could and have offered several reasons for thinking that total or average utility will be maximized if people give special attention to their own affairs. Sidgwick (1874, p. 431) wrote that "each man is better able to provide for his own happiness than for that of other persons, from his more intimate knowledge of his own desires and needs, and his greater opportunities of gratifying them." Furthermore, since "it is under the stimulus of self-interest that the active energies of most men are most easily and thoroughly drawn out", it would "not under actual circumstances promote the universal happiness if each man were to concern himself with the happiness of others as much as with his own".

Sidgwick's remarks in the preceding paragraph have to be treated delicately, more delicately I think, than Scheffler has treated them. They can be read virtually as a licence to practice ethical egoism, which would certainly be contrary to Sidgwick's intention. They should be read merely as empirical claims indicating the likely consequences of people being the way they are and doing what they are inclined to do. Read this way, the remarks are consistent with the remarks I made earlier about morality not being an exclusive interest, although it is a supremely comprehensive interest. Scheffler seems to accept Sidgwick's remarks as a good reason to make it morally permissible for "people to devote energy and attention to their projects, commitments, and personal relationships out of proportion to the weight from an impersonal standpoint of their doing so" (Scheffler 1982, p. 85). In another place (p. 21), he grants "the question of *how much* greater weight the agent may give to his own interests than to the interests of other people" involves issues that "are certainly not neat or simple, hut they are unavoidable for almost anyone whose moral outlook is neither egoist nor consequentialist."

Thus, Scheffler accepts the fact that people are more interested in themselves and their own projects than in others and their projects, and attempts to construct a moral principle that accommodates this fact. However, since he is unable to offer any way to calculate maximum allowable departures from the impartial weighting of one's own interests, he has opened the door to ethical egoism so wide that only the grossest of egoists could fail to pass through. While a utilitarian or a pragmatic moralist has a principle of impartiality to appeal to in order to arrest or constrain rampant egoism, Scheffler has nothing going for him but exhortations to moderation. Instead of providing an ideal standard that might be used in the selection of human aspirations or in the guidance of conduct, Scheffler provides a sympathetic principle of acquiescence. To make matters worse, he has rejected consequentialists' insistence and reliance upon trying to calculate the probable benefits and costs of particular departures from impartiality in order to prevent the grossest departures from this standard. So he has provided the morally faint of heart with a practically irresistable slippery slope.

2. *Distributive Justice.* A distribution of goods or services is generally regarded as just or equitable insofar as everyone gets what is due to him or her. Thus, if all other things were equal, just or equitable distributions would also be equal. In such a world, no departures from egalitarian distributions could be justified. In our own world, of course, all other things are seldom equal. So equitable distributions may fail to be equal. In this world, distributive justice may be achieved by beginning with the assumption that every person deserves the same treatment as every other person unless there are good reasons for some other sort of treatment. In other words, the interest of equity or distributive justice is best served by equal distributions unless there are legitimate warrants for unequal distributions.

It has been argued that insofar as a moral theory focuses on the maximization of some kind of good (e.g., welfare, happiness, etc.) regardless of any other aims or interests, some people may fail to obtain distributive justice. As Scheffler (1982, p. 10) put it, "classical utilitarianism will frequently require us to ignore the misery of a few people and concentrate instead on increasing the pleasures of the many simply in order to maximize aggregate satisfaction."

Insofar as the pragmatic moral theory that I am recommending prescribes the maximization of objective value, it may be expected to share the problems that utilitarian theories have with distributive justice. Although my theory does not have the unacceptable feature specifically cited by Scheffler, it has involved similar problems which I have tried to solve along the lines of some of my utilitarian predecessors. In particular, my definition of moral value (D8) includes several provisions for distributive justice.

In the first place, some account of distributive justice is taken by requiring every affected person to have the same estimated chances of obtaining objective value. Although one cannot foresee and guarantee all of the consequences of one's action, one can and ought to be responsible for one's probability estimates. Moreover, by equalizing people's chances of obtaining objective value, one is giving quantitative expression to their a priori equal value as persons.

Secondly, and similarly, by requiring the maximization of the average amount of objective value going to each person, further account is taken of distributive justice. A priori, according to D8, every person ought to obtain as much objective value as every other person, which is another way of expressing the view of the equal status of all persons as persons.

These first two provisions preclude one of the unacceptable consequences Scheffler cites, namely, that of ignoring the misery of a few people. By insisting upon the maximization of average amounts of objective value instead of, say, the idiosyncratic pleasures or satisfactions of particular individuals, some provision has been made to prevent inequitable distributions from arising as a result of the peculiarities of certain people. My introduction and operationalization of the idea of objective value should make it unnecessary to appeal to distinctions of "manifest preferences" and "true preferences", and to exclude from consideration "all clearly antisocial preferences, such as sadism, envy, resentment, and malice" (Harsanyi

1982, pp. 55–56). At this point in time it has not been demonstrated empirically that sadism, envy, resentment and malice have negligible amounts of objective value. So I am expressing more hope than fact. Nevertheless, insofar as the hope is reasonable in the presence of what we know about human socialization, I think it is reasonable to regard the appeal to objective value in D8 as a third provision for distributive justice.

The allowance of Pareto optimal increments represents a fourth provision for distributive justice. Objecting to the alleged implausible rigidity of "distribution-sensitive forms of consequentialism", Scheffler (1982, pp. 30–31) claims that "egalitarian variants would appear to require that given a choice between a situation in which everyone is very badly-off but equally so, and a situation in which everyone is very well-off but slight inequalities exist, we must always choose the former". My definition of moral value prevents such anomalous choices. It also allows one to take advantage of special circumstances and abilities of certain individuals. To take a relatively straightforward case, suppose someone's productivity were such that, in exchange for slightly higher wages than other people in her trade, she would always produce enough objective value to increase the average levels of everyone else. Under the circumstances, if she were not given a bit more than the average, everyone else would have to settle for a bit less. (For those who like numbers, suppose the choice is between she gets 10 and the average is 8, or everyone gets 6.) Here we have the possibility of a Pareto improvement which, I think, it would be unfair and unwise to prevent. Why, one might ask, should everyone be deprived of a bit more simply to prevent the exceptional worker from obtaining a bit more than that? Put another way, one might ask: Why shouldn't everyone get as much out of life as it is possible to get, so long as no one else has to get less?

3. *Free-riders*. Economists draw a distinction between public and private goods on the basis of the former having either of two characteristics lacked by the latter. Public goods are said to have the property of jointness if using them does not entail using them up. For example, no matter how many people use information how often, the information is not used up. In this respect, information is unlike such natural resources as lumber or coal, which are therefore regarded as private goods. Public goods are also said to have the property of nonexclusiveness, indicating that even people who do not pay for them cannot be excluded from them. For example, whether or not a particular individual pays for a system of national defense, if one's country has such a system then one automatically enjoys its benefits. In this respect, a system of national defense is unlike such things as privately owned burglar alarms, which only benefit their purchasers.

The property of nonexclusiveness provides a necessary condition for the so-called free-rider problem. Generally speaking, the problem is that if any particular person is going to be able to enjoy the benefits of a public good whether or not that person pays for it, then every person has some reason to try to take a free ride. Every person might reasonably suppose that he or she could escape payment by passing on the full cost of the good to their neighbours. For example, since my country is going to have a system of national defense whether or not I make any contribution to it, I might try to avoid making such a contribution. I might, in short, try to take a free ride at the expense of my neighbours.

It has been argued that utilitarian moral theories may not only encourage but may even prescribe free-riding in a variety of circumstances, some of which involve clear cases of public goods. A utilitarian might argue that, since one's fundamental moral obligation is to act so as to maximize total or average utility and in certain circumstances whatever one does, the appropriate level of utility will be produced, in such circumstances it would be morally right to take a free ride. Hare (1982, pp. 36–38) mentions four kinds of cases that have been discussed in the literature. These are cases in which (a) one may abstain from voting, letting others bear the costs of becoming informed about relevant issues and candidates, and of standing in line to cast their votes; (b) one may consume more electricity to provide more comfort for oneself, allowing others to bear the discomfort costs of conservation; (c) one may pretend to be joining others pushing a stalled car, while they are doing all the work; (d) one may make death-bed promises without keeping them. The first two of these cases involve classic problems in the provision of public goods. The third involves a relatively limited public good, and the fourth represents at best an extreme case of a public good. In the latter case one is taking advantage of a single person's belief that one is acting in good faith. Still, because the dying person has that belief, one is able to maximize satisfaction at no cost to oneself.

Insofar as the pragmatic moral theory that I am recommending prescribes the maximization of average amounts of objective value for all people affected by an action, advocates of the theory are apparently subject to free rider abuses. What, if anything, is wrong with taking a free ride in the previously cited cases? According to Hare (1982, p. 37), the "clue" to a correct answer to this sort of question

> lies in the observation that to frustrate a desire of mine is against my interest even if I do not know that it is being frustrated, or if I am dead. … the dying man's interests <u>are</u> harmed if promises are made to him and then broken, and even more … mine are harmed <u>if</u> people are cheating me without my knowing it. In the latter case, they are harmed because I very much want this not to happen.

Thus, according to Hare, free riding is wrong because it harms people's interests. The latter is wrong because it violates the generally accepted moral maxim proscribing actions causing such harm. In Hare's terms, it violates a "level-1 principle". In other words, Hare's solution of free rider problems involves the familiar appeal to two levels of moral reasoning. As an act-utilitarian, he wants to maximize the chances of every act of every individual maximizing utility. His strategy can be to recommend calculation on every occasion, or rule-following on most occasions and calculation in extraordinary occasions. The former strategy would be costly in terms of time and other resources, and liable to abuse as a result of individual circumstances and peculiarities. The latter would be relatively less costly, would draw on the moral experience of others as codified in generally accepted moral maxims, but would still be liable to abuse. All things considered, then, a rational act-utilitarian ought to recommend precisely the strategy that Hare recommended, namely, act in accordance with the moral maxims and vote, consume less electricity, push the car and keep promises. Although the cases in question have been cooked to make the immediate effects of one's action redundant, such action is morally and rationally warranted as part of one's general strategy for realizing one's fundamental moral and rational aims.

Becker (1982) suggested another way to address free rider problems. Essentially he recommended that people try to become the sorts of individuals who find satisfaction not only in failing to take advantage of others, but in performing generally benevolent actions. What is required, he claimed, is "actually *becoming* a person who does not count the cost of cooperation in these cases, so as to be a persuasive example without cost to oneself." In other words,

> … one would have to plunge into cooperative acts with the dual intent of persuading others to do likewise and at the same time covering one's losses by reaping the rewards of conviviality, fraternity, and eventually, perhaps, solidarity that often accrue to the generous, friendly, and openhearted. (Becker 1982, p. 220)

Thus, according to Becker, one's motive for avoiding free riding need not be the purely negative consideration that it is wrong. He has not recommended a rule-utilitarian solution, although that solution might be perfectly acceptable. On the contrary, he proposed the avoidance of free riding on purely positive grounds, namely, that personal satisfaction can be maximized through generally benevolent action. Acts of good will can be personally satisfying precisely insofar as they are generally satisfying, provided that one has an appropriate sort of character. Those who see free rider problems as insuperable, have failed to take such character into consideration.

Although Hare's and Becker's proposed solutions both strike me as acceptable, Becker's is more congenial to my theory because it is likely that more objective value can be generated from people with generally benevolent characters than from people who merely try to abstain from harmful actions. In my view, the moral ideal is not that of patching cracks in the dike against moral evil, but of developing a moral character that is relatively resistant to such cracks. I think my preference for people with generally benevolent characters is fairly typical of consequentialists. However, the point I want to emphasize here is that the question of which sort is most likely to maximize average amounts of objective value for all people is an empirical question. In principle, it is possible to address this question experimentally, with the help of MDT and the operational definition of objective value proposed earlier.

4. *Human Rights*. Human rights may be regarded as special claims or entitlements that are usually correlated with special duties or responsibilities. There are national and international documents indicating general agreement that people have, for example, a right to life, liberty, property, education, employment and housing. One has a negative right to something if others are obliged to allow one to have it, i.e., if others have a duty to abstain from preventing one from having it. One has a positive right to something if others are obliged to provide it, i.e., if

others have a duty to provide it. For example, although there is general agreement that people have a right to housing and work, some people regard these as merely negative rights while others regard them as positive rights. Thus, what governments and ordinary people are obliged to do to ensure that everyone gets the housing and work that they are entitled to as a matter of human rights depends on how those rights are interpreted (among other things).

A variety of answers have been given to the question: What is the justification, basis or warrant for human rights? Appeals have been made, for example, to natural law (Locke 1961), social contract (Rawls 1971), the meaningfulness of life (Nozick 1974) and utilitarianism (Hahn 1982). Virtually all nonutilitarian theorists believe that utilitarians have insoluble problems accommodating human rights. Some go so far as to define rights in an anti-utilitarian way. For example, Sartorius (1985, p. 2) wrote that "A claim of right is one the satisfaction of which takes priority over the satisfaction of competing claims based upon considerations concerning the promotion of the general welfare." Granting that "few would be willing to claim that there are any moral or political rights that are absolute", he added the following "escape clause"; "Failure to satisfy a claim of right may be justified if the consequences of satisfying it would be extremely severe."

Since anti-utilitarian definitions of rights are explicitly question—begging with respect to the issue of whether or not utilitarian theories can accommodate rights, nothing else has to be said about them. Accordingly, I will direct my attention to apparently more moderate theorists.

The views of Rawls (1971) are the most well-known among contemporary writers. Rawls (1982, p. 182) wrote that

> … since utilitarianism starts from an independent and prior conception of the good, no restrictions founded on right and justice are imposed on the ends through which satisfaction is to be achieved. All restrictions on ends arise only from what is necessary in the design of institutions if they are to realize the greatest good under given circumstances. But it is easy enough to describe realistic social situations in which the pattern of a people's desire and preferences are such that the greatest satisfaction would not be achieved by securing the basic equal liberties. Hence, these liberties are most secure when the possibility is recognised of many determinate conceptions of the good each constrained by the principles of justice.

Following Nozick (1974), Sen and Williams (1982, p. 19) claimed that "different people's rights stand incommensurable with each other—each imposing its own constraints on the actions of all." Furthermore,

> Even if rights are made a part of *consequential* evaluation, … the moral goodness of states will not correspond to some descriptive magnitude of the same type as 'total utility'. Indeed, consequential evaluation including goals of rights-fulfilment among other goals could even admit a great deal of incompleteness and restricted comparability, leading to no more than partial orderings of states of affairs. (Sen and Williams 1982, p. 19)

According to Hammond (1982, p. 88), the idea that people have rights precluding government interference may "lead to a restricted or constrained form of utilitarianism in which social welfare is maximized subject to the constraint that nobody's rights are infringed, and each individual chooses what he wants whenever he has a right to do so."

Since Rawls urges us to recognize the possibility of many "determinate conceptions of the good each constrained by the principles of justice", he must imagine enough comparability among all these conceptions to rank order the principles of justice above everything else. In fact, he uses five categories of "primary goods to make interpersonal comparisons" that will allow him to determine whether or not "the greatest benefit of the least advantaged members of society" is being achieved by any particular public policy (Rawls 1982, pp. 161–164). Having admitted this, it is unclear why he insists that in his "well-ordered society in justice as fairness … citizen's conceptions of the good are not only said to be opposed but to be incommensurable" (Rawls 1982, p. 179). If in principle it is always possible to decide whether or not "the greatest benefit of the least advantaged members of society" is being obtained, then there must be no benefit (no good) that is in principle incomparable with others. Insofar as there were such goods, there would be at best partial orderings of goods and no determinate greatest benefit for anyone.

Sen and Williams did not tell us which rights would take precedence over which others, although they were more consistent than Rawls in their insistence on the "incompleteness and restricted comparability" of consequential evaluations involving rights-fulfillment. Hammond apparently envisaged complete utilitarian evaluations (i.e., involving complete rather than merely partial orderings of all states of affairs) constrained by human rights.

Thus, we have three different but comparable views concerning utilitarian or consequentialist problems with human rights. No clear-thinking utilitarian would be troubled by any of them. After all, utilitarians propose a utilitarian account of the foundation or warrant for human rights. Just as moral maxims are designed in the interests of promoting happiness or well-being, so are human rights. In fact, from the point of view of likely consequences, it makes little difference if, for example, one endorses a maxim proscribing killing people or a right to life. It is easy to think of an appropriate maxim for every proposed right and vice versa. Sometimes, as in the case of killing, we have general agreement on the right, a correlative moral maxim and a body of criminal laws and sanctions. Whether we have one or more of such things, they may be given a utilitarian justification. So utilitarians have no fundamental problem with human rights.

I think my pragmatic moral theory is even better equipped than utilitarian theories to account for human rights. Clearly the latter are valuable things and my theory includes everything necessary to empirically determine the objective value of such things. In response to Rawls, I would say that instead of giving an a priori assignment of infinite utility to basic liberties (making them absolutely valuable and priceless in terms of any other combination of utilities), it would be wiser to measure the objective value of such liberties a posteriori. Rawls's basic liberties include such things as "freedom of association" and it is easy for me to imagine a starving person quite happy to trade some of this freedom for food. However, in my view it is a serious methodological blunder to attempt to resolve such issues by philosophical analysis and the invention of stories when they are resolvable by empirical research. Things like the freedom of association will have some tendency to generate some levels of satisfaction under controlled experimental conditions. So our research should be focused on the design of experiments that will allow us to generate reliable and valid lawlike statements about the objective value of such freedoms and all other things that we regard as valuable. In the name of liberty Rawls would have our understanding of human rights and other values laid finally to rest in a procrustean bed. This is precisely the sort of danger that the original pragmatists rose up against at the turn of the century, and they were absolutely right!

My response to Sen and Williams is now predictable. They too would have us settle issues of comparability on the basis of speculation and tradition, instead of on experimentation. Although Hammond's view is more limited than these other authors, he accepts their assumption that rights can constrain utilitarian calculations but cannot generate utilities. This is precisely what Hahn (1982, p. 190), for example, denied. "One may derive utility from rights" he wrote. In my view, human rights are clearly objectively valuable and the main problem they create is that of measuring exactly how valuable they are.

[Note: In my review of Sen and Williams's *Utilitarianism and Beyond* (to appear in *Teaching Philosophy*) I briefly identified nearly 40 objections to various forms of utilitarianism. In the final draft of this treatise I will consider all other apparently reasonable objections.]

Epistemic Value

According to C.I. Lewis (Goheen and Mothershed 1970, p. 112), "pragmatism might almost be defined as the contention that all judgments of truth are judgments of value: that verification is value-determination, and the criterion of truth is the realization of some kind of value." I call the species of value alluded to in this quotation epistemic value, and define it thus:

D11: Any belief has *epistemic value* exactly insofar as it maximizes the objective probability of maximizing the objective value of the total set of beliefs of all believers through the realization of a maximally coherent set of maximally descriptive beliefs.

A shorter and perhaps misleading formulation of D11 might run thus: A belief has epistemic value insofar as it maximizes the chances of obtaining a maximum amount of objective value from a set of beliefs.

Several features of D11 require explanation. First, although I have referred to beliefs in this stipulation, I might as well have referred to judgments, propositions, statements, sentences, hypotheses or theories. In general, anything that may be regarded as having a truth-value may be regarded as having epistemic value.

Second, although I have referred to "descriptive beliefs" at the end of D11, analytic beliefs may also be appraised for epistemic value (supposing one were able to draw some sort of a reasonable distinction between analytic and synthetic claims). By mentioning descriptive beliefs explicitly in my definition, I have tried to assign empirical knowledge some epistemic priority. I have tried to suggest that beliefs individually and collectively exist in the interests of understanding, predicting and controlling the world in which we live. Stipulative definitions and other sorts of analytic or logically true propositions have epistemic value insofar as they contribute to the empirical knowledge and practical interests on which our very survival depends.

Third, the reference to "maximally descriptive beliefs" in D11 is intended to encourage the reduction of redundancy and vacuousness in the total corpus of our beliefs. The idea is explained more thoroughly in Michalos (1971).

Fourth, a view of the maximal coherence of a set of beliefs has been fairly well developed in Rescher (1973). At this point I do not know how much of Rescher's machinery will be appropriate to articulate the idea I have in mind. Rescher contends, among other things, that while Tarski's formula ('p' is true if and only if p) provides an adequate meaning analysis of truth; coherence provides a criterion. This is very much in the spirit of Lewis and earlier pragmatists. As suggested in the first paragraph of this section, my notion of epistemic value is supposed to provide an explication of the idea of a criterion of truth. Following other pragmatists, I also accept the Tarskian formula (which of course antedates Tarski).

Fifth, D11 is designed to indicate that the maximization of coherence in our total set of beliefs is a *means* of obtaining a maximum amount of objective value from that set for all who accept that set. The assumption is that beliefs are generally obtained and maintained in clusters through communal activity in the general interest of maximizing objective value. Put negatively, it is being denied that knowledge is acquired or maintained through the activity of lone researchers pursuing single isolated propositions in the sole interest of those propositions.

Sixth, as in the case of moral value (D8), D11 includes a reference to maximizing the objective probability of obtaining certain aims instead of simply maximizing the attainment of the ends themselves. Given the vast number and variety of more or less unknown and unintended implications of beliefs and consequences of actions, the most one can plausibly ask of anyone is to try to maximize the chances of realizing their aims. (To simplify sentences, I frequently omit any reference to such probabilities.)

It may be instructive now to consider D11 in relation to some of William James's relatively famous pronouncements about his pragmatic theory of truth. I think the following two sentences reveal the heart of James's view and the similarity of that view to mine better than any other sentences I have seen. James (1907, p. 101) wrote that "Between the coercions of the sensible order and those of the ideal order, our mind is thus wedged tightly. Our ideas must agree with realities, be they facts or be they principles, under penalty of endless inconsistency and frustration." In these remarks James seems to be affirming that his theory appeals to both coherence and correspondence. Thayer (1982, pp. 537–550) shows considerably more textual evidence that James did indeed regard his theory as

> … a remolding rather than a renunciation of older ideas. He was concerned with clarifying, deepening, and extending the application of the more familiarly received conceptions, and with accounting for the function of the concept of truth in contexts which remained ignored or inexplicable by traditional theories. Thus, occasionally he will claim that his doctrine includes, absorbs, and supports others; that 'Pragmatic truth contains the whole of intellectualist truth and a hundred other things in addition'.

At another place, James (1907, p. 222) wrote that "*'the true' … is only the expedient in the way of our thinking, just as 'the right' is only the expedient in the way of our behaving*." I interpret this as follows. To talk of expediency is to talk of usefulness for some purpose. What is true is precisely analogous to what is right insofar as both are *means* to obtaining something else. A pragmatist is thoroughly consequentialistic, pursuing truth and performing morally right actions in the interests of objective value. But the criterion of truth is epistemic value. So maximization of the latter becomes the immediate aim. That is, the acquisition of a maximally coherent set of maximally descriptive beliefs is "expedient in the way of our thinking" because insofar as, "our thinking" has these characteristics it will maximize objective value for us.

In the same book, James (1907, p. 76) wrote that "*the true is the name of whatever proves itself to be good in the way of belief.*" One way to interpret this remark is to say that, so far as beliefs are concerned, their goodness or value is epistemic. Thus, to talk of a belief's goodness is simply to talk of its epistemic value. According to D11, a belief's epistemic value is just its contribution to the maximization of the objective value of the total corpus of beliefs. The latter, in turn, is determined by its contribution to a maximally coherent set of maximally descriptive beliefs.

Finally, there are the rather famous remarks for which James was accused of confusing truth and verification. According to James (1907, pp. 201–218), "the truth of an idea is not a stagnant property inherent in it. Truth *happens* to an idea. It *becomes* true, is *made* true by events. … Truth is *made*, just as health, wealth, and strength are made, in the course of experience." Rather than revealing any confusion in James, I think these remarks expose a fundamental and widely held mistaken view of the nature of the "discovery" of truth, including those truths regarded as scientific. Just as one performs actions that result in wealth and health, one does things that result in making some beliefs (propositions, etc.) true. The process of *verification* is essentially a process of *legislation*. This is the crucial pragmatic assessment of truth and verification. What scientists and others typically regard as discoveries, the pragmatist regards as legislated policies or proposals. People must agree to formulate an idea or belief in some way, must agree to use it some way, to try to make it fit some appropriate corpus of beliefs in some way and they must agree that the fit is adequate or acceptable. All of this is policy making. It is epistemic legislation. Thus, to say at the end of such a series of more or less informal acts of legislation that the output is "discovered" is to completely misperceive and misdescribe what actually occurred. As the pragmatist sees it, truth-seekers have an immediate epistemic aim, namely, the acquisition of a maximally coherent set of maximally descriptive beliefs. Pursuing the truth means doing what is required in order to achieve that aim. That is, it means getting a community of truth-seekers (Dewey's "inquirers") to agree on proper formulations of beliefs, proper methodologies, and so on. Insofar as truth or true beliefs are produced by such activities, James's characterizations seem to be profoundly accurate.

Rationality

Given D11, the following definitions seem plausible.

D12: A belief is *rational* exactly insofar as it has epistemic value.
D13: A belief (rationally) *ought to be held* (is *epistemologically warranted*) insofar as it is rational.

That is, since epistemologically speaking, beliefs are generally characterized as rational when they are given the highest approbation, and they merit such praise precisely insofar as they have epistemic value, D12 follows immediately. D13 is, I think, trivial.

[To be continued …]

Acknowledgements Several people have given me helpful suggestions about various parts of earlier versions of this paper, some of which I have used and some not. I would like to express my thanks to A.J. Bahm, H. Bakker, D. Brock, T. Carson, B. Carter, P.T. Durbin, J. Leslie, J. McMurtry, D. Odegard, and J. Simmons. Thanks are also due to Leo Mos and the Center for Advanced Study in Theoretical Psychology, University of Alberta, for generously providing assistance in the preparation of the manuscript.

References

Andrews, F. M., & Inglehart, R. F. (1979). The structure of subjective well-being in nine western societies. *Social Indicators Research, 6,* 75–90.

Andrews, F. M., & Withey, S. B. (1976). *Social indicators of well-being*. New York: Plenum Press.

Becker, L. C. (1982). The free-rider problem. In H. B. Miller & W. H. Williams (Eds.), *The limits of utilitarianism* (pp. 217–224). Minneapolis: University of Minnesota Press.

Dewey, J. (1939). *Theory of valuation. International encyclopedia of unified science* (Vol. II, No. 4). Chicago: University of Chicago Press.

Goheen, J. D., & Mothershed, J. L. (Eds.). (1970). *Collected papers of Clarence Irving Lewis.* Stanford: Stanford University Press.

Hahn, F. (1982). On some difficulties of the utilitarian economist. In A. Sen & B. Williams (Eds.), *Utilitarianism and beyond* (pp. 187–198). Cambridge: Cambridge University Press.

Hammond, P. J. (1982). Utilitarianism, uncertainty and information. In A. Sen & B. Williams (Eds.), *Utilitarianism and beyond* (pp. 85–102). Cambridge: Cambridge University Press.
Hare, R. M. (1982). Ethical theory and utilitarianism. In A. Sen & B. Williams (Eds.), *Utilitarianism and beyond* (pp. 23–38). Cambridge: Cambridge University Press.
Harsanyi, J. C. (1982). Morality and the theory of rational behaviour. In A, Sen & B. Williams (Eds.), *Utilitarianism and beyond* (pp. 39–62). Cambridge: Cambridge University Press.
James, W. (1907). *Pragmatism: A new name for some old ways of thinking*. New York: Longmans, Green and Co.
Lewis, C. I. (1946). *An analysis of knowledge and valuation*. La Salle: Open Court Publishing Company.
Locke, J. (1961). *Two treatises of government* (1690). In P. Laslett (Ed.). Cambridge: Cambridge University Press.
Michalos, A. C. (1969). *Principles of logic*. Englewood Cliffs: Prentice-Hall.
Michalos, A. C. (1971). *The Popper-Carnap controversy*. Hague: Martinus Nijhoff.
Michalos, A. C. (1976). The morality of cognitive decision-making. In M. Brand & D. Walton (Eds.), *Action theory* (pp. 325–340). Dordrecht: D. Reidel.
Michalos, A. C. (1978). *Foundations of decision-making*. Ottawa: Canadian Library of Philosophy.
Michalos, A. C. (1979). Life changes, illness and personal life satisfaction in a rural population. *Social Science and Medicine, 13A,* 175–181.
Michalos, A. C. (1980a). Satisfaction and happiness. *Social Indicators Research, 8,* 385–422.
Michalos, A. C. (1980b). Philosophy of science: Historical, social and value aspects. In P. T. Durbin (Ed.), *A guide to the culture of science, technology, and medicine* (pp. 197–281). New York: The Free Press.
Michalos, A. C. (1982). The satisfaction and happiness of some senior citizens in rural Ontario. *Social Indicators Research, 11,* 1–30.
Michalos, A. C. (1983a). Satisfaction and happiness in a rural northern resource community. *Social Indicators Research, 13,* 224–252.
Michalos, A. C. (1983b). *Job satisfaction, marital satisfaction and the quality of life: A review and a preview*. Paper presented at the Fourth Annual Founders Symposium Honoring Angus Campbell, Institute for Social Research, University of Michigan, February 18, 1983.
Nozick, R. (1974). *Anarchy, state and utopia*. New York: Basic Books.
Perry, R. B. (1926). *General theory of value*. Cambridge: Harvard University Press.
Rawls, J. (1971). *A theory of justice*. Cambridge: Harvard University Press.
Rawls, J. (1982). Social unity and primary goods. In A. Sen & B. Williams (Eds.), *Utilitarianism and beyond* (pp. 159–186). Cambridge: Cambridge University Press.
Rescher, N. (1973). *The coherence theory of truth*. Oxford: Oxford University Press.
Sartorius, R. (1985). Utilitarianism, rights, and duties to self. An undated paper written for a summer seminar sponsored by The Reason Foundation and Liberty Fund, Inc.
Scheffler, S. (1982). *The rejection of consequentialism: A philosophical investigation of the considerations underlying rival moral conceptions*. Oxford: Clarendon Press.
Sen, A., & Williams, B. (Eds.). (1982). *Utilitarianism and beyond*. Cambridge: Cambridge University Press.
Sidgwick, H. (1874). *The methods of ethics*. London: Macmillan.
Thayer, H.S. (1982). *Pragmatism: The Classic Writings*. Hacket: Indianapolis.

Chapter 15
Creating a Culture of Support for the Social Sciences: Lessons from the First Forty Years of the Social Science Federation of Canada

Alex C. Michalos

Introduction

The primary aim of this essay is to review some of the history of the first 40 years of the Social Science Federation of Canada in order to discover strategies that one might use today to create a stronger culture of support for the social sciences. While my methods are historical, reflective and analytic, my fundamental aim is practical and the main assessment of the value of this essay should be pragmatic. Although I am not going to try to prove it here, I believe there is considerable evidence showing that social scientific research has improved and still has a great capacity to improve the quality of people's lives. I would like Canadians to understand and appreciate these facts, and I would like them to show their appreciation in a very materialistic way, namely, by demanding greater governmental financial support for social scientific research. If my essay helps to bring about such support, it will have been worth the effort writing it. If not, it will not have been worth the effort, though it might have been worth some effort. I would be the last person in the world to underestimate the value of working in solidarity with good people trying to solve

Michalos, A.C.: 1997. Creating a culture of support for social sciences: lessons from the first 40 years of the Social Sciences Federation of Canada. Paper written for the Conference on Science and Culture at Trent University, May 1997.

I would like to thank UNBC's Cataloguing Librarian, Rudi Traichel, for his considerable effort and success in tracking down some historical figures, both human and mathematical. The initial research material for this paper was circulated among members of the Social Science Federation of Canada in March 1983 under the title "The Social Science Federation of Canada from 1938 to 1980". This version of the paper was written for the Conference on Science and Culture at Trent University, May 1997.

A.C. Michalos (✉)
University of Northern British Columbia, Prince George, BC, Canada
e-mail: michalos@brandonu.ca

A.C. Michalos, *Philosophical Foundations of Quality of Life*,
DOI 10.1007/978-3-319-50727-9_15

important problems. The great positivist Hans Reichenbach said it is better to try in uncertainty than to not try at all and be certain of failure, and the great anti-positivist Karl Popper told me that he was always optimistic about the future because pessimism leads only to despair. Of course, regardless of their occasional antithetical rhetoric, these two philosophers agreed on more besides the virtue of a valiant effort, but they certainly agreed on the latter and that is enough agreement for our purposes.

The structure of the essay is historical. It begins with a review of an ad hoc meeting of scholars in 1938 as that meeting was described in the first of 18 volumes of official Minutes of the Social Science Federation of Canada. By the time we reach the penultimate section of the essay, we will have visited and drawn something from every one of the volumes, each of which averages about 200 pages. Our focus will be on the perceived purposes and the sources of financial support of the Federation according to its Executive Officers in its first 40 years of existence. Following the historical excursion, I will provide a brief summary of some of the critical choices facing the Officers, and I will conclude with some reflections on how all this stuff might be useful for advocates of the social sciences today.

Ad Hoc Meeting 1

On a Sunday afternoon on May 22, 1938, a group of 12 scholars met at the Chateau Laurier Hotel in Ottawa "to discuss ways of improving the organization of social and economic research in Canada".[1] The group included:

J.F. Booth, Agricultural Economics
R.H. Coates, Statistics
C.A. Dawson, Sociology
C.L.P. Grant-Suttie, Geography
D. Jenness, Anthropology
N. MacKenzie, International Law
J.E. Robbins, Education
R. MacGregor Dawson, Political Science
H.A. Innis, Economics
G. Lanctot, Archives
R.G. Trotter, History
C.F. Wilson, Agricultural Statistics

Trotter acted as Chairperson and Robbins acted as Secretary. The head of the Dominion Bureau of Statistics, R.H. Coates, opened the discussion by informing the group that "he was interested in research that relied on quantitative data and statistical method", and that "there was no use collecting information except insofar

[1] *Social Science Research Council Minutes 1940–44*, Minutes of first meeting, September 16–17, 1940, Appendix 1. All quotations are from this Appendix until a change is specifically noted.

as it was of value in helping to solve problems." He wanted to see more collaboration between university teachers and the Bureau, and hoped to see the latter "becoming what might be called a national laboratory for research in the social and economic sciences".

MacKenzie said that "law ought to be altered from time to time in the light of its consequences on the individuals who come into conflict with it, and it should be a part of the interest of the legal profession to study these consequences". Coates immediately replied that the Bureau had "a record of all criminal offences in Canada since Confederation", apparently waiting to be analyzed.

At this point Trotter observed that "all comments seemed to point to the need of a better means than yet exists of focussing the varied interests in social problems". Then MacGregor Dawson "raised the question of how a central council for coordinating interest could be financed" and Lanctot "wondered whether such a body would best be a council with a paid staff or a consultative committee with membership from each of the Dominion Government Departments interested in social research".

Trotter thought that any such body should have representatives from various national organizations that had a scientific interest in social and economic problems, e.g., the Canadian Political Science Association, the Canadian Historical Association, etc. Wilson thought that "a good deal of preliminary work in studying the possibilities of co-ordination could be done by a temporary committee that would require little or no finance, and that the inauguration of such a group ought to be the immediate objective".

Innis noted that psychology was not represented at the meeting, but he knew its "followers would be interested". Professor E.A. Bott had informed him that in June the Psychology Section of the American Psychology Association meeting in Ottawa was going to consider the question of forming a "Canadian Association of Psychologists". "If formed", he said, "this would be another national organization that would be interested in participating in any movement for the coordination of social research". Robbins then suggested that "educationists as well as psychologists could probably be added to the number of interested groups".

Dawson "appealed for careful study of the problem of organization before making any recommendations. He thought…that any body which might be constituted ought not to be dependent on the government for support."

The meeting adjourned with formal agreement on a single point, namely, to meet again the following Wednesday. But informally there was considerably more agreement. Above all else, it is clear that most of those who came together for that first meeting had a very pragmatic view of the tasks before them and of the social sciences. MacKenzie's emphasis on evaluating laws by examining their consequences on the lives of individuals put him squarely in the pragmatic tradition. Coates and Trotter wanted social scientific information in order to solve social problems, and they seemed to see their primary task as institutionalizing this view. Without indicating any disagreement with this basic agenda, Lanctot asked what form the institutionalization should take (a separate body versus an interdepartmental committee), Trotter asked who should do the work, and MacGregor Dawson asked how it should be financed. Wilson saw the advantages of having a small group of like-minded people design the foundations of an organization and Dawson saw the advantages of having the organization independent of government support.

Although no one said that anyone had been sent by any organization, some of those present seemed to have thought of themselves as representing organizations. They talked as if "other organizations" should be "represented", and Innis and Robbins suggested adding representatives from disciplines not already present. Curiously enough, the minutes do not tell us who actually engineered the meeting. Who first asked who to do what?

The participants shared the view that there was both a legitimate division of labour among the diverse social sciences and a need for co-ordination among them. It was not made clear why there was a perceived need for co-ordination, but it was taken for granted and along with it there was a perceived need for funding to sustain their efforts.

Ad Hoc Meeting 2

Three days later, on May 25, 1938, when the group met the second time, they picked up D.C. Harvey, but were missing Booth, Lanctot, MacKenzie and Wilson. The issue of the representative status of everyone present was immediately addressed. Trotter began "by asking for a record of the appointments to the committee that had been approved by national organizations since the previous meeting". The Canadian Political Science Association sent Innis to represent economics, Dawson for sociology and MacGregor Dawson for political science. The Canadian Institute of International Affairs sent MacKenzie, and the Canadian Historical Association sent Trotter.

It was agreed that the question of further representation would be raised by Grant-Suttie at the Canadian National Committee of the International Geographical Union, W.A. MacKintosh at the Royal Society of Canada, Booth at the Canadian Agricultural Economics Society and Robbins at the Canadian Education Association. If the Canadian Psychological Association was formed in June, a representative would be invited from it.

There was a discussion of the possibility of having representatives from Government Departments. It was agreed that some "heads of certain branches of the public service" were essential, but they should "be given a special status as consultative members, and as such be exempt from responsibility for formal decisions of the committee". In the presence of Coates, the group could hardly have done less, and it is surprising that there is no record of serious dissent. Robbins's carefully selected phrase "exempt from responsibility" really meant that people like Coates could come and talk but they could not vote. So, they were clearly going to be second-class citizens in that community.

It was also agreed that Robbins and Trotter should carry on for a year as Secretary-Treasurer and Chairperson, respectively. To defray mounting expenses, Innis "proposed that the participating organizations each be asked to contribute ten dollars for incidental expenses of correspondence, etc. …and his proposal was endorsed".

Two important research initiatives were begun at this second meeting. Robbins was asked to prepare a "memorandum" on the "organization of social research in several countries", giving "the structure of individual national organizations, ... their inter-relationships in countries where there are several, and to mention the type of work undertaken by each". Second, Dawson proposed and the group agreed that there should be "a statement of the social and economic research in progress in Canada.... With this before it, the committee would be better able to determine... the topics in most need of further attention".

The following people accepted responsibility for reviewing their fields:

Agricultural Economics, Booth; Anthropology, Jenness; Economics, Innis; Education, Robbins; Geography, Grant-Suttie; History, Trotter; International Affairs, MacKenzie; Political Science, MacGregor-Dawson; Sociology, Dawson.

The several statements were supposed to be in the hands of Robbins by December 1, 1938, i.e., in 7 months. The meeting ended with agreement to meet when several national associations were meeting in Ottawa in the fall.

As in the first ad hoc meeting, although it was not made clear why there should be co-ordination among the several social science disciplines, it was assumed that there should be such co-ordination. Apparently some participants knew that some co-ordination existed in other countries. As we learn below, some were familiar with the work of the U.S. Social Science Research Council, which began in 1923 (Karl 1974). Since there has always been a tradition in science that advocates a kind of laissez-faire or free enterprise approach to scientific investigation, it is surprising that there is nothing in the committee minutes indicating that anyone spoke out in favour of this tradition or suggested that any efforts at co-ordination might constrain or be perceived to constrain the free flow of research and ideas. In later years when the Social Sciences and Humanities Research Council introduced the idea of thematic research, there were plenty of voices raised in behalf of the laissez-faire model.

Ad Hoc Meeting 3

On November 6, 1938, the third meeting of the ad hoc committee took place at the Chateau Laurier. Present were Bott, Coates, J. Coke, Dawson, Grant-Suttie, Innis, Jenness, Lanctot, MacKintosh, Robbins and Trotter. "The purpose of the meeting was to confer with Dr. Wesley C. Mitchell of Columbia University", who had been a President of the American Association for the Advancement of Science (AAAS), Chairman of the U.S. Social Science Research Council and President of the American Statistical Association.

Mitchell explained that the U.S. Council "was not an operating body, but a planning body, i.e., that it did not undertake investigations itself but that it rather directed and supervised the expenditure of funds in aid of social research" provided mainly by the Rockefeller Foundation and the Carnegie Corporation. The Council had started like the Canadian group, "by the representatives of several associations coming together for joint action on their common interest in research". Various foundations had given the Council funds for regular meetings, a permanent office and research grants. "Its purpose was not to control or centralize research in a single body, but to keep the whole range of the social sciences under review, and to assist research in sections where the gaps were most obvious".

Mitchell pointed out that although the U.S. Government "had not given financial-assistance to the Council, he believed that it had done things that were equivalent", e.g., improving statistical services for researchers as a result of "petitions of the Council". He also insisted that "the desirable consequences of the Council's existence…could not by any means be all written into its reports. There were many intangibles. There could be little doubt, for instance, that the associations which the Council made possible were having effect in reducing the excessive departmentalization of the social sciences within the universities". Finally, he "advised against administrators or the representatives of administrative bodies being included in the personnel of a committee or council of this kind. Persons whose interest was essentially 'practical' rather than scientific might tend to obscure basic issues with the plea of immediacy". The meeting adjourned after 3½ h.

Given the close and generally friendly relationships between scholars in Canada and the United States, the invitation to Mitchell was predictable. His cautionary remarks about the potentially conflicting 'practical' and 'scientific' interests of administrators and academics, respectively, suggest that his views on this score were similar to those of his Canadian hosts. The Minutes do not tell us much about the history of the U.S. Council, but there was a remarkable similarity in the intentions and actions of the founders of the two Councils.

Charles Merriam had addressed the December 1921 annual meeting of the American Political Science Association on the need for "cooperative enterprise". With Merriam in the Chair of an APSA committee struck in 1922 to explore the nature of political research in the United States, the first report of the committee

> …surveyed existing research agencies and methods. The surveys were divided into studies of recent advances in political methods, the work of government research bodies, legislative and municipal reference agencies, research and equipment in universities and colleges, and research carried on by social and industrial agencies bordering on the field of government. …Merriam was sharply critical of the state of research in the universities. Classwork and administrative duties made time available for research 'wholly inadequate.' Most institutions failed to provide stenographic or clerical aid, research assistants, or allowances for field work and provided only inadequate research and publication funds. 'It may therefore be concluded,' he stated flatly, 'that the time available for political research and the equipment for intensive inquiries is deplorably inadequate in view of the needs of scientific inquiry.' (Karl 1974, pp. 119–120)

Three years later, Merriam wrote

> If there were a benevolent despot of science, he would compel the union of all the scientific agencies centering around the welfare of the race. Geneticist and environmentalist, psychologist, anthropologist, biologist, social scientist would all be brought together to consider the fundamental social problems in which they are all concerned and which cannot be effectively solved without their joint consideration and action (Quoted from Karl 1974, p. 123).

According to Karl (1974, pp. 130–131), while Merriam "led the negotiations" with foundations to get funding for council meetings and travel expenses for members, thus getting recognition of "the existence of the council itself as an acceptable object of support", the initial demand for resources came from a research project of the American Sociological Society. Finally, it was the Laura Spelman Rockefeller Memorial which provided the operating grant and the recognition. As we will see below, in these latter respects too, the Canadian experience was similar to that in the United States.

Ad Hoc Meeting 4

When the group met again, on May 24, 1939, at McGill University, it had become "the Committee on Research in the Social Sciences". Robbins wrote a brief Secretary-Treasurer's report for the period from May 1938 to May 1939, which included the following instructive remarks on the proposed survey of research (which, you may recall, was to have been completed 4 months earlier).

> Completion of contributions to the survey of research was in most cases considerably behind schedule. Although it meant delaying their assembly into a single document until the middle of May, a fairly rounded survey at the later date seemed preferable to an earlier one with several omissions. There was a good deal of variation in the detail with which the different contributions were done, and they could not all be reproduced in full without obvious lack of balance. The compromise represented by the document mimeographed and put in the hands of committee members is not entirely satisfactory but may be excused as a first attempt under circumstances in which it was not possible to consult with others.
>
> A question for the meeting to decide will be whether the survey ought to be revised and improved in the light of the experience gained on it, or whether it should have some distribution in its present form. It might be decided to carry the investigation in some subjects further and let others stand. Consideration might also be given to the possibility of a similar survey with emphasis on the teaching of the social sciences in the universities, where the emphasis in this one is on research.

Besides these remarks, Robbins scrupulously recorded the following financial statement.

> In the lack of specific instructions, an account at the Bank of Montreal was opened in my name, in trust for the committee. Transactions have been as follows:

Deposits		*Withdrawals*	
Historical Assn.	$10.00	Guest and gratuities at	
Agric.Econ.Soc.	$10.00	November meeting	$2.50
Geograph.Ctte	$9.85		
Educ.Assn	$9.85		
Interest to May	.23		
	$39.93		$2.50
		Balance, May 1, 1939	$37.43

> In case larger sums of money should come into possession of the committee,…the Treasurer ought to…know whether the participating associations are to be asked to repeat their ten-dollar contribution this year, and I would ask the committee in making a decision to remember that it is easier to persuade others to help financially when there is some evidence that we are helping ourselves.

The McGill meeting included Booth, Dawson, Grant-Suttie, Innis, J.D. Ketchum (replacing Bott), MacKintosh, Robbins and Trotter. It was agreed that the committee should continue for another year and that before any associations were asked to contribute yet another ten dollars, "similar contributions from the others should be received". Then the question of the survey arose again and, after some discussion and failure to find anyone to take on the task, "the problem was left unsettled and the members asked to submit to the Chairman or Secretary suggestions that might seem worthwhile on further reflection after the meeting".

The discussion then moved to the possibility of finding funds for a more elaborate survey. Grant-Suttie "thought it would be an act of courtesy to make any request first of Canadian sources, and the meeting commended this suggestion". It was agreed that Trotter should "approach the Massey Foundation". As it turned out, "a first-hand approach could not be made" to the Foundation and since "any other kind did not seem worthwhile", none was made. However, since Innis was going to be in New York, he agreed to call at the Carnegie Corporation offices. About $2000 was apparently required.

In September, Innis met with a representative of the Corporation and, given "the probable influence of the outbreak of war on the Committee's position,…asked that the application be left in abeyance for the present". That seems to have been where it was left permanently.

Apart from the tiny sums of money scrupulously accounted for in Robbins's reports and the use of professorial titles in references to committee members' remarks, there is much in this report of the fourth meeting that has a familiar ring. For examples, regarding the surveys, deadlines for survey reports were not met. Reports varied in quality. The question was then raised as to how they should be distributed. The answer was first to distribute modestly according to need, which meant to executive members of represented associations. Then perhaps some willing and able scholar could be found to use the surveys to write a proper publishable report of the state of social science research in Canada.

Regarding funding sources, it is unclear to me why the group thought that requesting support from Canadian sources first was regarded as an "act of courtesy". Perhaps they thought that such a request would be perceived by a potential funder as an opportunity for a Canadian foundation to display its patriotism. In any case, there does not seem to have been much of a commitment to courtesy, since when there appeared to be no volunteer to visit only one Canadian foundation, nothing else was done on this score. Apparently not even a phone call or a letter to a Canadian foundation was attempted before the group turned its attention to our relatively wealthier neighbours to the south.

Ad Hoc Meeting 5

The group met at Queen's University on November 4, 1939, including Booth, Bott, Coates, Innis, Jenness, MacKintosh, Robbins, Trotter, C. Humphrey (a second psychologist) and H.M. Torr of the Royal Society. On the subject of the survey of research, Trotter

> reported that an article by him on historical research, substantially the same as the one done for the Committee's preliminary survey, had been published in the September number of the Canadian Historical Review, and that Professor Innis had arranged with Professor Bladen, editor of the Canadian Journal of Economics and Political Science, for an announcement concerning the Committee's work on the survey in a forthcoming issue of the Journal.

That seems to be how the survey was completed and what came of it. As I will report later, it was an idea whose time had come and gone in about 18 months, and come and gone several more times. It came again at the end of the period reviewed in this study in 1982.

The question of establishing a "permanent social science research body" was also discussed at this meeting, but no details were recorded. It was simply recorded that Trotter, "Innis and any further Committee members they may wish to co-opt" would draft a constitution to be discussed at the next meeting. At the McGill meeting 6 months earlier, Trotter had raised the question of the need for a full-nine director for such a body, and Innis had expressed the view that "available money should rather be diffused among research workers in the universities". It was not clear where the "available money" was going to come from anyhow or even how it would be pursued. Nor was there any record of any ideas about how such money might be systematically dispersed should any be obtained. It was clear, however, that *ad hockery* tended to breed *ad hockery*, i.e., a committee sitting at its pleasure would search for funds at its pleasure, would be greeted by potential funders at their pleasure, and so on. I would have thought that the appearance of permanence would have been a necessary condition of being taken and of taking oneself seriously, and that may have been in the minds of Trotter and Innis when they agreed to write a draft constitution for some sort of potentially permanent institution. Supposing that they had such plans, the remark that Innis would rather have seen any funds spent on "research workers in the universities" than on a permanent director/administrator suggests that, for him at least, organizational requirements were still subordinate to research.

Ad Hoc Meeting 6

Booth, Coates, MacGregor-Dawson, de Glazebrook (for MacKenzie), Innis, Liddy (for Bott) and Trotter met at the Hotel London, Ontario, May 22, 1940. A draft constitution for a "Canadian Research Council in the Social Sciences" was presented, discussed and adopted. It was agreed:

> That the Secretary be instructed (a) to report to the sponsoring bodies named in the constitution, asking for approval of the names of their members proposed as "representative" members on the Council, (b) to invite other persons, listed in the schedule attached to the constitution, to become members of the Council, (c) and to summon a meeting of the Council when possible.

The "sponsoring bodies" cited in the constitution included the Canadian Historical Association (CHA), the Canadian Committee of the International Geographical Union (CCIGU), the Canadian Psychological Association (CPA) and the Canadian Political Science Association (CPSA). For the CPSA, a note was added that "as the representative…is chosen from economics, politics or sociology, the remaining two may be represented by members at large". From these four groups came B. Brouillette (CCIGU), Bott (CPA), Innis (CPSA) and Trotter (CHA). Members at large included MacGregor-Dawson, MacKenzie, T.F. McIlwraith, H. Angus, Dawson, R.A. MacKay, F.C. Cronkite and W.B. Hurd (about whom much more will be said later). Associate members included Coates, Lanctot, Booth and MacKintosh, with Robbins as Secretary-Treasurer.

The minutes of this sixth meeting of the group contain not only the constitution, but a "Summary of Individual Views Presented Regarding Council Policy".[2] They provide us with excellent insights into the minds of the SSFC's founders.

Trotter saw "two fields of opportunity" for the new Council. "(1) the improvement of facilities, materials, personnel and organization of research in Canada" and "(2) the use of available research possibilities or capacities to serve the needs of society".

> "If planning is to be intelligent" he said, "we must know as much as we can about how the present institutions of society function and how they affect peoples' lives, and we must know more about human nature, about man as a social animal….As quickly as possible the Council should map out a programme which it might further, a programme partly of work already going on and partly of work to be initiated under Council auspices".

These remarks by Trotter, exactly 2 years to the day past the first ad hoc meeting, reveal that he remained squarely in the tradition of the turn-of-the-century reform-minded social scientists. Soffer (1978, p. 253) summarized the ethos of the earlier period thus.

> While nineteenth-century positivist theorists had gone beyond observable reality to postulate an essential unity of knowledge and experience, the new social scientists between 1880 and 1914 repudiated the grandiose ambitions of the predecessors and attempted instead to measure reality only as it appeared in such concrete problems as poverty, trade, and local government. Their methods and concepts introduced a behavioral social science designed for the analysis and solution of social problems. First [Alfred] Marshall 'recast' political economy as 'the Science of Social Perfectibility'; [William] James then tried to identify the psychological state of mind essential to social progress; and [Graham] Wallas combined their perceptions into a science of politics that would enable people to participate in progressive planning.

---

[2] *Ibid.*, Appendix 3. All quotations are from this Appendix until a change is noted.

While Trotter was in the reform tradition, it is not clear that this was true of Brouillette. The latter expressed the view that "the Council must stay as appointed —a purely academic body. To prove its existence," he thought, "the Council should face certain responsibilities. If anybody knows them, we, as members, should know in what fields social research must be carried on". In particular, he emphasized the "idea of planning for our own needs—to speak about it from a French-Canadian point of view". A "purely academic body" focused on "planning for our own needs" might well be committed to little more than the promotion of the social sciences themselves rather than to improving the quality of everyone's life.

Cronkite's focus was sometimes narrowly and at other times broadly pragmatic. He believed that "the matter of most immediate concern is the organization of the Council itself, especially with reference to its relations to public and quasi-public bodies". Specifically, he wanted "to see the Council achieve and maintain a position independent in fact". "If there is to be support from the Government" he said, "care must be taken that the Council is not to become the tool of any political party or group….On the other hand, support from Foundations or wealthy individuals may have strings attached".

When he shifted focus to the question of what sort of research the Council should plan, Cronkite thought that it "must in the first instance be fact-finding in its nature". But he saw the work on social conditions beginning "where the Bureau of Statistics leave off—that is by organizing the results of the Bureau with reference to social significance".

> "It has been remarked" he contended, "that sensitiveness to a reasonably well informed and intelligent public opinion is the criterion of democratic government and it would seem to me that the research work of this Council must be concerned with it. I would go further and say that the Council cannot stop short with what its members might call "reasonably well informed and intelligent public opinion" for it might thereby beg the whole question and become a dictator. The Council should be informed as to all public opinion, all desires or felt wants of any appreciable portion of the community".

Then, in a strikingly revealing passage indicating the technological distance of at least one member of the founding group from ourselves, Cronkite said that "a new technique seems to be arising in the development of public opinion polls, using statistical sampling methods to get a quick and accurate picture of what the people are thinking….It seems to me that the Council might, at some time in the future, undertake such surveys". "Personally", he went on, "I would be interested in finding out the underlying philosophy of life of the public without reference to matters which have already been brought into political issue. This, I admit, is very difficult, but in my opinion it lies at the heart of research work in the social sciences".

Humphrey's concerns seemed to be narrowly professional. He was interested in "finding more post-graduate scholarships" in order to get more "able students into social science research". He also recommended research professorships, since there were "only a few in Canada and none in social science fields so far as had been learned".

On the other hand, Booth's concerns seemed to be broadly professional. He wanted the Council to be a "clearing-house for information on research under way, a coordinating agency for research, an agency to "popularize social science research", and a pressure group, to get "sabbatical leave for university and government employees". Still, he believed that it should sponsor research on "problems that have political implications and which on that account civil servants may be inclined to avoid".

MacKay thought that the Council might also "concern itself with library facilities and other physical aids to research…particularly in the colleges at some distance from Central Canada". He also "expressed serious doubt as to the wisdom of the Council undertaking too far-reaching responsibility such as suggested in… Brouillette's statement". The basis of the last comment is unclear to me because Brouillette's focus seemed to be primarily on developing the social sciences themselves.

Like Dawson in the first ad hoc meeting, Innis "urged the need for independence from government finance for the social scientist".

Instead of approaching the subject of research funding from the perspective of trying to find additional resources, Hurd approached it from the perspective of using currently available resources in a different way. In particular, he suggested that university professors might seek release time from their teaching responsibilities in order to undertake more research. In his view, "support or request from Council would strengthen the case of an individual university teacher with his authorities… to obtain some reduction in teaching load". It is difficult for me to see any significant advantage in this approach because any government that had been providing funding with the understanding that a certain amount of teaching was required in some area would at least want to know why the same amount of teaching was no longer required or what additional funds would be required to pay for a substitute teacher.

While others had talked about the need to coordinate work in the different social science disciplines, McIlwaith seems to have been the first person in the ad hoc groups to advocate a multi-disciplinary approach to problems. The minutes note that he "was especially interested in the possibility of bringing scholarship from two or more "disciplines" to bear on a single problem, and in studying the combination of training that would produce well-equipped workers in the border line area between social and natural sciences". It is a remarkable fact that 57 years later there are still relatively few multi-disciplinary programs designed to train scholars for research in this "border line area".

Reflections on Directions

Reviewing all these suggestions regarding the functions of the proposed Canadian Research Council, it seems that they fall into three broadly defined classes which are not mutually exclusive and probably are not exhaustive of all alternatives. The three classes may be characterized as that of a Professional Trade Union, a National Planning Board and a Research Foundation. While the minutes indicate that certain members of the ad hoc groups recommended only one or another of these kinds of institutions, we have no way of rank ordering the three kinds according to their importance or desirability for a majority of members. However, I suspect that there would have been less support among the various members for a council designed to carry out the activities of a National Planning Board than for either of the other two institutions.

Functioning as a Professional Trade Union, the proposed Council would be limited to academic members and would lobby for research professorships, reduced teaching loads, sabbatical leaves, greater library facilities and other physical resources, and generally popularize the work of social scientists.

Functioning as a National Planning Board, the Council would undertake the sorts of coordinated planning that was recommended in the 1930s by groups like the National Planning Association in Canada and the United States, and the League for Social Reconstruction in Canada. Such planning would be informed and facilitated by the Council's third function.

As a Research Foundation, the Council would carry out fact-finding basic research to determine the functions of social institutions, the needs of Canadians and their "underlying philosophy of life" in Cronkite's phrase. In the present context that phrase would seem to designate an account of Canadians' views about a good quality of life, about what they wanted or perhaps thought they deserved or ought to get out of life. In its capacity as a Research Foundation the Council would also provide a clearing-house for information from different social sciences, coordinate the work of different disciplines, cultivate multidisciplinary research, and provide funding for research and post-graduate scholarships.

Although some members of the group issued warnings about the dangers of being captured by governments, political parties, wealthy individuals and private foundations, it was inevitable that funds would be sought from all these sources in order to carry out the wide variety of tasks that the group regarded as appropriate. It was also inevitable that some of the potential funders would refuse to support some of the proposed tasks. Obviously none of the listed potential funders would have been interested in funding a Professional Trade Union. So, insofar as Council members chose to advertise themselves as just that or primarily that, their only source of funds would be the academics that they purported to represent. In order to attract funds as a National Planning Board for ordinary citizens, the Council would have needed some kind of a mandate from the latter, which it did not have and did not seem inclined to seek. Apparently, then, the Council's best hope for attracting operating funds rested on identifying itself with those tasks appropriate to a Research Foundation.

While there were good reasons for the Council to become primarily a Research Foundation, the consequences of moving in this direction were not all favourable. Some members of the Council and many of the academics they represented would have lost their enthusiasm for the new initiative if it was not going to serve their professional union and/or national planning interests. Apart from that, there was an obvious conflict of interest involved in the idea that the Council would attract funds to do research and to fund others to do research. Serious questions would be raised about who was going to decide to spend what on what, using what criteria, and to give what to whom for what. Perhaps more importantly, it should be remembered that these were ad hoc groups for which the first year's budget was carefully calculated to have a balance of exactly $37.43.

Canadian Research Council in the Social Sciences, First Meeting

The first meeting of the new Council was on September 16, 1940 at the Chateau Laurier. The group mentioned above in Meeting 5 as members agreed to conduct its affairs according to the draft constitution. Among other things, a letter was read from the Carnegie Corporation asking the Council to "act as sponsor for a study of differential fertility in Canada which Dr. Enid Charles" had discussed with them. It was the policy of the Corporation and other major Foundations to fund agencies rather than individuals, and apparently there was no other available agency to play the sponsor's role in Canada. Being the "sponsor" meant simply receiving and disbursing funds allocated by the Trustees.[3]

The Council struck a committee to look into the matter, and another to look into the matter of incorporation with a view to handling "considerable sums of money". In other words, at the first official meeting of the Council, consideration was given to being a laundry for American Foundation money.[4] Apparently, then, to some extent the now familiar strategy of providing operational funding for a wide variety of organizations, from independent think tanks to universities, using "overheads" was adopted very early in the life of the Council.

Attention was also given to the question of allowing "social welfare and social service groups" to be represented on the Council. Several had asked for such representation. Another committee was struck to think about it.

The question of financing the next year's work arose again and MacKay was asked to draw up a budget of probable costs.

It was then moved "that the Chairman and Secretary nominate a Committee to make a survey of actual research projects in progress, and to suggest projects that should be undertaken".[5] Recall that the final word on the previous state-of-research survey had been uttered just about a year earlier. (See Meeting 5 above.)

[3]*Ibid.*, Minutes of the first meeting, pp. 2–3.

[4]*Ibid.*, p. 4. In a fine collection of essays, Arnove (1982) claimed that Foundations "have a corrosive influence on a democratic society". The evidence provided here indicates that from the point of view of those enjoying the Foundations' largesse, the "corrosive influence" may be acceptable, insofar as it is perceived at all.

[5]*Ibid.*, p. 5.

On the second day of the meeting, Hurd recommended that the Council "sponsor" the Charles project. Dawson recommended that social welfare and service groups should not be represented on the Council, though certain committees might appoint some members from such groups. The reasons for Dawson's recommendation were not recorded but, given his commitment to research and to strengthening universities' research capacities, he was probably worried that the addition of social welfare and social service groups to the Council would shift the focus of its activities away from things he regarded as central to its interests.

A committee was struck to consider "a survey of the post-graduate training field", the Chairperson was instructed to ask the Carnegie Corporation for $5,000 for "organizational purposes", and the Secretary proposed the following press release (which was approved).

> The new Canadian Research Council in the Social Sciences has concluded its first sessions, held at the Chateau Laurier, Ottawa, Monday and Tuesday, September 16 and 17. The purpose of the Council is to promote research in the social sciences in Canada. As a result of its broadly representative character, the Council hopes to further the cooperation of scholars in the numerous branches of the social sciences. Arrangements have been made for an immediate survey of the research now in progress, of the needs for additional research, and of the possibility of facilitating the training of Canadian research workers.[6]

While it was significant that the group had enough confidence in itself to issue a press release, it was perhaps even more significant that the Carnegie Corporation helped to legitimize its Research Foundation status by officially recognizing it as a Canadian research sponsor. Indeed, the Minutes leave the distinct impression that at the time there was no other organization in the country with greater visibility or legitimacy as a social science research sponsor. By agreeing to exclude "social welfare and social service groups" from official representation on the Council, the group's academic status and research focus was reinforced again.

CRCSS, Second Meeting

At the second meeting of the Council, at the University of Toronto, February 8, 1941, Trotter reported that the Carnegie Corporation had given them $4800 for the Charles project and a $5000 "sustaining grant" for Council operations that year, with "a like amount in January 1942". In fact, the Corporation supported the Council during the war years from 1941 to 44 and from 1948 to 50.

The state-of-research survey called for at the September 1940 meeting was apparently brought forward at this meeting, although it is dated December 1940.[7] The author/editor, McIlwraith, acknowledged having "the advantage of the report

[6]*Ibid.*, pp. 7–9.

[7]*Ibid.*, Minutes of the second meeting, February 8 and 9, 1941, Appendix 2.

edited by Dr. J.E. Robbins in May 1939". (The report is included with the Minutes of the First Annual Meeting: see footnote 11.)

It was at this meeting that Innis and Hurd asked for a "Committee on Publication of Results of Social Science Research in Canada".[8] The First Executive Meeting, April 19, 1941, appointed Dawson (Chair), Brouillette, Cronkite, Innis, and MacKay to this committee.[9] When this committee gave its report to the Council meeting of May 24–26, 1941 at Queen's University, Dawson informed the Council of "two immediate needs…(1) financial support for the Canadian Journal of Economics and Political Science and the Canadian Historical Review to enable them to maintain and improve their bibliographical service; (2) a publication fund to enable publication of certain manuscripts completed or near completion". Dawson and Innis then moved "that the Chairman inform the Rockefeller Foundation of the need for $500 in support of the bibliographical service and $4500 for a publication fund to meet immediate needs".[10] The motion was passed.

The Official First Annual Meeting of the CRCSS

When the First Annual Meeting was held at the University of Montreal, November 8, 1941, Trotter informed the Council that the Rockefeller Foundation had granted them "$4,500 for completion and publication of manuscripts and $500 for bibliographical work of the Canadian Historical Review and the Canadian Journal of Economics and Political Science".[11] In an Executive Session of that meeting, Dawson said that he would ask "each of the Council's four sponsoring bodies…if they would be willing to assist in the selection of reading panels….It was suggested that preference be given, at the outset at least, to the works of younger writers, though more mature authors should be encouraged to apply so the Committee would be able to plan with fuller knowledge".[12] Originally, publications and research grants funds were put in the same pot, a pot that was mainly filled by the Rockefeller Foundation in the 13 years from 1941 to 1953.

At the Executive Meeting of January 9, 1943, Brouillette proposed that "the Council should interest itself in the problem of obtaining a national atlas".[13] This

---

[8]*Ibid.*, p. 5.

[9]*Ibid.*, Minutes of First Executive Meeting, April 19, 1941, p. 1.

[10]*Ibid.*, Minutes of meeting held at Queen's University, May 24–26, 1941, p. 3.

[11]*Ibid.*, Minutes of First Annual Meeting, held at University of Montreal, November 7, 1941, p. 1. Exactly why the third meeting of the Council should have been called the "First Annual Meeting" is not clear to me.

[12]*Ibid.*, p. 4.

[13]*Ibid.*, Minutes of Executive Meeting, January 9 and 10, 1943, p. 2. There is no record of full Council or Executive meetings in 1942 or of full Council meetings in 1943. Presumably, the war interrupted schedules.

was the beginning of a massive and certainly necessary project which occupied the attention of the Council until its completion 3 years later in 1946.

The first joint Executive Meeting of the CRCSS and the Humanities Research Council (HRC) occurred on May 27, 1944. (The two councils formally combined in April 1996.) At that point in time, the latter "was not yet in funds but anticipated a Foundation grant for a Canada-wide survey of the position of humanities research. ...The possibility of a joint committee of the two Councils on sources of finance was raised by members of the Humanities Research Council, but it was not considered feasible by members of the Social Science Council".[14] There is no indication of why it was not considered feasible. The Chairperson of the HRC was made an ex-officio member of the other Council.

CRCSS Executive Meeting, November 4, 1944

At the Executive Meeting on November 4, 1944, it is recorded that "there was some discussion of the question of establishment of a permanent fund for support of the Council's administration, and of the advisability of establishing a reserve fund which might eventually become an endowment fund".[15] An endowment fund would have provided exactly the sort of independence and guaranteed permanence that several members of the Executive wanted.

CRCSS Annual Meeting, December 15, 1945

At this meeting "Hurd pointed to the desirability, to which reference had been made at previous annual meetings, of taking steps to secure a sum of $75,000 or more, the interest on which would be sufficient to meet the administrative expenses of the Council".[16] Hurd, Dawson, Innis and MacGibbon formed a committee "to explore the possibilities of raising such a sum".

Hurd was absent from the next Executive Meeting, March 16, 1946, but "the Chairman and Secretary had word that Mr. Hurd and Mr. MacGibbon had both been active toward the end of obtaining an endowment for the Council".[17] On May 18, 1946, Hurd told the Council that "the committee favoured attempting to raise needed funds from one or a few people, rather than attempting a campaign. Various

[14]*Ibid.*, Minutes of Meeting, May 27–28, 1944, p. 2.

[15]*Ibid.*, Minutes of Annual Meeting, November 4–5, 1944, p. 2.

[16]*Social Science Research Council Minutes 1945–49*, Minutes of Annual Meeting, December 15–16, 1945, p. 1. Notice that the name of the Council seems to have changed since the 1940 press release.

[17]*Ibid.*, Minutes of Executive Meeting, March 16, 1946, p. 1.

consultations had been held to this end. The committee was examining particularly the idea of establishment of a trust, corresponding to a collateral trust bond, in which the donor during his lifetime would maintain control of the securities placed in trust. Mr. Brebner drew attention to the procedure common at Columbia University—a deed of gift with undertaking to pay interest during the life of the donor".[18] Subsequently, "Mr. Hurd was complimented on his vigorous activity as chairman of this committee." So far, of course, the committee had not raised a dime.

CRCSS Annual Meeting, November 1, 1946

Hurd "reported progress in consultations with certain individuals" and the "Chairman expressed the Council's appreciation of Mr. Hurd's activity in this connection."[19] Still no money.

On February 8, 1947, Hurd "reported calling at the office of the Carnegie Corporation and discussing the affairs of the Council at some length on a recent trip to New York."[20] A couple months later (May 24, 1947), he "reported on a meeting of his committee with Mr. Shepardson of the Carnegie Corporation, in Toronto on February 14". Hurd thought that "more publicity should be given to the Council's work. Among other suggestions was one from Mr. Lamb for an exhibit of the books, publication of which the Council had aided, at the June meeting of the Canadian Library Association."[21] Apparently no funds were promised as a result of the Shepardson meeting.

The call for more publicity regarding the Council's work probably indicates that by 1947 some members felt that enough important work had been accomplished by the Council to seek broader recognition for it.

CRCSS Annual Meeting, October 25, 1947

At this meeting Hurd reported (through the Secretary) that he had "called at the office of the Carnegie Corporation the previous week" and "his (Hurd's) advice was that the Council should proceed to formulate a written request of the corporation".[22]

About 2 years after Hurd's committee had been struck, its ship came in, though it was admittedly a very small ship. The Chairperson, J.A. Corry, told the Executive Committee on February 21, 1948 that

[18]*Ibid.*, Minutes of Council Meeting, May 18–19, 1946, p. 3.

[19]*Ibid.*, Minutes of Annual Meeting, November 1–2, 1946, p. 1.

[20]*Ibid.*, Minutes of Executive Meeting, Feb. 8–9, 1947, p. 1.

[21]*Ibid.*, Minutes of Meeting of Council, May 24–25, 1947, p. 2.

[22]*Ibid.*, Minutes of Seventh Annual Meeting, October 25–26, 1947, p. 3.

> a grant of $2500 per year for three years had since been received from the Carnegie Corporation for administrative expenses, on the understanding that the Council would, during these three years, make every effort to obtain future administrative funds within Canada. ...Innis said that...the Rockefeller Foundation was willing to allow the Council to apply $2500 per year, of the grant for expenses of the Council's program, to administrative costs.[23]

It was agreed that Corry would ask the Foundation for $10,000 per year for 2 years.

CRCSS Annual Meeting, June 12, 1948

Corry told the Council that the Rockefeller Foundation had awarded them "$10,000 for 1 year, 1948–49...for the various aspects of the Council's program...$15,000 in 2 years, 1948–50, for fellowships...[and] from the Carnegie Corporation $15,000 for...Anglo-French studies".[24] Although these were encouraging signs of support, Corry was not particularly optimistic about the Council's financial prospects. He had written to all present and past members of Council about their views, and reported some of the results. Personally, he "expressed...doubt that funds could be raised for endowment of the Council". He noted that the U.S. Council "had some members without academic connections", presumably with attractive financial connections instead.

> The Secretary reported having obtained a ruling from the Department of National Revenue that donations to the Council would be considered as charitable donations for income tax purposes....Mr. (A.G.) Bailey hoped that in seeking funds the Council would not feel compelled to put too much emphasis on its furtherance of research in 'practical' problems. Mr. (G.A.) Elliott thought the real question was only one of admitting or publicizing 'practical' aims more, in order to obtain more funds to assist all scholarship in the social sciences.[25]

CRCSS Executive Meeting, January 22, 1949

Corry gave the Council "a draft brochure" at this meeting. "His thought was that it might be published in the autumn, when the budgetary needs of the Council became more certain, and presented personally by members to a number of people who

---

[23] *Ibid.*, Minutes of Executive Committee, February 21–22, 1948, p. 1.

[24] *Ibid.*, Minutes of Council Meeting, June 12–13, 1948, pp. 1–2.

[25] *Ibid.*, p. 3.

could be influential in securing funds for the Council. There were 'favoured' comments on the draft, and it was agreed the procedure proposed was sound."[26]

The question of hiring a secretary to assist the Secretary-Treasurer seems to have arisen for the first time at an Executive Meeting on June 11, 1949. "Discussion indicated general willingness for the Secretary-Treasurer to engage a full-time secretary, with something like two-thirds of the cost being borne by the CSSRC and one third by the HRCC."[27] At that meeting Corry also announced "preparation for a financial campaign in the coming year". He would chair a new Financial Campaign Committee, including D.A. MacGibbon, G.V. Ferguson, V.W. Bladen, M. Lamontagne and E.J. Tarr.

> The objective for the campaign should be $50,000, but could be set higher by the Committee without consulting Council. Grants over a period of years would be acceptable, also contributions through provincial government agencies. The Secretary was asked to express to Hurd the Council's gratitude for work of the earlier finance committee of which he had been chairman.[28]

CRCSS Annual Meeting, October 29, 1949

The Finance Committee reported that it would ask for "statements from the Carnegie Corporation, Rockefeller Foundation, and Universities Conference, expressing confidence in the Council, for inclusion in the campaign literature that was being prepared. It was not proposed to make an appeal to the universities in the first stages of the campaign at least."[29]

There is a note from Robbins at the end of his 1949 Treasurer's report that will strike a familiar cord in the hearts of anyone who has ever served as volunteer Treasurer of anything.

> "Total payments" he wrote, "made during the year approached $30,000, involved the issuing of more than 200 cheques, 100 receipts, purchase of several dozen money orders, making of two dozen deposits, etc., and keeping record of it all in a manner satisfactory to the auditor. The average item of business resulting in the issue of a cheque involves the writing of two or three letters, frequently a circular to the members of a committee rather than a single letter. This is by way of explanation to Members of Council as to why communications from the Secretary-Treasurer are short, infrequent, and come as circulars rather than as individual letters".[30]

The month after the Annual Meeting, the Council submitted a Brief to the Royal Commission on National Development in the Arts, Letters and Sciences (Massey

---

[26] *Ibid.*, Minutes of Annual Meeting, January 22–23, 1949, p. 5.

[27] *Social Science Research Council Minutes 1949–52*, Minutes of June 11–12, 1949, p. 3.

[28] *Ibid.*, p. 5.

[29] *Ibid.*, Minutes of Annual Meeting, October 29–30, 1949, p. 1.

[30] *Ibid.*, Report of the Treasurer to the Annual Meeting of 1949, p. 4.

Commission), which is included in the volume containing the Minutes of this meeting. A list of its recommendations suggests something of the ethos in which the Council and academic social scientists worked. The Council Brief said:

1. Federal grants for post-graduate fellowships, scholarships, research grants are, in the Council's view, both desirable and practicable.
2. The speedy establishment and development of the National Library is urgently needed as a research centre for Canada.
3. Public records of government departments should be under the control of the Public Archives and available for research.
4. Printed government documents need to be better distributed as tools of research.
5. Administrative re-organization of the National Museum is advisable under a Board of Trustees.
6. Canada should set up a UNESCO National Commission.

By the end of our period of investigation, 1980, every one of these recommendations had been implemented.

Executive Meeting, February 25, 1950

At this meeting the new Chairperson, T.F. McIlwraith, announced the death of W. Burton Hurd. As I read through the minutes, I felt I had become a friend of old Hurd. It was easy to imagine him tracking through cold, snowy, blowing days in Toronto and New York, hustling money for the folks back home. His virtually endless reports of discussions leading to nothing but more discussions sometimes struck me as comical. And then he was gone, and it was not funny anymore. In fact, Hurd was the first Council member whose death was announced in the minutes. Others followed, Trotter, Innis, etc. It is a sobering experience to follow these fellows year after year, meeting after meeting, and then to have their deaths announced. I think one faces one's own mortality and the likely limitations of one's own lifetime contributions. Here are the Chairperson's remarks for Hurd in full.

> With the death of W. Burton Hurd, O.B.E., M.A., F.R.S.C., the Canadian Social Science Research Council suffered the loss of one who contributed to the work of the Council in his sound judgment, scholarly activity, and administrative ability. Not only was Professor Hurd one of the first members of the Council, he was one of those who shared in the informal discussions that led to its formation. Hurd was a regular attendant at Council meetings, carrying his full share of the discussion in his own quiet, unassuming way, with every observation marked by common sense.
>
> Professor Hurd's greatest contribution to the Council was in the organization of the Publications Committee. When funds became available for publication, it was obvious that a committee had to be set up which would formulate a policy to ensure rigorous appraisal of all manuscripts from the standpoint of scholarly achievement; but at the same time to protect authors in their dealings with a publisher, and to ensure that the money entrusted to the Council should be expended to the full benefit of scholarship. The chairmanship of this Committee was a difficult assignment, and it was a tribute to Hurd's scholarship as well as to his organizing ability that he was selected. It was Hurd who formulated the policy of the

> Committee and set up the efficient system of reading panels and of business consultants to safeguard an author. The publications brought out through this system are one of the most significant achievements of the Council; in their publication Hurd contributed broadly and effectively to Canadian scholarship. He also won and perhaps this gave him greater satisfaction - the gratitude of scholars whose works were thus brought to publication. Hurd accomplished a definite task for the Council. He gave unsparingly of his strength, and we regret his death, not only as a collaborator, but as a loyal friend and colleague.[31]

Annual Meeting, June 3, 1950

Further progress on the fund-raising campaign was reported. Corry mentioned a "booklet entitled 'The Canadian Social Science Research Council, 1940–1950', which had been prepared by the Committee. …He also passed in review the preparations which have been made for the campaign in Montreal, Edmonton, London, Ottawa, Hamilton and other centres".[32] At the Executive Meeting on October 28, 1950 he happily reported that "Edmonton was the first centre to produce returns. Several cheques had come in…from there".[33] Four months later, February 10, 1951, the Secretary-Treasurer "reported receipt of cheques totalling $500 from Edmonton, and $100 from Crano Ltd., Montreal".[34]

Unfortunately, the Minutes do not contain any description of the nature of the campaigns or of the booklets. However, with the information that we already have about the activities of the Council, it is not difficult to imagine what the contents of a booklet might contain. It would have had some information about the Council's history and aims, its sponsored projects and publications, its potential benefits for individual social scientists and the social sciences in general, its past sponsors and its future needs. From the fact that the Council accepted a contribution from Crano Ltd. and from other businesses (see below), we may conclude that businesses were targeted, as well as foundations and individuals.

Annual Meeting, June 3, 1951

The most remarkable fund-raising event in the history of the Council was announced at this meeting at McGill. Robbins conveyed the "following verbal message" to the Council:

---

[31] *Ibid.*, Minutes of Executive Meeting, February 25, 1950, pp. 1–2.

[32] *Ibid.*, Minutes of Meeting, June 3–4, 1950, p. 2.

[33] *Ibid.*, Minutes of Meeting, October 28–29, 1950, p. 5.

[34] *Ibid.*, Minutes of Executive Meeting, February 10–11, 1951, p. 3.

> Mr. Howard W. Winkler of Morden, Manitoba, a mutual friend of Burton Hurd and myself, has authorized me to offer to the Council an annual contribution for five or more years, for the establishment of a W. Burton Hurd Memorial Fund to be used in furtherance of the Council's purposes. The gift would have no conditions attached other than that it be used to advance or continue the work that was so close to Burton Hurd's heart, the work to which he so unsparingly devoted his energy and talent. It would be the wish of the donor that the capital sum contributed to the Fund should remain intact for a period of years, though not necessarily in perpetuity.[35]

Naturally, "the members of the Council expressed delight at the prospect of the continued association of the name of Burton Hurd with its work", and accepted the gift with the specified conditions. The first $1000 was "received...within a week". By 1980, the end of the part of the Council's life under review here, the Ruth and Burton Hurd Memorial Fund was worth over $200,000. So Hurd, with the help of his generous brother-in-law, Winkler, and other members of the family, was able to generate more funds for the Council after he died than while he was living! Andrew Carnegie claimed that "Men who leave vast sums in this way [i.e., in their wills] may be thought men who would not have left it at all had they been able to take it with them" (Michalos 1984, p. 85). However, because very few other scholars have followed Hurd's lead in bequeathing funds or other assets to the Council, this is potentially a very big source of revenue.

At the same meeting, Corry reported further progress in the campaign. The Edmonton contribution had risen to $600, "the *Montreal Star* promised to contribute $500 for 7 years if others would participate" and "J.S. McLean of Toronto affirmed his willingness to help but favoured routing contributions through some Ontario university".[36]

In November it was agreed to have Corry

> proceed with his direct appeal to the Principals of the various universities, starting with University of British Columbia, Toronto and McGill and providing them with copies of relevant Council literature...with documents outlining direct benefits provided by Council to the scholars of the various institutions. ...It was formally approved by Council that the Administrative Fund be placed on a permanent basis, and that the appeal be made primarily and in the first instance for an annual grant from the Universities, rather than as formerly assumed direct to private individuals.[37]

This, then, was the first time the Council pressed the point of obtaining annual university grants. From 195 1 to 1980 the Council had support from some universities every year.[38]

---

[35] *Ibid.*, Minutes of Meeting, June 2–3, 1951, p. 8.

[36] *Ibid.*, p. 9.

[37] *Ibid.*, Minutes of Meeting, November 17–18, 1951, p. 5.

[38] *Ibid.*, Minutes of Meeting of Council, November 8, 1952, p. 3.

Meetings from November 1952 to March 1956

Robbins told the Council on November 8, 1952 that the "Carnegie Corporation had expressed a readiness to provide $2000 yearly for 3 years to provide secretarial services for the CSSRC and the HRCC. This grant would permit the employment by the two Councils of a half-time assistant who would, under direction of the Secretary-Treasurer, assume much of the detailed work".

In September of the following year it was announced that "Mrs. Hurd died during the winter, leaving $10,000 in her Will to the Fund",[39] increasing the Council's small endowment again.

The new Chairperson, W.J. Waines, told the Executive on February 20, 1954 that "he had spent the better part of a week in Toronto during January, calling on prospective donors, and had since written a number of letters formally presenting them with a request for assistance on a 3 year basis, enclosing a two-page mimeographed account…of the record of the Council to date. The first response (a cheque for $500 with promise of two more annual contributions of this amount) had just reached the secretary".[40] The fact that the requests for aid went out with "a two-page mimeographed account" may be taken as evidence that the "booklet" used in the campaigns of 1950–51 was also probably fairly modest. It seems unlikely that if a glossy publication had been produced only a few years earlier that it would have been abandoned in favour of an obviously very modest sort of document. Since the Council had more funds in these years than it did in 1950–51, it probably would have put its best advertising foot forward.

When the Council met on November 20, 1954, there was some discussion of its relation to the new

> Canada Council which, it appeared from the Prime Minister's address of the previous evening, would shortly be established. There was agreement that the CSSRC should in any case continue in existence as an independent body, prepared to receive funds from Government as well as from other sources, and willing to undertake or assist in making awards of fellowships and aid to research and publication, which might be provided from Government funds.[41]

It is a pity that the Minutes from this meeting do not provide more information about the content of the discussion of the new Canada Council. Since the Prime Minister had just announced his government's intention to establish and fund an agency that would function as a Research Council, some members of the CSSRC must have perceived the possibility of the latter becoming redundant. Indeed, since

[39]*Social Science Research Council Minutes 1953–56*, Treasurer's Report to the Annual Meeting for the year ended September 30, 1953, p. 2.

[40]*Ibid.*, Minutes of Executive Meeting, February 20, 1954, pp. 2–3.

[41]*Ibid.*, Minutes of Annual Meeting, November 20, 1954, p. 1.

most of the Council's backers outside of the academy regarded it as primarily a Research Council and provided it with funds on the basis of that understanding, some of them must have had second thoughts about its role given the new Canada Council. All we know from the Minutes of the meeting is that the CSSRC members had some discussion and apparently decided to simply carry on as before, which seems a bit naive given the changes that were probably coming.

Robbins suggested in his Secretary-Treasurer's Report of September 30, 1954 that one way to save money would be to reduce full meetings of the Council from two to one a year. "The main problem," he thought, "other than those looked after by the standing committees, is one of assuring continued financial support, and it does not seem to be one that discussion twice a year will solve".[42] He also reported that $500 had been received from the Hurd's son, Donald.

At the end of his May 31, 1955 report, Robbins informed the Council that

> the present is the third year of the Carnegie three-year grant ($2000 a year) for a joint CSSRC-HRCC secretaryship. We had hoped, in arranging this in 1952, that by 1955 a solution to the problem of the secretaryship of the two Councils would be found. What a hope! It was seventeen years ago today that this secretarial "life sentence" began. How about commuting it?[43]

He and Waines told the Council in March 1956 that "they saw no hope remaining of assistance from the Government in 1956 for the Council's program", although "a substantial private contribution…($5,000) had been received from Mr. Walter Koerner of Vancouver".[44]

In case it was not already clear, Robbins's remark about his "life sentence" suggests the extent to which the success of the Council in its early years depended and probably always depends on the size and strength of its volunteer workers. Robbins in particular was a man of extraordinary talents, the sort of volunteer whose presence can make and whose absence can break an organization. According to his biographer, McLeish (1978, pp. 19–20), Robbins

> …was one of the moving spirits–some of his fellow-builders finally called him *the* moving spirit–behind the foundation and growth of the Canadian Social Science Research Council and the Humanities Research Council of Canada. …he employed his post at Ottawa as a kind of intervention centre in aid of dozens of Canadian cultural and social causes. He became one of the legendary matchmakers of Canadian life as a result of the large network of men and women whom he had come to know from across the nation. On numerous occasions he brought together various people on behalf of cultural projects, and many times facilitated the appointment of able people for pivotal vacancies.

---

[42] *Ibid.*, Secretary-Treasurer's Report to the Annual Meeting, September 30, 1954, p. 1.

[43] *Ibid.*, Report of Secretary-Treasurer to Meeting of May 31, 1955, p. 2.

[44] *Ibid.*, Minutes of Executive Meeting, March 10, 1956, p. 3.

Meetings, June 9, 1956 to November 30, 1957

S.D. Clark informed the Council that "It should be the objective of the Executive to secure assurance of further funds for Council purposes before the next annual meeting, because, practically speaking, present resources would be exhausted when the annual awards are made next winter".[45]

A working arrangement was made with the new Canada Council in 1957. The latter would "advertise the competitions and receive applications itself (for scholarships, fellowships and grants)…proposing to turn over five copies of applications to HRCC and CSSRC to be judged".[46] It was also suggested that Canada Council would give the two councils about $10 for each application processed.

At this meeting the new Chairperson, G.E. Britnell, took pleasure in announcing

> a grant of $150,000 from the Ford Foundation. …It is a three-year grant - $80,000 in 1957-58, $40,000 in 1958-59, and $30,000 in 1959-60 - for 'general support' of CSSRC. The Council is free to use it in such ways as it thinks best, but presumably keeping in mind the purposes for which the Foundation had been asked to make a grant. At the head of the list of purposes, the chairman noted, was the establishment of an office and employment of an executive officer, such as the present secretary-treasurer. The secretary indicated that… sometime within the next year, he would be free to accept employment by CSSRC. He also mentioned that the Executive of the HRCC…had expressed the hope he might continue to serve HRCC in the same capacity.[47]

It was agreed that CSSRC would pay half of Robbins's salary in 1958, that he would lease an office after December 31, 1957 and hire a secretary. Perhaps the most interesting aspect of this new grant is its size compared to the $2500 donated by the Carnegie Corporation only a decade earlier. From 1947 to 1957 the Council was able to increase its worth 32 times.

With the passing of about two and a half years since the Prime Minister's announcement of the new Canada Council, substantial changes in emphasis of the CSSRC's activities had been introduced, even though initially it looked as if members of the CSSRC intended to carry on as if nothing new had happened. Here it is simply reported that "Since it appeared that the main financial burden of the CSSRC program of fellowships and grants would now be born by the Canada Council, the CSSRC would be free to devote more of its resources to planning and projects….Mr. Clark was asked to assume chairmanship of a Research Planning Committee to put proposals before the Council Meeting".[48] Among the first tasks performed by this Committee was the preparation of "recommendations for the meeting of the Canada Council scheduled for the first week in February. The

---

[45] *Ibid.*, Minutes of Annual Meeting, June 9, 1956, p. 3.

[46] *Social Science Research Council Minutes 1957–59*, Minutes of Executive Meeting, September 6, 1957, p. 1.

[47] *Ibid.*, p. 2.

[48] *Ibid.*, p. 3.

Canada Council had already referred to CSSRC for advice several requests from organizations for large sums".[49]

The Minutes from this 1957 Council meeting report the preparation of the first formal set of recommendations from a group that was becoming a Planning Council of academics to a government sponsored Funding Council, i.e., from what the CSSRC was at the end of our period in 1980 and is now, and what is now the Social Sciences and Humanities Research Council of Canada (SSHRCC). At least the main functions of the two Councils can be seen this way. Since the current Federation distributes funds granted to it in blocks from SSHRCC, the former is not only a Planning Council. Moreover, since SSHRCC can not just spread money around without thinking about what it is doing, it is not only a Funding Council. Still, the main emphases, expertise and responsibilities of the two Councils seem to divide fairly well between the two functions of planning and funding. Furthermore, that seems to be a reasonable division of labour.

It was also "agreed that the Council's Reserve Fund should be combined with the W. Burton Hurd Memorial Fund and that the Treasurer should ask Mr. Winkler to let his name, the maiden name of his sister (Mrs. Hurd) be associated with that of Mr. Hurd in the name of the fund".[50] Another contribution of $2,500 from Winkler in 1957, matched by the Rockefeller Foundation, brought the Fund up to over $42,000. Robbins reported that he personally would "like to see it reach $100,000 before it is put to use. ...Such a sum", he thought, "treated as an endowment, would provide a substantial guarantee of permanence in the Council's operations".[51]

In the report of the Research Planning Committee at the November 1957 meeting, written by S.D. Clark, there appears the recommendation that "the condition of (research grant) support should be the worth of the scholar not the nature of the study in which he is engaged". Over the years, Canada's main research funding agencies have tended to swing back and forth between Clark's suggestion to give more weight to a scholar's track record versus more weight to a scholar's particular project proposal. By the 1990s, Clark's suggestion was being followed at SSHRCC.

Clark also provided a very clear account of how he saw the future. He said that,

> ...what is clear is that the Canada Council Programme will meet almost all those needs which were formerly met by the Canadian Social Science Research Council programme and on a basis much more adequate financially. It is our [i.e., his] view that the Canadian Social Science Research Council should not now attempt simply to supplement the kind of help offered by the Canada Council. It is time to remind ourselves of our name. Ours is a research council. Yet if we review our past programme, we are forced to the conclusion that much of what we have been doing has been only indirectly or remotely related to research. Under the circumstances this was inevitable. These other kinds of support of social science scholarship were vitally necessary. With the assurance now that this work will be carried on by the Canada Council, however, it would appear important that our council carefully

[49] *Ibid.*, Minutes of Council Meeting, November 30, 1957, p. 5.

[50] *Ibid.*

[51] *Ibid.*, Report of the Treasurer to Meeting of November 1957, p. 2.

consider what are the most effective means by which it can accomplish the things for which it primarily exists.[52]

From the point of view of financial stability, given the healthy level of support from the Ford Foundation and government support for the Canada Council, it is fair to say that the social sciences had never had it so good as they did when Clark wrote those words in November 1957. While it may be unfair to say that one might have expected to see a substantial endowment built up beginning around this time, that never seems to have happened.

Meetings, 1958

As suggested above, it would have been unreasonable and politically unwise for the new Canada Council to try to faithfully serve the interests of Canada's academic researchers without giving the latter some sort of an institutionalized voice in their deliberations. Accordingly, a relatively formal institution or practice was created. The first appearance of what came to be called Liaison Meetings with SSHRCC was announced at the Executive Committee Meeting of March 22, 1958. The Chairperson, G.E. Britnell, "read a copy of an invitation to attend a one-day meeting of humanists and social scientists to be convened by Canada Council in Ottawa during Easter week, on April 9th. It was expected that about a dozen members of Canada Council and staff would attend, and about an equal number of others. The purpose was to discuss the Council's program in the humanities and social sciences."[53]

In the fall of 1958, the Council sent V.W. Bladen to New York to visit Foundations about funds. He wrote to the Chairperson, E.F. Beach, on November 4, 1958 that,

> The Ford Foundation is clearly the best bet. But even here there was an inclination to suggest that after the foundation of the Canada Council projects from Canadians would be considered as parts of their North American program and that grants for rather general purposes in Canada would not be likely to be made. …their interest is in Economics rather than Social Science in general. …The Sloan Foundation…had moved over pretty completely to Cancer and mathematics and physics.…The Rockefeller Foundation has had a drastic change of policy. Its Canadian grants were pretty clearly terminal… . The Carnegie Corporation similarly seemed unlikely to make any block grants, or indeed any substantial grants.[54]

It would appear that the biggest American Foundations came to regard the Canadian academic establishment as secure enough that attention could be diverted

---

[52] *Ibid.*, Report of the Research Planning Committee, November 1957, p. 10.

[53] *Ibid.*, Minutes of the Executive Committee, March 22, 1958, p. 3.

[54] Letter from V.W. Bladen to Chairman of SSRCC, November 4, 1958.

elsewhere. Reflecting on the 20 year period from 1938 to 1958, it is clear that these Foundations played a key role in the development of the CSSRC and academic social scientific research in Canada. On the whole, these Foundations contributed more money than Canadians.

Judging from the remarks just quoted from Bladen's letter, it is equally clear that members of the Council's Executive were quite prepared to continue drawing upon the Foundations. While one's (my own at least) national pride is a bit wounded at the thought of Canadian scholars shamelessly going cap-in-hand to rich American benefactors in the interest of developing Canadian social science, one must remember that then, as now, we live in a world in which the public purse tends to be squeezed in order to allow some private purses to be inflated. In the absence of a system of fair taxation according to individuals' and corporations' ability to pay, followed by a reasonable redistribution of revenue, those seeking funds for worthy causes must go where the money is, and a lot of it is still in Foundations. The big difference between then and now is that today a search for Foundation funding would be guided by well-designed Directories including potential sources from countries all over the globe.

Although things in the south had gone sour, things in the north were increasingly sweet. Seven months after Bladen's letter, Robbins reported that Winkler had "undertaken to raise his contribution to the Fund from $20,000 to $50,000 on the understanding that the name of the Fund would become The Ruth and W. Burton Hurd Memorial Fund."[55] The Executive decided in November 1959 to "allow the fund to accumulate for at least another year before using it". It was then worth $104,071.[56] At that same meeting it was agreed to make a "3 year request to the Ford Foundation for general purposes".

Meetings, 1960–1962

As Chairperson of the Joint Committee of HRCC and SSRCC, Britnell sent a letter to the Director of the Canada Council, A.W. Trueman, dated February 5, 1960. The letter is especially instructive in indicating the perceived functions of the two planning Councils in contrast to the funding for Canada Council. Among other things, Britnell wrote that in "the opinion of our Councils…the fellowship program by itself does not meet all the needs of scholarship in the humanities and social sciences". In particular, he pointed out that,

> The Humanities and Social Science Councils should also take the initiative in promoting and setting up research projects. Here a clear distinction must be made between the need of support for the well and fully planned research project and the need of support for that research project which may not yet have got off the planning board. It is not hard to

---

[55]*Ibid.*, Treasurer's Report to Council Meeting, June 7, 1959, p. 1.

[56]*Ibid.*, Meeting of the Executive, November 14, 1959, p. 4.

demonstrate the need to support the well and fully planned research project. Here presumably a group of scholars have settled upon the objectives of their study. The initiative can be taken by them in seeking support. They know what they want in the way of financial assistance and are in a position where they can demonstrate the need for such assistance.

The other kind of project is more difficult to appraise. An offer of support must be made before the project is fully organized and the personnel determined. Yet if such an offer of support is not made the project fails to achieve its purpose which is that of stimulating scholarly work on the part of persons who have not yet demonstrated their worth or are not wholly clear what they want to do.[57]

After some details about current levels of funding, Britnell indicated "many things which are not being done or which are being left undone". They included the following:

(a) The searching out and stimulation of research and scholarship which, as described above, is a continuous and demanding task;
(b) Planning and development of larger projects, similar to the Canadian Frontiers of Settlement Series, the Canadian-American Relations Series, and the Social Credit Series;
(c) Vigorous projection of the current projects of our two Councils, e.g., the Morton project on the History of Canada, the Literary History of Canada…;
(d) Explorational and experimental work, i.e., surveys of need and exploration of points of new departure; (e.g., Chairs in the History and Philosophy of Science; History of Art; History of Literature and Literary Scholarship)…
(e) Planning and development to meet the increasing pressure and needs of an expanding academic community… Entirely new talent must be recruited into the academic profession and, once recruited, must grow and flourish there…[58]

In conclusion, he argued that,

The main task of supporting Canadian scholarship in the humanities and social sciences must be left to the Canada Council. That support is assured by the fellowship program. What we seek is not a major diversion of Canada Council funds to the support of the work of our Councils but, rather, a modest appropriation which would, in our view, enormously strengthen and further the program of work being carried on by the Canada Council.[59]

It seems to me that Britnell carved out a precise niche for the two Councils versus the Canada Council. Indeed, it appears that the two Councils successfully occupied this niche over the years in spite of some very difficult economic constraints. Although I have not made a detailed examination of the two Council's output of Council-initiated major research projects, my guess would be that more of such projects have come from independent scholars who increasingly have had direct access to our various funding agencies. However, it would be worthwhile for someone to make a careful examination of this question. If some capacity to

[57] *Social Science Research Council Minutes 1960–62*, Letter from G.E. Britnell to the Director of Canada Council, February 5, 1960.

[58] *Ibid.*

[59] *Ibid.*

generate major projects or series of projects has been lost, it would be helpful to know it and to be able to take appropriate remedial action.

The new Chairperson's (Beach) report to the Annual Meeting of June 1960 is also instructive, especially on the matter of funding. He began with the comment that he felt "somewhat like an unsuccessful business man who thinks he knows the answers but has very little material success to show for it. The funds of the Council are at a very low point. …the creation of Canada Council seems to have assured the existence of this Council, at least in the short run, but it has on the other hand cast great shadows over our ability to achieve an independent existence". He then recorded the results of the Bladen trip mentioned earlier.

> Our main problem is, as alway's, funds. …The raising of funds must be the work of all of us, along with the appraising of and assisting in, and sometimes the creation of projects. We must build up in this Council a group of people who have the interest and vigour to undertake such work. And in doing so there will be created in the public mind a rather different picture of the Council and its activities… . Even the academics feel that this Council is a very aloof and non-responsible (if not irresponsible) organization of which they seldom hear, and some of what they do hear is not good.
>
> The improvement of this 'public' image is a very complicated task, and we must give it adequate thought. Of more immediate importance is the reformulation of its activities so as to assure its vitality. Indeed, I think that this transformation may be necessary for the long-run existence of this Council.
>
> In closing, let me emphasize that this report is a purely personal one. These ideas are thrown out almost as cries of anguish, but the suggestions will, I hope, be the subject of serious consideration by all members of the Council.[60]

As this chronicle has shown, Beach's remarks were similar to those of many earlier members of the Council in all its incarnations. There have always been some members who have given serious consideration to sources of funding, purposes, public images and planning. The trouble is, their efforts have always seemed to be barely adequate. In general and in fact there are always new tasks to perform, new projects, new social needs and demands for better information about this or that social issue which, given the typical level of knowledge and expertise of the typical Council participant, are well-known. In such circumstances, it is virtually inevitable that demands will outrun supplies of resources.

Granting these general points, we should emphasize the following particulars. First, the first contributions for administrative purposes came from Canada Council in 1958 and for what is now the Aid to Scholarly Publications program in 1959. Second, although Beach recommended "assisting in…the creation of projects", he did not seem to be suggesting that funding for administrative purposes might be drawn from research overheads. Today there are many organizations that sustain themselves on such "soft money". Third, nearly 40 years after Beach's letter, the social sciences in Canada still have a relatively low and misunderstood profile. If one judges their profile from discussions of science and technology in government

[60] *Ibid.*, Report of the Chairman, Annual Meeting, June 1960.

agencies like Industry Canada or the Science Council of British Columbia, it is clear that social sciences are practically invisible as "sciences". There is still a lot of room for image-building and information dissemination.

The minutes of the Executive Committee of August 6, 1960 report that Bernard Ostry would assist the Secretary-Treasurer, Robbins, until J.R. Kidd would assume Robbins's office.[61] The records show that Kidd and Ostry undertook the most exhaustive funding campaign the Council ever had. At least they left us the most detailed account of their campaign. Kidd reported to the Executive Committee in January 1962 that he had prepared

> lists of possible donors, including,
>
> i) Canadian Foundations (15)
> ii) Canadian corporations (selected on a basis of average earnings and the record of donations to education: 186)
> iii) American Foundations considered most likely to be interested in the work of the Council (16).

It was agreed to let Kidd "seek the active support of a number of businessmen who are interested in scholarship and in planning fund-raising for the Council….[A model was]…the National Bureau of Economic Research".[62]

At an Executive Committee meeting the following month, Kidd reported that "a brochure describing the functions and program of the Council to be used in requesting grants from corporations and Foundations has been prepared in draft form". It was suggested that "a meeting with a selected number of businessmen be held in Montreal. …It was also agreed that requests should now be made to universities to increase (recommended double) the size of their grant to SSRCC as has been proposed at the Annual Meeting last June".[63]

At the June 1962 Annual Meeting, Kidd reported that he had "visited ten Foundations during the year and has been in touch with others". Moreover, "about two hundred corporations" had been given information resulting in interviews with corporation executives.[64] The Treasurer reported at that meeting that

> While no request was made for funds, this [i.e., Kidd's activities] has resulted in several cheques… . Talks have been initiated for the purpose of having a small advisory group of businessmen who are seriously interested in scholarship and who will meet periodically to advise the Executive about finances and investments.

Universities were invited to increase their contributions and several did. His general conclusion was that "our financial position is strong".[65]

---

[61] *Ibid.*, Minutes of the Executive Committee Meeting, August 6, 1960, p. 1.

[62] *Ibid.*, Minutes of the Executive Committee Meeting, January 21, 1962, p. 7.

[63] *Ibid.*, Minutes of the Executive Committee Meeting, February 25, 1962, p. 2.

[64] *Ibid.*, Minutes of the Annual Meeting, June 9, 1962, p. 2.

[65] *Ibid.*

In November 1962, the new Chairperson, J.H. Aitchison, informed the Executive Committee that although the Council finances seemed to be "stabilized", there were no funds "for entertaining or initiating new projects. …Efforts will be made in the next 2 years", he said, "to secure substantial additional funds, from government, corporations and Foundations".[66]

Meetings, 1963–1965

At the January 1963 Executive Meeting, the Treasurer reported that it had not yet been possible to arrange a meeting with the businessmen. However, Aitchison said that he had discussions with the Chairperson of the HRCC about joint fund-raising efforts.[67] In February a joint meeting of the Executives of both Councils was told that "Copies of reports of activities and the needs of the Councils have been sent to 150 corporations in Canada, 40 Foundations in Canada and 40 Foundations in the United States".[68] Apparently, then, the discussions of a joint campaign resulted in precisely such a campaign.

At the Executive Committee meeting of June 8, 1963, members present were informed that the ground rules for all grants for administrative purposes had been changed. According to the Minutes,

> The Chairman informed the Executive that on June 3, just a few hours prior to the meeting which had been planned between members of both Research Councils with members of the Canada Council, he and the Chairman of the Humanities Research Council and the Secretary-Treasurer had been invited to a luncheon arranged by two members of the Canada Council. At this luncheon it was announced that Canada Council had decided to take over complete responsibility for all phases of the Canada Council competitions, including the arrangements for appraising the qualifications of the applicants. The reasons given for the action are:
>
> 1) that the Canada Council has statutory and legal responsibilities for the competitions which were not fully met under the arrangements existing over the past 6 years;
> 2) that some additional fields of study such as law and business administration should now be included;
> 3) that greater flexibility is needed with respect to categories.
>
> No explanation was given for the lack of consultation before the decision was announced.[69]

At the Council's Annual Meeting on the same day (June 8, 1963) "It was agreed unanimously that the time had come for a full review of these developments and for a reconsideration of the role, function, structure and financing of the Research

[66]*Ibid.*, Minutes of the Executive Committee, November 24, 1962, p. 2.

[67]*Social Science Research Council Minutes 1963–65*, Minutes of Executive Committee, January 4, 1963, p. 3.

[68]*Ibid.*, Minutes of a Joint Meeting of Executives of HRCC and SSRCC, February 16, 1963, p. 2.

[69]*Ibid.*, Minutes of the Executive Meeting, June 8, 1963, p. 2.

Council itself". A motion was then passed to strike a sub-committee to conduct the review.[70]

The ex-Chairperson, Beach, offered the following observations to Aitchison in October 1963, concerning the usefulness of businessmen to the Council.

> "I have made several approaches to businessmen" he said, "to discuss the problem in general terms. I find them cautious. They are afraid of commitments of unknown consequences. … It should be possible indeed, not overly difficult, to obtain small amounts – say up to a thousand dollars a year from each of ten to twenty-five businesses for support of a limited program. One suggestion is that the Council set up a clearing house on what research is going on in this country in the social sciences. This could take the form of quarterly reports consisting of lists of books, government reports, articles, those finished or in preparation, classified in various ways so as to be as helpful as possible. Additional reports on special topics of current interest, such as pension plans could be considered; and provision for special requests must be considered."[71]

Beach's comments seem to me to have been worth serious consideration. Some organizations have been and are able to provide sustainable funding by putting together a small set of industrial donors, just as the two Councils were able to get annual funding from universities to support their administrative costs. Given the largely apolitical aims and activities of the Councils, there might have been some businesses willing to make regular, if very modest, contributions. There may yet be some such businesses today.

In spite of the apparent difficulties forming an advisory council of business-people, the finances of the two Councils were improved with a Ford Foundation grant of $85,000 each over a 5 year period.[72] Nevertheless, the Secretary-Treasurer was "authorized to make approaches from the office for increased donations by universities and for donations from corporations. …he pointed out that, unless more than this was done, there would be a substantial deficit at the end of the year".[73] In fact, the Ford grant was seriously restricted. It was "to be used for the development or extension of scholarly exchanges and relationships with scholars and academic organizations in other countries".[74]

The "Chairman's Review" to the Annual Meeting of the Council in June 1964 indicated that relations between the two Research Councils and Canada Council were still strained. In any case, Aitchison said:

> The major concern of your Executive Committee throughout the year has been to explore the means of implementing the decision made by the Council last June that the time had come for a full review of the changes that had taken place affecting social science research in Canada and for a reconsideration of the role, function, structure and financing of the Research Council itself. … I am happy to be able to announce that Dr. Mabel F. Timlin, Professor of Economics (now emeritus) of the University of Saskatchewan has agreed to

[70]*Ibid.*, Minutes of the Annual Meeting, June 8, 1963, p. 2.

[71]*Ibid.*, Minutes of Executive Committee Meeting, October 19, 1963, pp. 3–4.

[72]*Ibid.*, Minutes of Executive Committee Meeting, December 14, 1963, p. 6.

[73]*Ibid.*, p. 7.

[74]*Ibid.*, Minutes of Executive Committee Meeting, February 15, 1964, p. 2.

> undertake the task. I need hardly say how grateful we all are to Dr. Timlin, who is here with us today. She has already discussed the project with many Canadian social scientists and other academics and has been greatly encouraged by them. Like myself, she has found them to be unanimous about its great urgency and importance.[75]

The report was published in May 1968 by the SSRC and called simply *The Social Sciences in Canada: Two Studies*. Two authors were listed on the title page, Mabel F. Timlin and Albert Faucher. Faucher's contribution was called "La recherche en sciences sociales au Quebec: Sa condition universitaire".

Meetings, 1966–1968

In the Minutes of the Executive Committee of April 16, 1966, it is recorded that a representative from the Canadian Sociological Association would be added to the Council.[76] Some revision of the Constitution also took place at that time. The report of the Chairperson, J.R. Mallory, to the Annual Meeting in June of that year included a section on the "Future Role and Constitution of the Council." Mallory said that,

> We felt that before redesigning the constitution we had to ask ourselves what role, if any, the Council might play in the future. It was clear to us that the initial role of the Council, twenty-five years ago, in encouraging research and publication through its own resources for a small community of scholars, hampered by isolation and low salaries, could no longer justify its existence. ...
>
> Nevertheless, we feel that a body such as the Social Science Research Council still has a necessary and vital role to play, not so much in identifying individuals worthy of support, as in finding new and important areas of inquiry, in fostering the development of the social sciences as such, and in making special studies of new facilities and new techniques of research. For example, among the many matters which require such initiative and study are the encouragement of the improvement and elaboration of census data of use to social scientists, and the development of census monographs....[77]

On the question of the Council's relation to Canada Council, Mallory wrote that "Our relations with the Canada Council in particular have been good. ... In particular, it has set up an Academic Panel, which now has a strong voice in the development of policy. While this Panel is made up of individuals, rather than representatives of other bodies, its membership includes those who are at the same time members of both Research Councils."[78]

The Advisory Academic Panels to which Mallory just referred were structural features of the Canada Council that were carried on at least to the end of our period of study. Assuming that governments and bureaucrats make appointments to their

[75]*Ibid.*, Minutes of Annual Meeting, June 9, 1964, pp. 1–4.

[76]*Social Science Research Council Minutes 1965–67*, Minutes of the Executive Committee, April 16, 1966, p. 4.

[77]*Ibid.*, Minutes of Annual Meeting, June 11, 1966, pp. 3–4.

[78]*Ibid.*, pp. 6–7.

advisory councils with reasonable assurance (but probably no guarantees) that they will get the sort of advice they want to hear, it is likely that appointed advisory panels will not rock the boat. It would appear, then, that a relatively independent advisory group should exist which is fairly representative of the broad spectrum of social science interests. Strategically, I think it would have been better for the two Research Councils to have been pressing for that sort of role rather than embracing the idea of allowing their voices to be mediated through the Advisory Academic Panels. Nevertheless, the existence of such things as census monographs and access to census data tapes for academic research scientists suggests that the Panels provided some means of bringing ideas from the Research Councils to Canada Council.

Considering the strains between the Canada Council and the Research Councils mentioned earlier, it must have been gratifying indeed for Mallory to report good relations with the Canada Council. He went on to say that,

> The Social Science Research Council of Canada began as a body providing a few graduate scholarships and modest support to individual scholars. This programme of ours was taken over, without significant change in conception, by the Canada Council nearly ten years ago. Far from feeling that the Canada Council was in effect putting us out of business, as some of us thought at the time, we should have realized sooner than we did that, when a programme of ours has proven sound enough to be taken over on a larger scale by some other body, we should then turn our whole energies to finding new frontiers to develop.[79]

This sounds eminently reasonable to me. He wound up his remarks on a high note of optimism.

> The last two years in the life of our Council have been critical ones, in which our usefulness, and indeed our future, have been daily in doubt. Yet I feel that we are now out of the woods, and ready to take up the opportunities which exist for us. If this is so, it is due to the loyalty, energy, and imagination of the Executive Committee, the members of the Council, and its Committees, to all of whom I am thankful beyond words.[80]

The most striking and far reaching new development in the recorded Minutes of the June 11, 1966 Meeting occurred without comment. For the first time ever a French version of the Minutes was written. Except for an occasional French phrase or sentence, the business of the Council (so far as it was recorded in Minutes of all previous Meetings) had been entirely in English. By the end of our period of study, it was common practice for people to speak either official language in SSFC Meetings and for Recording Secretaries to take notes in the language of the intervention. Clearly, some progress toward the acceptance of bilingualism had been made.

Mallory's report to the Annual Meeting in June 1967 included useful comments on relations with the federal government. He said that,

> Public policy, particularly the policy of the federal government, has and will continue to have the greatest importance for the future of social science research in Canada….All the evidence suggests that, for self-protection, the community of scholars in the social sciences

---

[79] *Ibid.*, p. 9.

[80] *Ibid.*, p. 13.

> and the humanities need a strong and flexible presence in Ottawa which can influence decisions which affect us before they become irrevocable. Such a presence, for reasons of both economy and strength, must be a unified one, and we have been concerned, in the Social Sciences Research Council, with the difficult exploratory steps to bring it about.[81]

To this summary, the new Executive Secretary, W.J. Waines, added that "There is, in Canada, no organization representing Canadian scholars apart from the Canada Council, which is regarded primarily as a funding body, to press governments and others for support of scholarship".[82]

In these two statements by Mallory and especially Waines, we have forceful re-articulations of the idea that the two Research Councils should perform the functions of Professional Trade Unions. These passages also indicate that the Councils were being forced into a defensive position. Instead of being primarily planners and catalysts, events seemed to have driven Council Members to focus on self-protection. That mode seems to have prevailed to the end of our period of study, and probably continues today. Insofar as this mode tended to become paramount, the chances of getting business support for annual operating expenses decreased. On the other hand, the chances of getting support from individual scholars should have increased. That greater levels of support from individuals was not forthcoming indicates some problem either in the Councils' performance of their primary tasks or in persuading scholars that the tasks being performed really warranted their support, or both.

The Social Sciences in Canada (Timlin-Faucher Report)

As indicated earlier, the Timlin-Faucher Report came out in May 1968. In their introduction, the two authors tell us that "by 1963, appointments made by the government to the Canada Council had been such that its membership contained no social scientist (or humanist) members".[83] What is worse, Canada Council

> proceeded to set up competitions and administrative machinery to distribute the funds made available to it by government, and the two research Councils were left without funds to carry on their own research programs. The only funds forthcoming from the Canada Council for the research Councils were certain accountable grants to be used as subsidies to ensure publication of scholarly books in their respective fields. In default of financial support from the American foundations, private sources in Canada, or government funds through the Canada Council, the two research Councils found themselves virtually isolated from the communities of scholars whose interests they had once been able to serve.[84]

---

[81]*Social Science Research Council Minutes 1967–1968*, Minutes of Annual Meeting, June 13, 1967, pp. 4–6.

[82]*Ibid.*, p. 10.

[83]M.F. Timlin and A. Faucher, *The Social Sciences in Canada: Two Studies* (Ottawa: Social Science Research Council of Canada/Conseil canadien de recherche en sciences sociales, May 1968) p. iii.

[84]*Ibid.*, pp. iii–iv.

In response to this situation, Timlin and Faucher were asked to write a report describing the sources of support for social science in Canada and to "make recommendations for improvements". The authors claimed that

> evidence secured from some 106 social science departments throughout Canada – and from many more individual scholars – revealed (in the autumn of 1964) an almost universal frustration related not only to the limitations on financial support for research in the social sciences, but also to the conditions imposed on grantees respecting the administration of funds, such as they were.[85]

By March 1965, given increases in finances for and policy changes by Canada Council, things were "greatly ameliorated".[86]

They saw three basic problems: (1) an "enlarged need for communication among specialists over many disciplines"; (2) an organization "to ensure that basic research in the social sciences is not sacrificed in the search for short-term solutions to social problems"; (3) the identification of an appropriate kind of organization to bring about "effective cooperation among specialists".[87] In brief, the questions were who should coordinate and finance the cooperative efforts of social scientists, and how? Point (2) comes very close to being the antithesis of the remark attributed earlier in this paper to R.H. Coates at the first meeting of the ad hoc group in May 1938 that "there was no use collecting information except insofar as it was of value in helping to solve problems".

The authors were quite clear on the need for financial independence. They wrote that:

> The fairly liberal allowances made to the two Research Councils at the present time have eased the positions which they occupy in relation to the Canada Council, but they do not change their position of dependence or the implications it carries. It would be incredibly imprudent for Canadian social scientists to believe that under the present statute situations similar in some degree to those of 1963 could not recur. There is nothing to guarantee that some future government administration may not replace the very few social scientists presently among the twenty-one members of the Canada Council with quite other persons or that they may not appoint administrative officers to some dangerous degree ignorant of some of the disparate interests whose affairs have been entrusted to them.[88]

They recommended two distinct councils, one for planning (which became two, SSFC and HFC, and now one again) and one for funding (now SSHRCC). The former would be

> the agency which gathers, systematizes, and makes available all achievable information respecting the human resources in the social sciences and the research projects being pursued in these disciplines in Canada. In the second place, it should be the agency through

[85]*Ibid.*, p. 25.

[86]*Ibid.*, p. 26.

[87]*Ibid.*, p. 30.

[88]*Ibid.*, p. 78.

which the organization and planning of research projects would be carried out whose personnel needs outran the resources of the individual campus.[89]

In fact, given their additional recommendation to separate humanists and social scientists by setting up "separate secretariats…for each", there would be two planning councils. The social science research planning council was not supposed to "support the actual processes of research from its own funds" and "its central function should be that of research".[90] They imagined, then,

… two types of expenditures connected with research projects: there are those required by the planning of the project and those required in the course of the execution of the plan. The first are legitimate expenses of the research council itself; expenses connected with the second should be covered by funds secured from elsewhere. For the Social Science Research Council of Canada this means that it must have money enough from its own income to cover expenses of the first type but that once a research project has been successfully organized funds to meet the other expenses must come from other sources, typically perhaps from a government agency charged with the support of the social sciences in Canada, from a provincial or federal government agency charged with responsibilities for particular policies or services, or (hopefully,) from private sources of finance willing to provide funds on non-contract bases for independent research.[91]

Going into further detail, they listed the following specific functions for "a reformed Social Science Research Council".

1. To act as partner and adjunct to the universities and other research institutions in facilitating communication among specialists and helping to implement research and granting ventures that cannot be encompassed with a given institution
2. In connection with the carrying out of the preceding function, to institute gradually a structure of research-planning committees so open with respect to membership that the most highly qualified specialists in any area or areas of the social sciences may be brought together for the formulation of research projects important to Canada;
3. To arrange for surveys and studies of human resources in the various areas of the social sciences in Canada;
4. In conjunction with the organization which is the source of funds to establish a register of all current research projects being carried on in the social sciences in Canada and periodically to publish brief information about projects;
5. In accordance with the interdisciplinary character of the Council to foster such interdisciplinary conferences and interdisciplinary or multidisciplinary projects as may appear valuable to the social sciences in Canada. In discharge of this function to form any liaison with scholars and disciplines outside the social sciences which may promise to be conducive to the advancement of knowledge in the social sciences;
6. To keep constantly abreast of new methodological developments affecting the social sciences and through negotiation with the government organization offering grants to make arrangement for their dissemination.[92]

---

[89] *Ibid.*, p. 82.

[90] *Ibid.*, p. 117.

[91] *Ibid.*, pp. 117–118.

[92] *Ibid.*, pp. 118–119.

Of the six broad functions that Timlin and Faucher thought a "reformed" Council should perform, four seem to have been largely or entirely unachievable. At least since the year of their report, the SSFC and the HFC were not successful at implementing "research and granting ventures", establishing "research-planning committees" and keeping "abreast of new methodological developments". Although a national registry of social scientists, including some information about research in progress, was set up after some months of struggle in 1982, it never proved to be very useful for research purposes. I recall receiving flyers asking for information for the original set-up of the registry and for later updates, and I recall seeing some promotional material indicating that news media people searching cold for a Canadian "authority" on some subject were contacting the registry. However, regarding the usefulness of the registry for research purposes, I would say that it could only be a poor substitute for the great number of electronically accessible citation indexes and other data-bases currently available on the web. Typically a researcher's literature search would begin with a question like "What has been published on this topic?" rather than "What has been published in Canada on this topic?", unless the researcher had a specific reason to limit the search to Canadian authors. In any event, according to a telephone message I received this morning (March 27, 1997), the registry still exists but was last updated in 1987!

Given the wide variety of functions envisioned by Timlin and Faucher, it was clear that the form of the Council had to be broadly representative. "In an organized world" they wrote,

> it is highly important that there should be an organization capable in the interests of the social sciences to speak for the whole body of scholars engaged in them and that it should occupy such a position in relation to the different associations which represent the individual disciplines that it has a right to speak for them. This means that its own membership must be broadly representative of these associations and that the connections of the Council with the executives of these associations must be close enough to ensure that they appoint or elect their most out-standing research scholars to the Council's membership.[93]

The financing of the Council was to be secured by

> statutory authority…from the government requiring (its funding Council)…to pay over annually to the SSRCC and HRC some specific percentage of total funds made available for research support in each of the research areas of the two Research Councils. It would also be a measure conducive to better long-run planning if statutory authority were extended permitting funds unexpended in one year to be held over for a succeeding year. …Only a loose estimate can be made at this point but it is possible that if 3% of the total funds presently available for research support of the social sciences by the Canada Council were instead available for the uses of the SSRCC they might be sufficient to permit the SSRCC to discharge successfully the functions allotted to it here.[94]

The idea of having a specific percentage of the funding council's funds set aside for the research-planning councils would be very attractive to members of the latter

[93] *Ibid.*, p. 122.

[94] *Ibid.*, p. 134.

but perhaps less attractive to members of the former, although it would eliminate some decision-making costs in all councils. In fact, the research-planning councils had substantial support from the funding councils from 1971 to 1980.[95]

All things considered, I doubt that a single percentage of any funding council's expenditures should ever be set aside a priori for a research-planning council. My main reason for doubt is that I think it would invite lethargy. All volunteer organizations are populated by people with all sorts of personal agendas that are more or less consistent with the mandates of the organizations. Indeed, all human organizations may be similarly characterized. If a planning council had complete financial security from a funding council, the personal agendas of individual members might easily become more influential than one would prefer. The planning council might easily become a self-serving, old boy and girl club out of touch with its constituency and its original mandate. As we saw earlier, that complaint was raised against the Federations at various times in their history. As a mild buffer against such a state of affairs, I would recommend that about half of a planning council's expenditures should be met by a funding council or a direct government grant on an annual basis. The rest would have to be collected from donations or from regular fees (from associations, institutes, universities, etc.) paid by people who presumably receive something of equal value in exchange. If it were possible to decide exactly what percentage of a planning council's output were a pure public good and what percentage benefited only the social science community itself, it would be much easier to decide who should pay what. But I am not optimistic about our ability to measure these diverse outputs with much precision.

Meetings in 1968

At a joint meeting of the Executive Committee of HRCC and SSRCC with the Director of Canada Council, J. Boucher, in December 1968 (formally a Liaison Meeting), the latter gave his views of the difference between the Councils.

> Boucher emphasized that the Canada Council has avoided establishing priorities in research in the social sciences and humanities. Though not important at the present time, he saw the necessity of having priorities of this nature established. He believed that through the more effective organization of the academic community, scholars could make these decisions themselves. He emphasized that the Canada Council was neither equipped nor intended to make these decisions, and that they had not in the past. When the time came for the establishment of priorities the scholarly community would find it in their own interest to participate. With or without this participation, however, government would require the establishment of research priorities.[96]

---

[95]Social Sciences and Humanities Research Council of Canada, *Annual Report 1981–1982*, p. 206; Social Science Federation of Canada, *Annual Report 1981–1982*, p. 35.

[96]*Social Science Research Council Minutes 1967–1968*, Minutes of a Joint Meeting of the Executive Committees, December 12, 1968, p. 3.

The President of SSRCC, Hugh Thorburn,

> emphasized that the Research Councils had as their constituency the research community. This was a very different basis than the Canada Council. With a block grant not ear-marked for specific purposes, the Council could move quickly, assuring support for basic studies in certain areas. It would avoid the preparation of a full application to Canada Council, and the related psychological block that exists preventing requests for research ideas.[97]

At the same time, Gilles Paquet (then Co-director of Research for the Special Senate Science Policy Committee) "emphasized that though it may not seem accurate, the Science Council's responsibility was limited to the natural sciences. It was thus important for the Special Senate Science Policy Committee to have the views of social scientists, and all other interested parties".[98]

The next day (December 13, 1968) the Executive Committee of SSRCC met. Mallory told the group that it should tell the Senate Special Committee of "the need for direct funding of SSRCC to counter balance other sources of government funds, and to give the Council 'seed money' for projects and consequently additional flexibility".[99]

In an enclosure with a letter from Thorburn to the Council of Ministers of Education, he pointed out that there were several functions the SSRCC could perform,

> e.g., small meetings of specialists from time to time to review and discuss their research problems, meetings of scholars to plan interdisciplinary projects and to provide small amounts to assist scholars to complete research in preparation for publication support, interdisciplinary and other joint studies, the planning of regional research facilities such as data banks, survey centres, information retrieval centres, and the establishment of research centres. …The principle objective is to have bodies which can speak with authority to the Federal and Provincial Governments and to other bodies as to the research needs in the social sciences and as to their priorities. The combined voice of the Social Science Learned Societies speaking through the Research Councils, we believe, would be an appropriate means of communicating with government and other outside bodies.[100]

There are some now familiar themes in these suggestions that merit some comments. First, it is worthwhile to consider Bouchard's assumption, shared by some key players in our story, that a planning council would establish research priorities for the social sciences. Failing that, he suggested that some "government" would do the job. Has this happened? I think it depends on what research is counted. Regarding research undertaken by academics in universities, it seems to me that there has been relatively little collective establishing of priorities by any planning council or government. Indeed, it seems to me that such planning is usually resisted by academics in principle and that in fact it would be difficult to

---

[97] *Ibid.*, p. 4.

[98] *Ibid.*

[99] *Ibid.*, Minutes of the Executive Committee, December 13, 1968, p. 9.

[100] *Ibid.*, enclosure with letter from H.G. Thorburn to the Council of Ministers of Education, December 1968 (no date is given on the letter), pp. 5–6.

orchestrate. Because there are many different research problem areas within scientific disciplines and there are many different problems in each area, there are many different frontiers identified by the areas and problems. To take one example from the area in sociology with which I am most familiar, in social indicators research there are some people who specialize in issues related to subjective indicators and some who specialize in issues related to objective indicators. Among those who specialize in subjective indicators, there are some who focus on overall subjective well-being and some who focus on particular domains, like job satisfaction or marital satisfaction. Some work with very little direction from well-articulated theory and some are primarily motivated to elaborate and confirm specific theories. Clearly, the research problems and frontiers identified in these diverse areas will most likely be equally diverse, and this diversity would be multiplied many times if one were to attempt to map the frontiers of the whole discipline of sociology. So, I think it would be very difficult for any group of scholars from a broad-based council to set priorities for social indicators research in particular and it would be practically impossible for such a group to set priorities for the whole discipline.

Second, it is not likely that Thorburn's suggestion of block grants to the research councils to support basic studies would be preferable to the sort of operation currently run at SSHRCC. The latter has the virtue of having at least a modest amount of independence between the panels recommending funding and the people receiving the funds. Greater independence and lower likelihoods of conflicts of interest might be introduced by adopting some of the U.S. National Science Foundation procedures, but any moves in this direction would take us even farther away from Thorburn's suggestion.

Third, Thorburn's suggestions to the Council of Ministers of Education about the opportunities research councils provide for scholars to present and review perceived problems, and to construct collective positions and development strategies seem to me to be quite reasonable. It might have been possible at one time for such councils to determine where research centres, survey research centres and data banks should be located in order to minimize overall national costs and get the best geographic locations all things considered, but I think we are well past such time now. There seem to be so many experts so widely dispersed across the country that planning for research centres is and probably is best left to the various places where some people actually take it upon themselves to create specific plans. Even if one were going to try to undertake centralized planning for scientific research, one's best strategy would probably be to begin from recognized research centres and build upon those. As we will see below, this seems to have been what actually happened.

Meetings in 1969–1970

At the Annual Meeting in June 1969, there was some discussion of revisions of the Constitution of the Council. It is worthwhile to notice that the representative from the Dominion Bureau of Statistics, Walter Duffet, "emphasized the importance of involving non-university social scientists in the Council, either as members at large, or through the Consultative Assembly. Dr. Timlin emphasized as well, that through wise use of the members at large section, persons representative of funding agencies could easily be kept in touch with the Council's activities".[101]

The Director of the Canada Council, Boucher, offered further observations on the different roles of his Council and the others.

> "Essentially the Canada Council is a research foundation", he said, "and for this reason does not consider that its main responsibility is to assume a leadership role in the Academic community. The Council must respond to the demands of scholars. The SSRCC is the one body in the social sciences which can exercise leadership, and the Canada Council expects to receive comments from the members of the SSRCC".[102]

These were profoundly instructive remarks that remained relevant throughout our period of investigation and even today. The joint social sciences and humanities federation is today, as the SSRCC was in 1969, still "the one body in the social sciences which can exercise leadership", the single voice firmly rooted in the several voices of its constituent associations. It is easy for any appointed government agency, such as SSHRCC today, to play one disciplinary voice against another. If there were no combined single voice, an agency like SSHRCC would have to listen to all disciplines individually and arrive at its own view of a fair combination of all opinions, after all things are considered. "All things considered" would include all the peculiar constraints, biases and purposes of the agency itself. I would much rather have that smorgasbord of considerations brought to bear on a single voice than several. The more noise allowed into the system, the more difficult it becomes to understand and manage it.

Boucher also gave his opinions about the "establishment of a separate granting body for the humanities and social sciences". He thought first, that it might be proper to consider such a body "when the social sciences and humanities have developed and strengthened their ties with government". Second, he thought "that the Canada Council is better able to resist political pressures than other granting bodies".[103] Maybe he was defending his own turf. However, at a joint meeting of the Executive Committees of the HRCC and SSRCC in April 1968, Mallory (who may have been defending his own turf) said that

---

[101] *Social Science Research Council Minutes 1969–1970*, Minutes of the Annual Meeting, June 8, 1969, p. 4.

[102] *Ibid.*, Minutes of Annual Meeting, June 8, 1969, p. 6.

[103] *Ibid.*, p. 7.

> the modus vivendi which had been now attained with the Canada Council should not be overturned and new organizations with which the Councils were not familiar substituted. He urged that the current structure of the Canada Council be continued and indicated that it was more practical, he felt, to encourage the hopeful evolution of the Canada Council rather than to embark on a full scale argument with its basic structure.[104]

In a letter to Waines dated June 20, 1969, Boucher pointed out that "5 years ago, the natural sciences had almost twenty times more money at their disposal than the social sciences and humanities. Now they do not even have five times more".[105]

The General Council Meeting of February 27, 1970 began with a far–reaching report from the Policy Committee. Thorburn

> pointed out the need for the SSRCC to act as a more effective spokesman for the social science community in Canada. The Report recommended new and enlarged functions whereby the SSRCC could fulfill this role. These functions were:
>
> 1. Communications, with the social science community through a news-letter and by means of closer working relationships with the learned societies, as well as with government and other organizations through greater representation of social science views.
> 2. Catalytic, whereby interdisciplinary research could be encouraged, and learned societies could work together more easily on matters of common concern…
> 3. Funding, though one of the oldest roles of the Council, it was recommended that it not be expanded, as a function of the Council, and that it might at a later date be completely abandoned.
> 4. Research, for the preparation of briefs and other documents of direct interest to the Council's work.[106]

Thorburn also remarked that "an expanded secretariat of the Council" would be necessary to carry out these functions. As well, there would be need for an expanded committee system, additional secretarial assistance, a research officer and the

> employment of a full time senior person in Ottawa. …To provide for this increased staff in the Council's secretariat, it was suggested that the Council request learned societies to contribute to the financial support of the Council. As well support would be sought from the Canada Council and universities. The value of diversified financial support was emphasized.[107]

Although Thorburn's recommendations seem to provide a reasonable strategy for strengthening the internal workings of the Council as well as its ties to its constituency, the minutes record the fact that there were "some reservations about the Report, particularly that the proposed functions did not reflect the same priorities as set out in the Constitution of the Council. …It was also suggested that learned societies might not agree with supporting an increasing bureaucracy in the

[104] *op. cit.*, p. 2.

[105] *Social Science Research Council Minutes 1969–1970*, letter from J. Boucher to W.J. Waines, June 20, 1969, p. 2.

[106] *Ibid.*, Minutes of General Council Meeting, February 27, 1970, pp. 2–3.

[107] *Ibid.*, p. 3.

SSRCC".[108] However, "the Executive Committee later agreed that a full time Executive Director should be engaged for the Council." It was also agreed to set up a central office as recommended and to finance it, "in principle" by (a) a contribution of $3.00 per member of each member society; (b) existing revenue sources; and (c) Canada Council or similar external sources."

Once again the Council recommended that "each learned society appoint, as soon as possible, one representative to a Social Science Survey Committee; and that the Committee work closely with D.B.S. [Dominion Bureau of Statistics] representatives".[109] In addition, a Research Resources Committee was struck to

> consider resource and development needs for social science research in Canada. The Committee would look broadly at the bases for research in Canada, and might consider such matters as capital development for the social sciences, classification of national facilities, caps in the provision of funds for research, the adequacy of funding concepts in the Canada Council, the development of centres of excellence for research in Canada.[110]

I believe the phrase "centres of excellence for research" appeared for the first time in Council minutes in the passage just quoted from 1970, and it was nearly 20 years before the first competitions were held and grants for their establishment were awarded. The TriCouncil Network Centres of Excellence were initiated in May 1988 and the first awards were given in October 1989. Those who would initiate changes in public policy and programs might take note of the lead time required for this particular program to come into being. The suggested $3.00 per-member fee is currently from $6.00 to $7.00, depending on the size of the disciplinary organization.

The Minutes continued by indicating that each learned society was to be asked to form its own Research Resources Committee "to consider the needs, deficiencies, and priorities of research in their own disciplines and…collaborate with the Council's committee".[111] There then followed a report from Thorburn giving

> his impressions of the formative meeting of Scitec held in January. He questioned the scholarly research interests of the organization but recommended that there should be a social science membership. …(R.F.) Salisbury, drawing on his impressions of a meeting he attended, indicated that researchers whether in the physical and life sciences or the social sciences, had similar concerns and could probably work together easily. The other representatives involved in Scitec particularly those from industry, he considered, could make a useful contribution to the work of the organization. …Thorburn emphasized that there were misconceptions about the nature of the social sciences in the other scientific disciplines as well as in government. He suggested that by not joining Scitec the SSRCC would only help to continue these misconceptions. …It was agreed…in principle, the SSRCC join Scitec.[112]

[108] *Ibid.*

[109] *Ibid.*, pp. 3–5.

[110] *Ibid*, pp. 5–6.

[111] *Ibid.*, p. 7.

[112] *Ibid.*, pp. 8–9.

Although not much came of Scitec or of the Council's connection to it, the decision to join the organization was probably justifiable for the precise reasons mentioned by Salisbury and Thorburn. If one must error, it is better to error on the side of over rather than under exposure, and over rather than under connectedness to possible collaborators.

The President of the Council, M.Y. Dube

> reported that the Canada Council support for the social sciences had not been increased in 1970-71 because
>
> 1) of the current 'austerity' program;
> 2) other departments were offering funds through contracts and research grants for social science research;
> 3) Canada Council policies did not fit in with national priorities;
> 4) the federal government, through fiscal transfers to the provinces, was supplying universities with substantial funding. If universities did not devote enough of these funds to the support of social science research the government concluded that this research, in the eyes of the university community, did not have adequate priority;
> 5) the social sciences were in a disorganized state, which required improvement before the government would consider increased funding.[113]

It would be interesting to know why anyone had a perception that "the social sciences were in a disorganized state". There were particular disciplinary associations and a federation of the associations with representatives sitting on a co-ordinating Council, and there were 30 years of cooperative efforts with several surveys of resources, needs and priorities leading to some well-know publications. If the social sciences were "disorganized", which sciences were organized? Was there, is there yet, a well-organized federation of physical or life sciences? If so, perhaps the place to look for instruction on how to build a culture of support for social sciences is somewhere beyond the social sciences themselves.

Dube also reported that he had a meeting with Ian McTaggart-Cowan, Executive Director of the Science Council, and that "the work of the Science Council was making it more and more anxious to have some more formal connection with the social science community and especially the SSRCC".[114]

In the President's Report of the Council on June 7, 1970, Dube noted that "Mr. John Banks, who had been Assistant Executive Secretary since February 1968, was asked, and agreed, to accept the position of Executive Secretary of our Council as well as of the Humanities Research Council." He said he had attended the US Council's annual meeting and was "impressed with their elaborate Committee structure" and "by the involvement of the American Council in the social affairs of the country". Then he reviewed the Report of the Thorburn Committee mentioned above (footnotes 93, 94). Among other things, he said that the Committee recommended a grant of $50,000 should "be sought from Canada Council to help finance the operations of the new Council and increase its budget to $100,000, from

[113] *Ibid.*, pp. 11–12.

[114] *Ibid.*, p. 14.

the present $30,000." In fact, the Canada Council "indicated its willingness to support the SSRCC by a grant of $50,000, on the condition that the learned societies, which are members of the Council, also indicated their support of the SSRCC…by contributing to the financial revenues of the Council". Several associations had agreed in principle to support the Council, which led Dube to say that "though this support from the learned societies will be of obvious material advantage to the Council, it has an additional value. These contributions show clearly that the societies and their memberships have confidence in what the SSRCC is now doing, and has indicated it will do. The moral position of the Council is therefore now much stronger than it has ever been before."[115]

He went on to indicate his concern "to find a person who can serve the Council as its Executive Director", and to summarize the Briefs sent to the Special Senate Science Policy Committee and the Secretary of State. Among other things, the Council suggested "that the Science Council of Canada be made up equally of representatives from the physical and social sciences".

In the discussion of the President's Report, S.G. Peitchinis suggested that the Council "might urge that the Prime Minister have a social science advisor as a counterpart to his Science Advisor". Dube replied that "there were a large number of social scientists who occupied senior positions in government". Frank Milligan, then Associate Director of Canada Council,

> pointed out that it seemed that the climate of opinion in government was not too sympathetic to the social sciences. Administrators were looking for concrete, if not immediate, pay-offs for money invested in social science research. These pay-offs are at present not visible. …There was a growing doubt about the value of continuing support for the social sciences. He believed that the SSRCC should be concerned to provide a strong counter argument to this position.[116]

This is a remarkable quotation, and I think it is remarkably contemporary because there are probably many in government today who doubt "the value of continuing support for the social sciences". Considering the scope of the social sciences and the numbers of people trained in them working in government then and now, it is difficult to make sense of the charge that there are no visible pay-offs. What would be left of government bureaucracies if we eliminated the social statisticians, sociologists, economists, geographers, political scientists, urban and rural planners, demographers, educationists, psychologists and historians? Could a Finance Department or the Bank of Canada operate then or now without statisticians, accountants and economists? Of course there were finance departments and banks long before there were professional social scientists, but by 1970 it would have been unthinkable to run such organizations without professional expertise. So, granting that there is still a relatively oxymoronic perception of invisibility for social sciences among government officials, what could be its source? Off the top of my head, I would say that the social sciences are relatively invisible precisely

[115] *Ibid.*, pp. 1–11.

[116] *Ibid.*, Discussion, pp. 1–2.

because of their successful infiltration into virtually all aspects of government. Just as writers of research reports cease citing the publications that originally introduced concepts that are now part of everyone's English (e.g., the unconscious, correlation coefficient, gene, relativity theory), government officials cease taking account of all the social science that they routinely use. It might be worthwhile for someone to actually test this hypothesis.

1970–1973

At the Annual Meeting in October 1970, Dube recommended that the Council sponsor a conference related to the topic of the social sciences and their contribution to Science Policy. Sylvia Ostry, then Director of the Economic Council of Canada, suggested that the conference "should focus on social science research, its funding and its contribution to improving decisions of the government".[117]

David Hopper, President of the International Development Research Centre and Council Member at Large, addressed the Council.

> He noted that the Board of Directors would be meeting to consider the content of the Centre's programmes. …Concerning the social sciences, they were important aspects of the Centre's concerns since they could make contributions to the solution of problems which might be viewed as basically technical. As well a broader usage of the social sciences would help the Centre to see in clearer perspective what its concerns in development should be. …The IDRC could take advantage of the existence of the Committee on International Scholarly Affairs. He indicated that the Council possibly through this Committee might well assist the Centre as a catalyst in developing social science capabilities abroad.[118]

The offer of cooperation from IDRC was one of the most hopeful signs the Council had in this period of its development, but there is no evidence that anything came of it. Still, as a strategy for development in the future, it would be worthwhile to cultivate cooperative projects between the research councils and IDRC.

The Report of the Projects Committee to the Executive Committee Meeting of February 1971 discussed the development of a Directory of Social Scientists.[119] Since that proposal was first mentioned by Timlin and Faucher in 1968 and finally became operational in 1982, the project had a lead time of about 14 years. The Committee also proposed a review of the social sciences in Canada in the 70s.[120]

The Committee's recommendations were approved in principle. However, at the Annual Meeting two months later Jan Loubser, then Executive Director of the SSRCC, reported "that the proposal which had been circulated to the learned

---

[117]*Social Science Research Council Minutes 1970–1971*, Minutes of the Annual Meeting, October 9–10, 1970, p. 3.

[118]*Ibid.*, pp. 8–9.

[119]*Ibid.*, Minutes of the Executive Committee, February 6–7, 1971, pp. 5–6.

[120]*Ibid.*, pp. 7–9. The BASSS Report was the US Council's *Behaviorial and Social Sciences Surveys.*

societies had resulted in only one reply". Accordingly, the proposal was referred back to the Projects Committee "for further development".[121]

"Only one reply"! Why was there so little response to such a detailed proposal for a comprehensive needs assessment leading to an equally comprehensive strategy for developing the social sciences? At this point, all I can offer is speculation. In the light of the historical record already reviewed in this essay, the recommendations have sounded too familiar to those who may have received them nearly 30 years ago. Remember that these recommendations went out early in 1971 and that the Timlin-Faucher Report came out only 4 years earlier. Even though the material for the former Report was collected in 1964–65, roughly 6 years is not a long time considering the scope of the surveys involved. Maybe people felt that there had not been enough time and change from the previous Report to undertake another one in 1971. It is also possible that people were reluctant to invest time in a project that was so similar to projects that had not yielded great results in the past. No deluge of new government funding or spontaneous rallying behind the social sciences from most social scientists, let alone the general public, had followed the publication of the Timlin-Faucher report. Maybe the Council's constituents felt that the comprehensive survey followed by a report with recommendations was simply not an effective and efficient strategy for creating the kind of culture of support and real support that they hoped to see. At this point in time, we really have no way of knowing what caused the lack of support.

At any rate, the Minutes of the April meeting also contain a summary of a discussion with Milligan about grant application rates, success rates and comparisons among granting Councils. The report is not clear, at least not clear to me. It is clear that Milligan argued that there was no need for new funds because, among other things, "Canada Council supports only about 7% and receives requests from only 10%".[122] The Council responded to this claim by agreeing to "commission a scholar to analyze the measure of support, success rates, and criteria for assessing Canada Council grants as compared to NRC [the National Research Council] and other funding bodies supporting Canadian scholars".[123]

At the April 1972 meeting of the Executive Committee, the President, D.A. Soberman, informed the group that only three associations had contributed to the SSRCC in that year, namely, the Association of Canadian Law Teachers, the Canadian Association of Geographers and the Canadian Sociology and Anthropology Association. The Canadian Historical Association had promised payment and the Canadian Psychological Association "indicated its inability to pay". The President "noted that all associations had agreed in principle to the payment of this contribution". Then he reminded the group that "the lack of financial support undermines the influence of the Executive and the Council officers, and also could affect the support given by Canada Council since it was based

[121]*Ibid.*, Minutes of Council, April 24–25, 1971, p. 10.

[122]*Ibid.*, p. 14.

[123]*Ibid.*, p. 17.

on the understanding that financial support would be forthcoming from the member associations". He agreed to talk to the Canadian Economics Association and the Canadian Political Science Association.[124]

While the Minutes do not tell us why the nonpaying associations were not honouring their agreements in principle, it is difficult to avoid the conclusion that the members of those associations did not believe they would get good value for their money. This would be consistent with the general impression that the historical record gives of Council members over the years practically always searching for ways to involve more scholars, to launch comprehensive surveys in order to identify active researchers, and to find new sources of funding. One would think that given the great number of university scholars alone, if they were convinced that their research Councils provided valuable services, they would be gladly contributing the nominal $3.00 per year per individual requested and the Councils would not be starved for funds, volunteers and information.

When the full Council met, Mrs. J. Morrison (Head, Research Grants Section, Humanities and Social Sciences Division, the Canada Council) addressed it on the question of the establishment of a new council (SSHRCC), the Timlin-Faucher Report and status quo surveys. She thought most of the criticisms of the Canada Council in the Timlin-Faucher Report were "out of date and quite inappropriate". This was, after all, April 1972 and the SSRCC was again receiving operating funds from the Council. "She also questioned, as the SSRCC had done, the possibility of distinguishing between curiosity–oriented basic research and mission-oriented research."[125] Insofar as the distinction rests on someone's intentions, aims, goals or interests, one person's basic research can be another person's applied research. Insofar as the distinction does not rest on intentions, it will probably only be operationalized in fairly arbitrary ways to suit the different purposes of different people.

The most interesting part of Morrison's presentation was summarized in the Minutes as follows.

> With reference to the SSRCC recommendation that a funding body for the humanities and social sciences should be actively encouraging research activities, rather than just responding to applications, she pointed out that the Canada Council was working towards the development of consultative committees which are to serve as stimuli for the research community. The Council is also going to examine whether the current forms of support which are the same for the humanities and social sciences, are equally well suited to these two groups of disciplines. The Council is considering the possibility of studies on the state of the social science and humanities disciplines, in order that some of its funding activities might be directed into those areas where support in the eyes of the research community is most desirable.[126]

---

[124] *Social Science Research Council Minutes 1972–1973*, Minutes of the Executive Committee, April 17, 1972, pp. 1–2.

[125] *Ibid.*, Minutes of Meeting of Council, April 17–18, 1972, p. 3.

[126] *Ibid.*

Apparently, the SSRCC had recommended that Canada Council undertake some sort of catalytic or promotional function. That is odd because it is precisely the sort of activity which members of the SSRCC had routinely accepted as their own responsibility. The Council's consideration of status quo surveys would also have been an odd thing to have been recommended by the SSRCC, if that is what happened. But the main point here must be that once anyone gets serious about the growth and health of social science in Canada, someone has to begin reflecting on surveys of the total picture and programs of some sort of an agenda for action. Today, of course, some of the basic statistics about numbers of people enroled in university programs, graduates, labour force participation, employment status and alternative projected figures are routinely prepared and published by Statistics Canada. We even have statistics regarding publications of our scientists compared to those around the world in the Institute for Scientific Information's *Science Citation Indexes* of various sorts, as well as several others. So, status quo surveys that might be undertaken these days would be able to dig much deeper, much more rapidly than they were in the past. Although in principle the several disciplinary associations could collectively periodically strike ad hoc exploratory committees to prepare comprehensive surveys of all the social sciences, it is unclear that such ad hoc assessments would be as efficient as assessments routinely made by a permanent research council. Since there has always been a certain amount of ad hockery about the comprehensive surveys actually carried out by the councils over the years, there may be little to choose between the two approaches. Still, I suspect that permanent councils would have an edge over purely ad hoc survey committees. Admittedly, my suspicions are hardly decisive reasons for favouring the continued support of the Humanities and Social Science Federation as a public service, with public benefits justifying expenditures of public funds.

Following the discussion with Mrs. Morrison, there was a presentation and discussion with Dr. A. Beaulnes (Secretary, Ministry of State for Science and Technology). Beaulnes identified "five levels from which advice" to MSST might be received, namely, (a) "groups of wise men such as the Science Council and the SSRCC"; (b) "broad organizations such as SCITEC, the CMA [Canadian Medical Association] and the AUCC" [Association for Universities and Colleges of Canada];

> (c) Societies and individual groups which have been invited to spell out their views to the Ministry. He noted one drawback here, in that many of these groups did not have the facilities to provide advice at the level of sophistication which could be of use to the Ministry. He noted that if these organizations were to receive greater financial support they would be in a better position to have more effective input to the Ministry's activities; (d) Individuals who have been approached by the Ministry for assistance in developing points of view; (e) comments from interested citizens.[127]

His third point about individual societies with insufficient funds to prepare adequate cases in their own interests merits emphasis. It is one thing to open a

[127] *Ibid.*, p. 6.

secretariat in Ottawa. It is something else to be able to staff it in such a way that monitoring, planning and lobbying can emerge from it. At the end of the period under review, 1980, the biggest learned society in the social sciences was the Canadian Psychological Association with fewer than 3000 members. It could not afford much more than a staff big enough to manage its publications and membership services. Significant lobbying activities could not have been expected from its skeleton crew, and any monitoring and planning would have been carried out by academic volunteers who were probably teaching full loads and carrying out research. Quite apart from the disciplinary myopia that usually constrains the activities of individual societies, such groups have severe constraints resulting from limited resources. As a potential consumer of the output of such groups, Beaulnes's recognition of their limitations was important.

> Dr. Beaulnes indicated that in seeking social science advice the Ministry had spoken with such groups as members of the Canada Council, Rectors and Deans of Universities and heads of departments. The Ministry had not, however, approached the SSRCC or learned societies for advice.
>
> ...[He] noted that it was only recently that the Ministry had received authority to develop a concern with the social sciences and humanities. He realized that representatives of these disciplines had not shared in the formulation of advice. Alternatives which might be considered in order to improve this situation could be to expand the Science Council or the Economic Council or to establish a separate Crown Corporation. The effectiveness of such an organization for social science advice would be based on its representative nature, its ability to produce an impact on policy, and the quality of its output.
>
> ...It was agreed, in conclusion, that more regular links between the Ministry and the SSRCC were extremely desirable.[128]

These three quoted paragraphs constitute a strangely inconsistent triad. The first seems to express regret that the SSRCC had been ignored in the past. The third expresses an interest in not ignoring it in the future. But the middle paragraph seems to be written from a very abstract and hypothetical point of view, as if the author had not considered the possibility that the existing SSRCC might have provided useful advice to MSST about social sciences in Canada. Having granted the group status as a "group of wise men", it is curious that they seem to have so rapidly and completely fallen out of the picture.

When the Executive Committee met the following month (May 1972), Soberman informed the group that he had received a letter from the Canadian Psychological Association, indicating

> that CPA was unable at the present time to contribute financially to the Council. He emphasized that this was a particularly serious problem, not so much financially but, because if associations were to withdraw from the SSRCC, the actions would considerably undermine the effectiveness of the Council to act as a spokesman for all the social science disciplines.[129]

---

[128] *Ibid.*, p. 7.

[129] *Ibid.*, Minutes of the Executive Committee, May 25, 1972, pp. 3–4.

It was agreed that the President of SSRCC should urge the CPA to reconsider its position. So, the President wrote a long letter to the CPA President, Daniel Berlyne, in which he outlined the potentially "calamitous consequences of the psychologists'" withdrawal from the SSRCC.

"The effects of such a withdrawal", he wrote, "would be fourfold:

1. It would tend to demoralize the remaining members of the Council to find that a stalwart participant had withdrawn at a critical time. It might well make them think seriously of doing the same thing.
2. While the sum of money contributed by the CPA is not in itself large, it is part of a commitment upon which the Canada Council's $50,000 per year grant was based. The Canada Council might feel that a condition of the grant had been broken.
3. Despite all the difficulties of the CPA, a decision not to pay the per member fee to the SSRCC would be an implicit statement of priorities: it would signal that you have other higher priorities for your funds, whether it be publications or payments to other organizations. This decision could be interpreted by governments as suggesting that the SSRCC does not have a high priority among its own members and therefore cannot speak effectively for the social sciences. Such an interpretation would undercut our ability to influence governments.
4. It could be viewed by other organizations - in particular the physical and biological sciences - as disarray amongst the social scientists and evidence of their inability to co-operate in making a cogent case for their views on the ordering of research and science policy. Indeed, it might well encourage the natural scientists to presume to speak for the entire scientific community, social as well as physical."[130]

To make life a bit easier for the CPA, a lowered fee schedule was suggested. When the full Council met three months later, the CPA was represented by A. Doob, C.R. Myers and A.M. Sullivan.[131] There was no further mention of the issue in any other Minutes.

At the Executive Committee Meeting in November 1972, the question of relations with Canada Council was raised again. "There was some agreement that the SSRCC should be looking to alternative forms of support either through federal departments or provincial governments, so that it is not dependent on one granting body."[132] Then F. Maranda made several recommendations on behalf of a committee of the Canadian Sociology and Anthropology Association. These included the suggestion that Canada Council's Academic Advisory Panel "be nominated by SSRCC…that changes be made in the appointed Canada Council so that it would reflect more accurately the community which Canada Council serves. …that there be a larger number of social scientists on the Canada Council staff", and "that there be a liaison committee established with Canada Council".[133]

The problem of dependence on a single source of funding was not raised again for over 2 years. In February 1975,

[130] *Ibid.*, Letter from D.A. Soberman to D. Berlyne, June 2, 1972, pp. 3–4.

[131] *Ibid.*, Minutes of the Annual Meeting, September 28–29, 1972, p. 1.

[132] *Ibid.*, Minutes of the Executive Committee, November 28–29, 1972, p. 3.

[133] *Ibid.*

> Concern was expressed over the SSRCC reliance on Canada Council, as well as the possibility that the Council might become dependent on one department for support through a sustaining grant. More diversified support, it was agreed, would be desirable. On the other hand, it was noted that with a sustaining grant from either Canada Council or a department the efforts of the staff could be directed to the immediate objectives of the Council since the problem of raising funds would not be so pressing.[134]

The solution was to allow the Executive Director, J. Loubser, to "attempt to raise funds from various government departments in seeking to increase the revenue of the Council for 1975–76".[135]

The Annual Meeting Minutes of June 1, 1975 recorded the appointment of Rene Dickner as Finance Officer and then reiterated that "There is continuing concern with the heavy reliance of SSRCC on Canada Council funding. Efforts have been made to reduce the size of this support in relation to the overall revenues of SSRCC".[136] There was no indication of exactly what efforts or, more importantly, of any output to show from the efforts.

The biggest financial crisis in the SSRCC's entire history seems to have arisen in 1975. The November Council Minutes record the event as reported by the Finance Sub-Committee.

> Professor Myers, the Chairman of the sub-committee, reported that the sub-committee had at its meetings reviewed Council budgets, expenditures, and administrative matters. He reported that the revised 1975-76 budget, which the Executive had recently approved, envisaged a deficit of some $30,000. He also reported that at the present time it appeared that the budget for the National Conference would also have a deficit, possibly as large as $30,000. He noted that the Executive had also approved this budget.
>
> Dr. Loubser, the Director, pointed out that the expected deficit on the Conference arose from a lack of clarity on the size of the federal government's grant for the Conference. No written confirmation was received until two days before the conference and it was only after that, it became clear the total grant was intended to be $70,000 rather than $99,000 as earlier understood in telephone communications. He pointed out that attempts were currently being made to seek clarification and, he hoped, to secure the higher level of federal grant. Referring to the budgeted deficit in the operating fund, he noted that it arose from decreased revenues as a result of the current budgetary restraints imposed by the federal goverment rather than from increased expenditure. During the next six months expenditures will be monitored and controlled carefully in order to avoid such a large deficit.[137]

The remarkable thing about this event, apart from the size of the deficit, is the apparent fact that someone was able to go so far toward pulling off a national conference without having any written confirmation of a supporting grant. Two

---

[134]*Social Science Research Council Minutes 1974–1975*, Minutes of the Executive Committee, February 1, 1975, p. 4.

[135]*Ibid.*

[136]*Social Science Research Council Minutes 1975–1976*, Minutes of the Annual Meeting, June 1, 1975, p. 3.

[137]*Ibid.*, Minutes of the Semi-Annual Council Meeting, November 23, 1975, p. 2.

months later, the Executive Committee was informed that there was a revised budget with a deficit of $20,000 instead of the $41,000 envisioned in November.[138]

> In discussing the deficit position of the Council, it was noted that it was only the Operating Fund which was in a deficit position, and that the Project Grants Fund and the Hurd Fund provided the Council with sufficient funding to ensure the necessary cash flow. However, in the Operating Fund, it was pointed out that the accumulated deficit by the end of this fiscal year will be some $70,000 and that a deficit of some $8,000 might be anticipated on the National Social Science Conference.[139]

There was some discussion of increasing the fees from member associations, but it was decided to have the staff design a system of gradual increases.[140]

From January 1976 to February 1979, the Minutes record no special concern with finances. At the latter time, it is recorded that "the Finance Committee felt that it would be necessary to look into the possibility of raising funds for the Reserve Fund. Since no one on staff or any committee has such a mandate, it would be important to create a committee for that purpose". Accordingly, the "matter was referred to the Executive Committee".[141]

In September the Treasurer, W. Gillen, expressed some concern with funding and suggested some initiatives he wanted to take. In particular, he mentioned approaching Foundations, the possibility of an "advisory council on financing" and outside funding for committees. He agreed to make a proposal regarding costs of some of his initiatives.[142] The following month he "reported that letters introducing the Federation are being sent to various foundations". He said he would "be contacting Presidents of various corporations" and "would welcome names of direct contacts".[143] In the month after that he sadly reported that responses to his letters indicated that "they [whoever they were] will only be interested in financing projects". Moreover, J. Trent added "that he had held some discussions with provinces and foundations and had come to a similar conclusion".[144]

There are at least two curious facts about all this flurry of initiatives. First, the Council seems to have had no memory, since everything that was suggested had been suggested before and little had come of it. Second, no one seems to have suggested the possibility of a fund raising campaign directed specifically at social scientists themselves. It seems to have been taken for granted that those who would benefit most from the Council's activities were either unwilling or unable to make individual, tax-deductible contributions to the SSRCC.

---

[138] *Ibid.*, Minutes of the Executive Committee, January 29–30, 1976, p. 2.

[139] *Ibid.*

[140] *Ibid.*, p. 4.

[141] *Social Science Federation of Canada Minutes February 2, 1979 to June 5, 1980* (loose leaf binder), Minutes of the Meeting of the Board of Directors, February 2, 1979, p. 7.

[142] *Ibid.*, Minutes of the Meeting of the Executive Committee, September 14, 1979, p. 6.

[143] *Ibid.*, Minutes of the Meeting of the Board of Directors, October 12–13, 1979, p. 4.

[144] *Ibid.*, Minutes of the Meeting of the Executive Committee, November 30, 1979, p. 5.

In February 1980, the Treasurer reported that there appeared "to be a developing practice for larger universities to pay less than the full amount requested". The Finance Committee recommended "that future request letters to the universities be specific about the level of contribution and work out increases with the university representatives concerned".[145] It was also recorded that "several association members are delinquent in the payment of their fees" and that "there is no provision in our Statutes for non-payment of fees". It was then decided that "in case of non-payment of fees, the Board is authorized to take appropriate action".[146] There is no hint of what such action might have been, although it is clear from the CPA incident in May 1972 that the Council probably would have been very reluctant at best to drop any association from the Federation.

Four months after that "the Canadian Political Science Association informed the Council that the CPSA did not intend to pay its fees after October 1980".[147] There is no indication in the Minutes regarding any action that might have been taken. However, in February 1981, a representative of the CPSA, D. Stairs, reported that its executive intended "to propose to their Annual General Assembly the withdrawal of the motion to withdraw from the Federation".[148] As it turned out, the CPSA did not withdraw from the Federation.

Critical Choices

Forty years of history for an organization just turning 60 years of age ought to be enough to provide some useful guides to its future strategies for building a culture of support, including most importantly financial support. In fact, besides revealing many worthwhile suggestions for attracting financial support, the first 40 years reveal both actual and potential benefits and costs of implementing those suggestions. The following list of alternatives summarizes the critical choices that arose in the development of the Humanities and Social Sciences Federation up to 1980.

1. Government funding gave the councils some financial security and, although it created some dependency as some people predicted, it is not clear that it led to any manipulation that was also feared if not exactly predicted.
2. In the early years, funding from private American foundations provided more research funds than the Canadian government was prepared to provide and, although the funds available were for research that was perceived to be relevant and good from the point of view of administrators of the foundation funds, that point of view was apparently consistent with the aims of those who founded the Social Science Research Council.

---

[145]*Ibid.*, Minutes of the Meeting of the Board of Directors, February 8–9, 1980, p. 6.

[146]*Ibid.*, p. 17.

[147]*Ibid.*, Minutes of the Meeting of the Board of Directors, June 3–4, 1980, p. 2.

[148]Minutes of the Meeting of the Board of Directors, February 12, 1981, p. 3.

3. A federation of diverse disciplines was built upon the individual strength of each discipline and, although some people feared that such a federation would be a breeding ground for conflicts of interest and power struggles, there is little evidence that such conflicts and struggles occurred.
4. Giving civil service personnel full status membership on the council would have encouraged wide participation and strengthened the organization, but such status was never granted by the academic members of the council because they feared it would reduce their own relative impact in the organization.
5. Having some civil service personnel on the council probably provided it with greater access to information, but it might also have constrained the council's ability to publish controversial material that could compromise the government, the civil service itself or even individual privacy.
6. A council consisting only of academics would have been relatively free to publish controversial material, but it would not have had access to the full range of information available to civil service personnel.
7. The coordination of social science research could have helped eliminate duplication, identify gaps in research frontiers, and obtain efficiencies and opportunities for more diverse, multifaceted research, but it might also have stifled individual initiative and the free exploration of frontiers in specific disciplines.
8. As an operating body, the council could undertake its own research, but such undertakings would put it in direct competition with other researchers who might then have been reluctant to co-operate with the council.
9. As a planning body, the council could direct and supervise the funding of research into perceived gaps or to solve specific social problems, but the plans of such a body might have been and have been perceived to be limited to the pursuit of its own research aims and political agendas.
10. If the council focused its activities on research then that would have left a considerable amount of the working lives of academic researchers unaccounted for while, if it focused its activities on teaching (which was and still is what most academics are paid for) then that would have left the problem of co-ordinating research inadequately addressed and might also have turned the proposed research council into something closer to a trade union for university teachers.
11. Having social welfare and social service groups affiliated with the council would have expanded its membership and perhaps given it more influence in public issues and more political clout, but such affiliates would also have broadened the focus of the council's work, perhaps making it unmanageably broad by bringing in conflicting agendas.
12. By increasing publicity for the council's work, more people might have become interested in the council and its influence might have been increased, although such increases might also have created jealousy and stimulated other groups to organize, and in the end produced more competition for limited funds.

13. A council devoted to pure research might have been able to attract more tax-deductible donations, but it would also have had to avoid overt lobbying, while a council committed to lobbying probably would have lost some donations in exchange for greater freedom to try to influence public policy.
14. Targeting businesses and accepting funds from them would have opened up a very large source of potential funding but, because businesses are driven by the profit motive, it is likely that insofar as contributions were forthcoming, they would have been tied to some commitments and constraints regarding acceptable ways of spending the money.
15. Recommending research grants to those with proven track records would increase the prior probability of successful production, but it would also decrease the probability of funding good projects coming from relatively young scholars with short track records and it would contribute to the Matthew Effect (those with more tend to get still more and those with less tend to get less).
16. Organizations that deliver valuable goods and services to their members should not have difficulty attracting sustaining membership fees, although many unions do deliver valuable goods and services to their members and do have difficulty attracting fees as well as volunteer services.

Conclusions

I began with the candid admission that I hoped my essay would lend some support to the cause of increased financial support for the social sciences. As I reflect on the content of the essay, I wonder why on earth anything I have said here would have any impact on anyone's inclination to spend money on the social sciences or anything else. I have presented page after page of moaning and groaning about finances by some of Canada's most thoughtful social scientists, and I think some of it was interesting. But why should this move anyone to action, let alone action designed to redistribute funds from somewhere else to the social sciences?

Perhaps someone will be moved by the fact that so much effort has already been spent trying to create a culture of support for the social sciences. Maybe my efforts here can generate some sort of a bandwagon effect. Of course they can, but I find it hard to believe that they will.

It is also possible that someone might read about the funding strategies that have been used in the past and try to use them again. For all anyone knows, the current environment might be more hospitable than earlier environments have been, and strategies that were fruitless the first few times around might be fruitful today. We have noted more than one example of ideas that led to concrete initiatives and programs several years after they were first suggested. Maybe there is some ash in this historical dustbin with enough spark in it to ignite a new flame.

Reflecting on the contents of this essay, someone might be moved to ask why I think more funds should be spent on the social sciences when the historical record seems to have so little to show for all the money that has been spent so far. I think the assumption that there is little to show for the money that has been spent on the social sciences would require some justification and, as I remarked in the very first paragraph of this essay, I think it would be easy to provide a very substantial justification. The justification would necessarily be lengthy and time-consuming to be conclusive, but it would not require any complicated research or analysis. However, even if it is granted that so far the benefits from social scientific research have outweighed the costs, it does not follow that right now there should be some increase in the funds currently invested in such research. Indeed, no indication has been given of the current size of the social scientific research budget in Canada today, of the current needs or demands by any social scientist or anyone else, or of the perceived or real discrepancy between the former and the latter. Without such information, recommendations for increased funding can hardly be taken seriously.

Bad as the last couple sentences may sound, they are probably very helpful for our purposes. They carry the clear implication that anyone trying to extract more funding for social scientific research today would have to proceed along lines that are very similar to those followed by our predecessors in the first 40 years of the Social Science Federation. My guess would be that it would be practically impossible to attempt a comprehensive review of everything that might plausibly be referred to by the phrase "social scientific research", but certain limited areas might be carved out for very careful review and analysis. One model of what might be done is what was done a few years ago for the field of gerontology. A variety of meetings and consultations were held which identified some significant gaps in personnel and information, special funds were assembled for training and research, and new scholars and research frontiers were developed. Today, for my own field of social indicators research, it would be worthwhile to apply such a model to what some people call the aggregation problem. That is the problem of aggregating social, economic and environmental information in order to form one coherent accounting system of indicators of the quality of life. There are many people around the world working on this problem, but not so many (certainly not in Canada) that the numbers would prevent us from making a comprehensive review followed by a strategic plan for actually solving the problem. If such things happen partly as a result of this essay, all my labours would be adequately compensated.

References

Arnove, R. F. (1982). *Philanthropy and cultural imperialism: The foundations at home and abroad.* Bloomington: Indiana University Press.

Karl, B. D. (1974). *Charles E. Merriam and the study of politics.* Chicago: University of Chicago Press.

McLeish, J. A. B. (1978). *A Canadian for all seasons: The John E. Robbins story.* Toronto: Lester and Orpen Ltd.

Michalos, A. C. (1984). Review of Arnove. R. F. Arnove (Ed.), Philanthropy and cultural imperialism: The foundations at home and abroad. *Journal of Business Ethics*, *3*(1), 69–70, 84–89.

Soffer, R. N. (1978). *Ethics and society in England: The revolution in the social sciences 1870–1914*. Berkeley: University of California Press.

Chapter 16
Notes for a System of Scientific Research Reports Accounts

Alex C. Michalos

My aim is to model the production of scientific research reports along the lines of the National Income and Product Accounts. Originally I hoped to model the scientific and technological enterprises or some mix of science and technology into a single coherent system of accounts. I still have hopes for such a system, but here I am merely trying to design one part of it. Although the National Accounts have been significantly and correctly criticized throughout their existence on the grounds of a variety of built-in limitations and biases, they have also been enormously helpful in allowing governments to manage our national and international economies. Whether or not it makes sense to try to model the production of scientific research reports along those lines remains to be seen.

Virtually all of the literature on science policy or science and technology policy is a combination of material related to the production of research reports on the one hand or marketable industrial products (goods or services) on the other. In fact, there is much more literature devoted to industrial innovation and the role of scientific research in the interests of such innovation than there is to improving our understanding and the quality of scientific research in the interest of improving the quality of our lives. So, from that point of view, I suppose my focus on the latter implies there will be relatively less interest in my proposed project. Nevertheless, the successful development of this part of the full story will bring us closer to success for a full account later on. More about this later.

Although internally a System of Scientific Research Reports Accounts (SSRRA) relates all its components as inputs and outputs, viewed from outside, such a system

Paper presented at the 13th World Congress of Sociology, Bielefeld, Germany, July 1994.

Michalos, A.C.: 1994. Notes for a system of scientific research reports accounts. Paper presented at a Conference at the Berlin Institute for Social Research.

A.C. Michalos (✉)
University of Northern British Columbia, Prince George, BC, Canada
e-mail: michalos@brandonu.ca

A.C. Michalos, *Philosophical Foundations of Quality of Life*,
DOI 10.1007/978-3-319-50727-9_16

may be regarded as consisting entirely of the most salient output of the scientific enterprise, namely, scientific research reports. Whatever else scientific research produces, it certainly produces research reports.

Some scientific research reports are reproductive themselves while others are not. Our most highly valued reports are those that provide answers to pressing problems, new knowledge and new avenues of exploration leading to still more new knowledge. These are our most frequently cited reports.

Some reports provide obsolete or redundant results, giving less precise information than we already have or precisely what we already have. Then, some reports provide new knowledge that cannot be connected to any new research. Presumably reports with obsolete or redundant results would be characterized by random citation patterns, while those without connections to new research would never be cited.

There is no way to decide which papers that fail to have future connections today will continue to be disconnected in the future and there is no rule book to tell us how long we should wait to decide that a given paper will be forever disconnected. But there is some evidence showing that most of the papers that will be followed up by others tend to reproduce within 5 years. So there is some justification in designating reports that reproduced other reports within 5 years (operationalized as reports that have been cited by others in 5 years or less of the original production) as simply reproductive research reports. Those that fail to reproduce in this sense will be designated as nonreproductive research reports.

With these assumptions and explanations out of the way, we may proceed immediately to construct the SSRRA.

Our analog to the Gross National Product in the National Income and Product Accounts has the same name in the SSRRA, only here the GNP stands for a particular kind of product, namely, the sum total of the value of all scientific research reports produced by Canadians. Here the value of a research report is arbitrarily defined and measured by the number of citations it receives in the 10 years following its publication. Although there are a wide variety of reasons for people citing other research reports and. many reports are cited in order to criticize them, I think that more often than not people cite reports because the latter got something right than because they got something wrong.

Supposing that there are n reports, $p_1, p_2, \ldots, p_n$ produced in some year and that each one may be assigned a value equal to the number of citations, c_j ($j = 0, 1, \ldots, m$), it gets over the next 10 years, then the GNP for that year would be defined and measured by the sum:

$$\mathrm{GNP} = p_1c_1 + p_2c_2 + \cdots + p_nc_m. \tag{16.1}$$

Some of the citations a report receives will come in 5 years or less and some will come later or not at all. Since we cannot wait forever to capture the value of those that come later, I arbitrarily put our cutoff point at 10 years. So, we may define later citations as those that come in the sixth to tenth year following the original production of the report. Following our understanding of reproductive versus nonreproductive reports then, every research report will have a total value equal to the sum of its 10-years worth of citations = c, a reproductive value equal to the sum of its citations in 5 years or less = r, and a complementary nonreproductive value equal to the sum of its citations in 6–10 years = −r.

Since a report produced is a report available to someone (as a dollar produced is a dollar of income for someone), we may say that the GNP equals the Gross National Income (GNI), as in the National Accounts. So we have,

$$\text{GNP} = \text{GNI}. \tag{16.2}$$

It is likely that very little will be lost if we assume that all scientific research reports are produced by people connected in one way or another to one or more of three sectors, namely, universities and nonprofit research institutes U, private industry R or government V. So, letting U, R and V stand for the value of the reports in each of the three sectors,

$$\text{GNP} = \text{U} + \text{R} + \text{V}. \tag{16.3}$$

Following our decision regarding reproductive and nonreproductive reports, the value of the research report output of each sector can be divided into two complementary classes. For ease of reference to the different sectors, we will write

$$\text{U} = \text{Ur} + \text{U} - \text{r},\ \text{R} = \text{Rr} + \text{R} - \text{r and V} = \text{Vr} + \text{V} - \text{r}. \tag{16.4}$$

Collectively we may regard the set of nonreproductive reports as analogous to savings in the economic accounts. Some reports would be similar to relatively unmarketable wealth, like the proverbial priceless family jewels or church relics. Others would be like nest eggs set aside for a rainy day or investment at an opportune time. Examples of nonreproductive reports of both kinds may be found in noneuclidean geometries, some of which were interesting in themselves but had no consequences for future research while others became very provocative and useful in understanding the structure of physical space. So, we may define the value of research report savings S,

$$\text{S} = \text{U} - \text{r} + \text{R} - \text{r} + \text{V} - \text{r}. \tag{16.5}$$

Subtracting savings from the Gross Product, we get our Net National Product (NNP), which is equal to our Net National Income (NNI). That is,

$$\text{NNP} = \text{NNI} = \text{GNP} - \text{S} = \text{GNP} - (\text{U} - \text{r} + \text{R} - \text{r} + \text{V} - \text{r}) = \text{Ur} + \text{Rr} + \text{Vr}. \tag{16.6}$$

Since research reports produced by private industry and government laboratories are not typically published for public consumption the way university research reports are typically published, there is a rough analogy here to our economic accounts in which some of the GNP is retained by industry as profits and some of it is taxed away by governments. So, we may think of what is left as similar to our household, personal income (El). Thus,

$$\mathrm{El} = \mathrm{Ur} = \mathrm{NNP} - (\mathrm{Rr} + \mathrm{Vr}). \tag{16.7}$$

These, then, are the basic components of our SSRRA. Figure 16.1 illustrates the main relationships among them. Some of the relationships are simply true by the preceding seven definitions in Eqs. (16.1)–(16.7), while others are not. Assuming that the seven definitions constitute a self-consistent set, little more needs to be said about the relationships among these concepts. The remaining relationships constitute hypothesized consequences of the model that are empirically testable. It will take some time to work out all the procedures required to operationalize the key concepts, determine sampling frames for sectors and subsectors, time frames, appropriate analytic techniques and so on. But all I want to do here is first, emphasize again that the basic data to be manipulated would be numbers of scientific research reports of various sorts and their citations from the three productive sectors and second, note that I suppose the hypothesized empirical relationships would be tested using ordinary least squares regression equations, alone or with others.

Perhaps the simplest place to begin exploring relationships is to return to our basic assumption that the value of the GNP in scientific research reports is equal to the value of the sum of reports in savings plus the reproductive parts of the three productive sectors. Thus, regarding the GNP as a linear function of those four components, we can write,

$$\mathrm{GNP} = \mathrm{f}(\mathrm{S}, \mathrm{Ur}, \mathrm{Rr}, \mathrm{Vr}). \tag{16.8}$$

Assuming minimum measurement errors, close to 100% of the variation in the distribution of GNP figures for any period of years should be explained by the four predictors. More importantly, the standardized regression coefficients or beta values attached to each predictor will provide a measure of the percent of variance in GNP figures that is explained by each predictor on the assumption that the values of the others are held constant. In other words, the beta values give us a measure of the relative contribution of each predictor to the variation in GNP figures.

Instead of or in addition to this holistic analysis, one could effectively break up Eq. (16.8) to explore simpler relationships. For example, one might want to directly measure the impact of savings on GNP,

$$\mathrm{GNP} = \mathrm{f}(\mathrm{S}), \tag{16.9}$$

or the impact of the total university output on GNP,

$$\mathrm{GNP} = \mathrm{f}(\mathrm{U}), \tag{16.10}$$

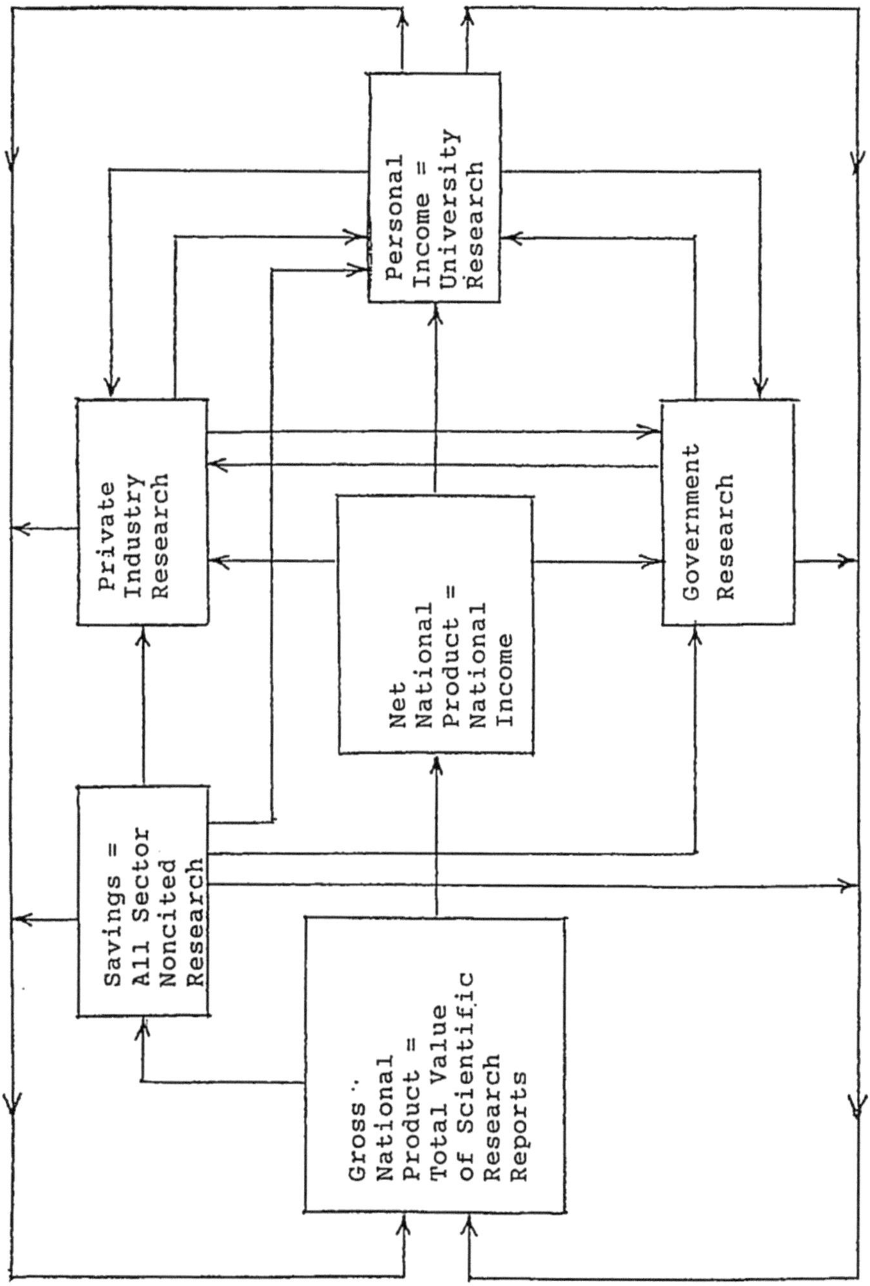

Fig. 16.1 Product and income flows of scientific research reports

or the impact of total savings plus the reproductive part of total university output on GNP,

$$GNP = f(S, Ur). \tag{16.11}$$

There are three sets of relationships whose exploration requires the use of simultaneous equations. I suppose that each of the three productive sectors has some influence on the others. So, in the broadest terms, the question is which sector benefits how much by which other sector. For example, one would want to measure the contribution of the scientific research output of private industry to the output of university researchers, and vice versa. That would require two equations:

$$U = f\ (R), \tag{16.12}$$

$$R = f\ (U). \tag{16.13}$$

Alternatively, of course, one might simply be interested in examining the relative impact of the reproductive parts of each of these two sectors on the other; i.e.,

$$Ur = f(Rr), \tag{16.14}$$

$$Rr = f(Ur). \tag{16.15}$$

Rough as this model of the SSRRA is and rough as its analogies are to our economic National Accounts, it seems (to me at least) to have some promising payoffs in terms of our understanding of the scientific research report production system. As in the latter case, one can get more out of the SSRRA by connecting it to other elements of the scientific enterprise. It will be worthwhile to make some of these connections now.

In the first place, one would want to connect our research report output figures to input figures for capital and operating expenditures, and personnel. So, for examples, in addition to exploring the aggregate relationships reviewed above, one would calculate the GNP, U, Ur and so on per employed scientist, and then measure the relative contribution of the various components on this sort of per capita basis. Such measurement provides one rough measure of the relative efficiency of the producers in our productive sectors.

One would expect to find some differences in the relative efficiency of producers in different sectors, with different kinds or levels of training (measured by degrees attained, years of experience or previous output), different disciplines or specific areas of investigation, different time commitments to research, different equipment and raw materials, different ages, sexes, incomes, religious, ethnic and linguistic backgrounds, and a wide variety of different personal and professional attitudes, motives and beliefs. Similar analyses may be undertaken to measure the research report output per dollar spent on research facilities, equipment and salaries for researchers in different sectors, with different training and so on.

Clearly, the final elucidation of the causal antecedents in a model of the production of typical scientific research reports would be considerably richer than those captured in the SSRRA. In economists' jargon, a relatively complete model of the production function for scientific research reports would be much more complicated than the model suggested in the SSRRA. Again, however, in this respect the SSRRA is similar to our National Accounts, though of course the former is much more tentative.

It is unclear how much of the preceding discussion could be pressed into service to explain the production of patents or, more generally still, industrial innovation in the form of marketable goods and services. At this point in our investigation, these are bridges that do not have to be crossed, though they merit some preliminary reflection. However, rather than speculate on these issues, I want to sketch some ideas about the design of an empirical test of the relationships in the SSRRA.

To begin with, it does not seem possible to just tap into the citation index data-base for our initial lists of research reports, because these data-sets do not include lists of most of the research reports produced by private industry and much, if not most, of the reports produced by government laboratories. Supposing that is the case, it would appear that we would have to undertake our own survey research in order to get a proper data-base. That, of course, would require significant agreements from some private industrialists and government agencies.

From the point of view of testing the model in the SSRRA, such agreements may be easier to obtain than one might imagine, because we do not need timely data. We could use data from practically any period in which there are reasonably accurate records of research report output. For example, I would recommend exploring the hypothesized relationships in the SSRRA using data from the base year of 1955 to 1975. That would require tracking the reproductive future of reports produced in 1975 all the way to 1985, which would probably be old enough that no proprietary advantages would be threatened by any of our results. Of course, our results might be embarrassing from some points of view. For example, people working in one sector or discipline may not want anyone to know that they are relatively less efficient than those working in another sector or discipline. So, one should not expect automatic acceptance and assistance. Still, we might be saved by a sufficiently long temporal distance from the events examined, although the length of this distance may be inversely related to the usefulness of this research for current public science policy-making.

Since twenty observations (one for each of 20 years) are barely enough to run useful regressions, it would be worthwhile to try to find some way to increase our data-base. Maybe we could examine several fairly specific research areas of one or more disciplines simultaneously over the 1955–1975 period, and do some kind of meta-analysis to increase the reliability and validity of our results.

Perhaps this is enough to provide some ideas for discussion. The fact that our most likely potential funding agency at this point (the SSHRCC through it Strategic Grants Program on Science Policy) specifically endorses cooperation among diverse sectors and disciplines makes our need for such cooperation a distinct advantage.

Appendix

History in Photographs

See Figs. A.1, A.2, A.3, A.4, A.5, A.6, A.7, A.8, A.9, A.10 and A.11.

A.C. Michalos, *Philosophical Foundations of Quality of Life*,
DOI 10.1007/978-3-319-50727-9

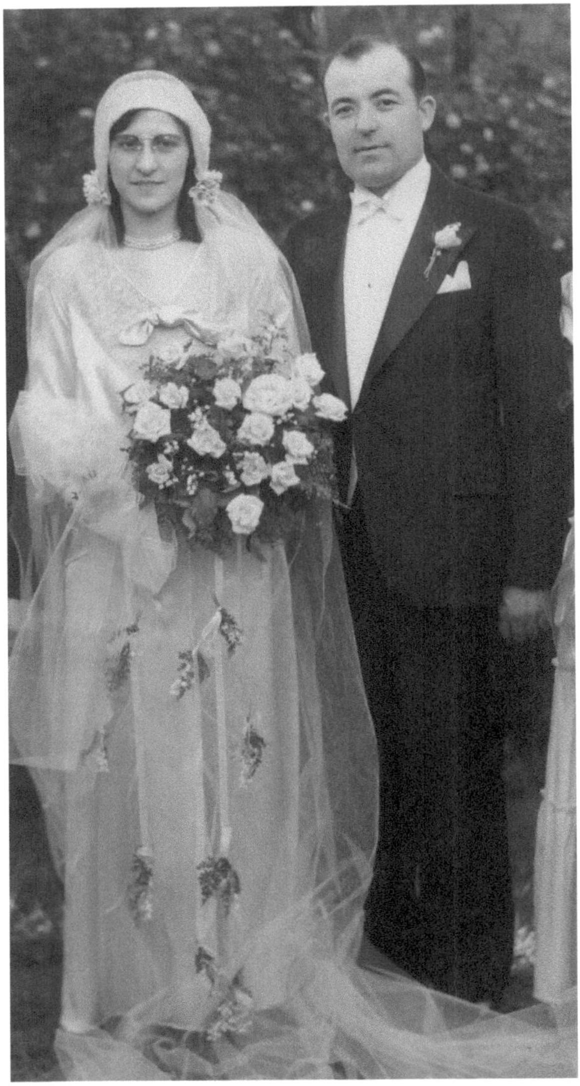

A.1 Josephine and Charles K. Michalos wedding June 1931

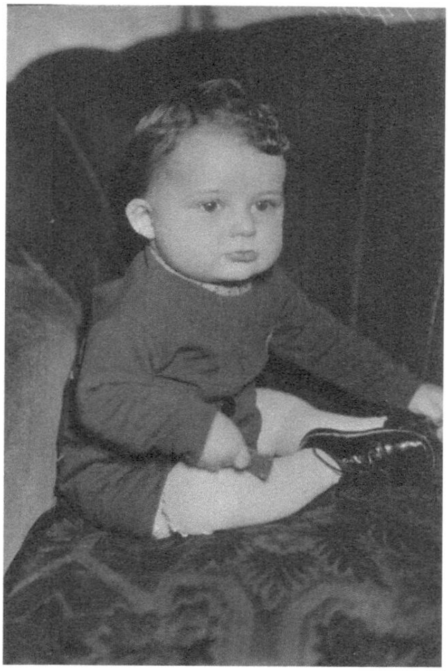

A.2 Alex C. Michalos around Easter 1936

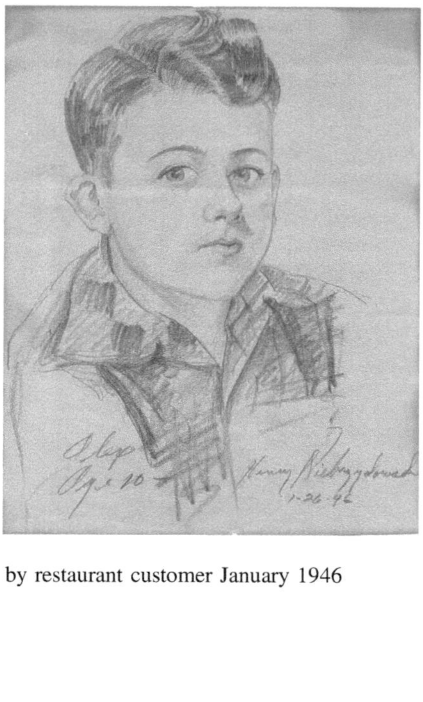

A.3 Alex portrait drawn by restaurant customer January 1946

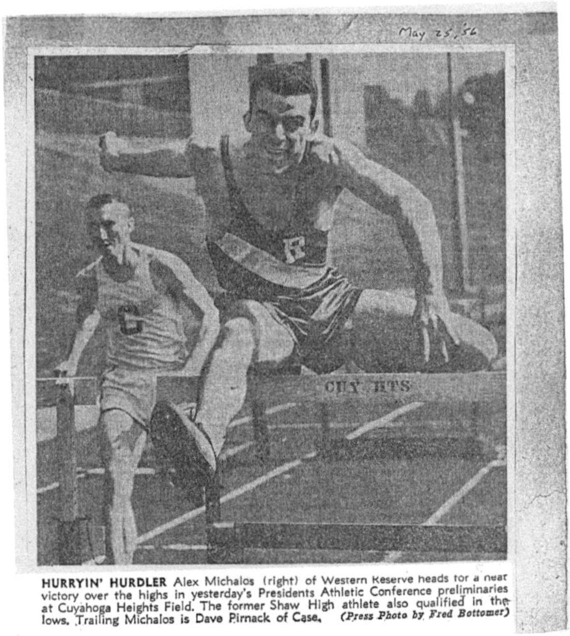

HURRYIN' HURDLER Alex Michalos (right) of Western Reserve heads for a neat victory over the highs in yesterday's Presidents Athletic Conference preliminaries at Cuyahoga Heights Field. The former Shaw High athlete also qualified in the lows. Trailing Michalos is Dave Pirnack of Case. *(Press Photo by Fred Bottomer)*

A.4 Alex at Western Reserve University in race with Case Institute of Technology May 1956

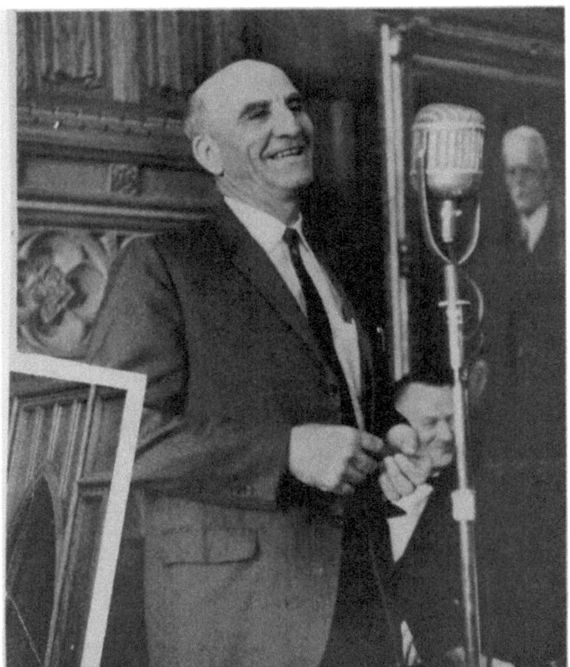

A.5 J. Coert Rylaarsdam at University of Chicago 1970

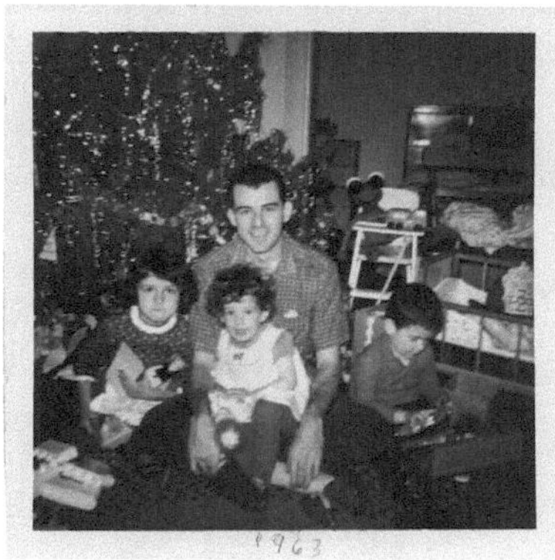

A.6 Alex, Cyndi, Stephanie and Ted in Saint Cloud, Minnesota December 1963

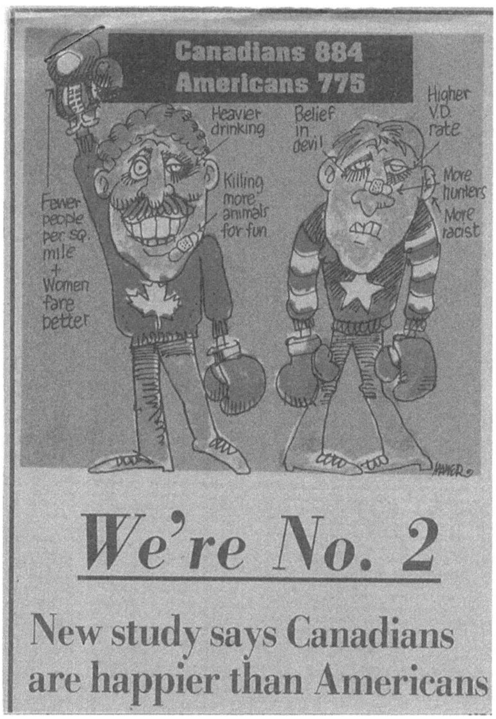

A.7 Cartoon accompanying article on *North American Social Report* in the Detroit Free Press April 1982

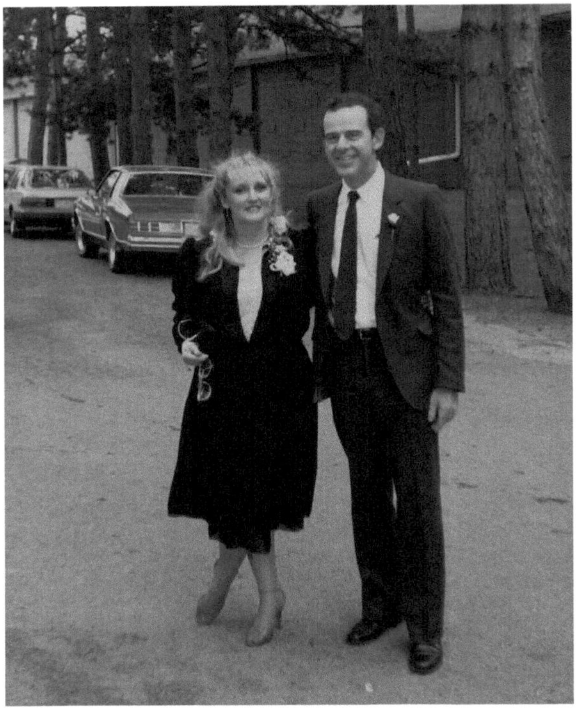

A.8 Deborah and Alex at Ted's wedding 1983

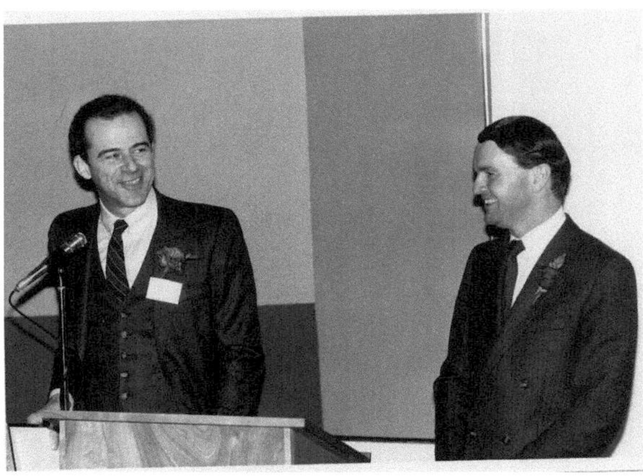

A.9 Alex receiving from Secretary of State Serge Joyal the Prize for Excellence in Interdisciplinary Research in Canadian Studies for *North American Social Report* 1984

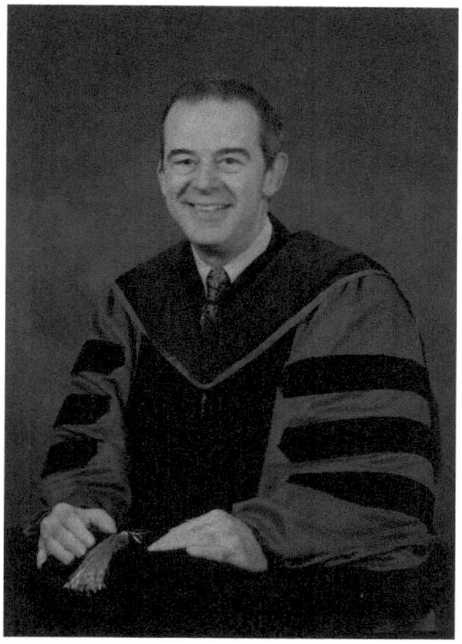

A.10 Alex at 60 in 1995

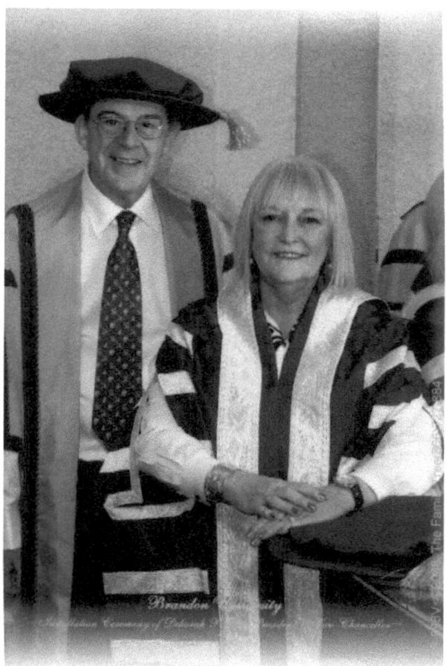

A.11 Alex as Chancellor of the University of Northern British Columbia and Deborah as President and Vice Chancellor of Brandon University at Deborah's Installation October 2009

MIX
Papier aus verantwortungsvollen Quellen
Paper from responsible sources
FSC® C105338

If you have any concerns about our products,
you can contact us on
ProductSafety@springernature.com

In case Publisher is established outside the EU,
the EU authorized representative is:
Springer Nature Customer Service Center GmbH
Europaplatz 3, 69115 Heidelberg, Germany

Printed by Libri Plureos GmbH
in Hamburg, Germany